Trends in Clinical Deep Brain Stimulation

Trends in Clinical Deep Brain Stimulation

Editors

Marcus L. F. Janssen
Yasin Temel

MDPI • Basel • Beijing • Wuhan • Barcelona • Belgrade • Manchester • Tokyo • Cluj • Tianjin

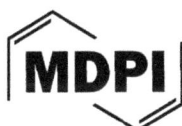

Editors
Marcus L. F. Janssen
The Netherlands University
The Netherlands

Yasin Temel
Maastricht University Medical Center
The Netherlands

Editorial Office
MDPI
St. Alban-Anlage 66
4052 Basel, Switzerland

This is a reprint of articles from the Special Issue published online in the open access journal *Journal of Clinical Medicine* (ISSN 2077-0383) (available at: https://www.mdpi.com/journal/jcm/special_issues/Developments_Deep_Brain_Stimulation).

For citation purposes, cite each article independently as indicated on the article page online and as indicated below:

LastName, A.A.; LastName, B.B.; LastName, C.C. Article Title. *Journal Name* **Year**, *Volume Number*, Page Range.

ISBN 978-3-0365-0336-3 (Hbk)
ISBN 978-3-0365-0337-0 (PDF)

Cover image courtesy of Geertjan Zonneveld.

© 2021 by the authors. Articles in this book are Open Access and distributed under the Creative Commons Attribution (CC BY) license, which allows users to download, copy and build upon published articles, as long as the author and publisher are properly credited, which ensures maximum dissemination and a wider impact of our publications.

The book as a whole is distributed by MDPI under the terms and conditions of the Creative Commons license CC BY-NC-ND.

Contents

About the Editors vii

Marcus L. F. Janssen and Yasin Temel
Special Issue: Trends in Clinical Deep Brain Stimulation
Reprinted from: *J. Clin. Med.* **2021**, *10*, 178, doi:10.3390/jcm10020178 1

Frederick L. Hitti, Andrew I. Yang, Mario A. Cristancho and Gordon H. Baltuch
Deep Brain Stimulation Is Effective for Treatment-Resistant Depression: A Meta-Analysis and Meta-Regression
Reprinted from: *J. Clin. Med.* **2020**, *9*, 2796, doi:10.3390/jcm9092796 5

Milaine Roet, Jackson Boonstra, Erdi Sahin, Anne E.P. Mulders, Albert F.G. Leentjens and Ali Jahanshahi
Deep Brain Stimulation for Treatment-Resistant Depression: Towards a More Personalized Treatment Approach
Reprinted from: *J. Clin. Med.* **2020**, *9*, 2729, doi:10.3390/jcm9092729 19

Sharafuddin Khairuddin, Fung Yin Ngo, Wei Ling Lim, Luca Aquili, Naveed Ahmed Khan, Man-Lung Fung, Ying-Shing Chan, Yasin Temel and Lee Wei Lim
A Decade of Progress in Deep Brain Stimulation of the Subcallosal Cingulate for the Treatment of Depression
Reprinted from: *J. Clin. Med.* **2020**, *9*, 3260, doi:10.3390/jcm9103260 39

Meltem Görmezoğlu, Tim Bouwens van der Vlis, Koen Schruers, Linda Ackermans, Mircea Polosan and Albert F.G. Leentjens
Effectiveness, Timing and Procedural Aspects of Cognitive Behavioral Therapy after Deep Brain Stimulation for Therapy-Resistant Obsessive Compulsive Disorder: A Systematic Review
Reprinted from: *J. Clin. Med.* **2020**, *9*, 2383, doi:10.3390/jcm9082383 89

Rose M. Caston, Elliot H. Smith, Tyler S. Davis and John D. Rolston
The Cerebral Localization of Pain: Anatomical and Functional Considerations for Targeted Electrical Therapies
Reprinted from: *J. Clin. Med.* **2020**, *9*, 1945, doi:10.3390/jcm9061945 99

Prasad Shirvalkar, Kristin K. Sellers, Ashlyn Schmitgen, Jordan Prosky, Isabella Joseph, Philip A. Starr and Edward F. Chang
A Deep Brain Stimulation Trial Period for Treating Chronic Pain
Reprinted from: *J. Clin. Med.* **2020**, *9*, 3155, doi:10.3390/jcm9103155 115

I. Daria Bogdan, Teus van Laar, D.L. Marinus Oterdoom, Gea Drost, J. Marc C. van Dijk and Martijn Beudel
Optimal Parameters of Deep Brain Stimulation in Essential Tremor: A Meta-Analysis and Novel Programming Strategy
Reprinted from: *J. Clin. Med.* **2020**, *9*, 1855, doi:10.3390/jcm9061855 131

Hye Ran Park, Yong Hoon Lim, Eun Jin Song, Jae Meen Lee, Kawngwoo Park, Kwang Hyon Park, Woong-Woo Lee, Han-Joon Kim, Beomseok Jeon and Sun Ha Paek
Bilateral Subthalamic Nucleus Deep Brain Stimulation under General Anesthesia: Literature Review and Single Center Experience
Reprinted from: *J. Clin. Med.* **2020**, *9*, 3044, doi:10.3390/jcm9093044 145

Michael J. Bos, Ana Maria Alzate Sanchez, Raffaella Bancone, Yasin Temel, Bianca T.A. de Greef, Anthony R. Absalom, Erik D. Gommer, Vivianne H.J.M. van Kranen-Mastenbroek, Wolfgang F. Buhre, Mark J. Roberts and Marcus L.F. Janssen
Influence of Anesthesia and Clinical Variables on the Firing Rate, Coefficient of Variation and Multi-Unit Activity of the Subthalamic Nucleus in Patients with Parkinson's Disease
Reprinted from: *J. Clin. Med.* **2020**, *9*, 1229, doi:10.3390/jcm9041229 . . . . **167**

Bethany R. Isaacs, Max C. Keuken, Anneke Alkemade, Yasin Temel, Pierre-Louis Bazin and Birte U. Forstmann
Methodological Considerations for Neuroimaging in Deep Brain Stimulation of the Subthalamic Nucleus in Parkinson's Disease Patients
Reprinted from: *J. Clin. Med.* **2020**, *9*, 3124, doi:10.3390/jcm9103124 . . . . **181**

Marc Baertschi, Nicolas Favez, João Flores Alves Dos Santos, Michalina Radomska, François Herrmann, Pierre R. Burkhard, Alessandra Canuto, Kerstin Weber and Paolo Ghisletta
Illness Representations and Coping Strategies in Patients Treated with Deep Brain Stimulation for Parkinson's Disease
Reprinted from: *J. Clin. Med.* **2020**, *9*, 1186, doi:10.3390/jcm9041186 . . . . **209**

Carlo Alberto Artusi, Leonardo Lopiano and Francesca Morgante
Deep Brain Stimulation Selection Criteria for Parkinson's Disease: Time to Go beyond CAPSIT-PD
Reprinted from: *J. Clin. Med.* **2020**, *9*, 3931, doi:10.3390/jcm9123931 . . . . **223**

About the Editors

Marcus L. F. Janssen MD, Ph.D., is a neurologist and clinical neurophysiologist with a special interest in movement disorders and neurophysiology. He currently works at the Maastricht University Medical Center and is an assistant professor at the School for Mental Health and Neuroscience, Faculty of Medicine and Life Sciences, Maastricht University. Dr. Janssen obtained his Ph.D. at Maastricht University in 2015. Since 2018 he has taken up the position of deputy director of the Department of Translational Neuroscience. His translational research line focusses on the development of novel neuromodulative therapies and the search for new insights into neurological diseases, such as Parkinson's disease and tinnitus, using electrophysiological approaches.

Yasin Temel MD, Ph.D., is head of the Department of Neurosurgery at the Maastricht University Medical Center. After receiving his Medical degree, he combined his training in Neurosurgery with his Ph.D. training at Maastricht University Medical Center. He obtained his Ph.D. cum laude from the faculty of Medicine of Maastricht University in 2007. In 2012, he was appointed as Professor of Functional Neurosurgery. His clinical and research topics include the neurosurgical treatment of patients with movement and psychiatric disorders and patients with skull base tumors. He has received several personal awards, including the science award from the Dutch Brain Foundation in 2011.

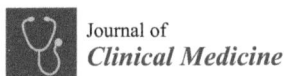

Editorial

Special Issue: Trends in Clinical Deep Brain Stimulation

Marcus L. F. Janssen [1,2,*] and Yasin Temel [2,3]

1. Department of Clinical Neurophysiology, Maastricht University Medical Center, P. Debyelaan 25, 6229 HX Maastricht, The Netherlands
2. School for Mental Health and Neuroscience, Faculty of Health, Medicine and Life Sciences, Maastricht University, Universiteitssingel 40, 6229 ER Maastricht, The Netherlands; y.temel@maastrichtuniversity.nl
3. Department of Neurosurgery, Maastricht University Medical Center, P. Debyelaan 25, 6229 HX Maastricht, The Netherlands
* Correspondence: m.janssen@maastrichtuniversity.nl

Received: 8 December 2020; Accepted: 11 December 2020; Published: 6 January 2021

Deep brain stimulation (DBS) has been successfully applied in several neurological and psychiatric disorders. A substantial number of patients suffering from a brain disorder either do not, or insufficiently, respond to pharmacological treatment. This results in increasing costs for public health systems and a growing burden for society. Fortunately, the number of approved indications for DBS keeps expanding, thereby improving the quality of life of many individuals. Nevertheless, defining the optimal target and stimulation paradigm for the individual patient remains a challenge. In this Special Issue, a series of twelve papers is presented by international leaders in the field on the current trends in clinical deep brain stimulation for a range of neurological and psychiatric disorders.

One of the most common psychiatric disorders considered to be treated using DBS is depression. Unfortunately, recent randomized controlled trials show disappointing results of DBS for treatment-resistant depression (TRD). Contrary to these findings, the meta-analysis conducted by Hitti et al. shows that DBS is an effective treatment for TRD [1]. This promising finding should serve as an encouragement for future studies to optimize patient selection, stimulation settings and target selection. In line with this, Roet et al. also plead for a more personalized treatment approach for patients suffering from TRD [2]. They conclude that depression should not be considered as one disorder and patients should be subtyped. Target selection would depend on specific patient characteristics assessed by a variety of biomarkers, such as clinical characteristics and findings from (functional) imaging studies. The authors argue that postoperative monitoring using momentary assessment techniques could be helpful in optimizing DBS therapy for the individual patient suffering from major depressive disorder. Khairuddin et al. conducted an in-depth literature review on DBS treatment of the subcallosal cingulate in patients with TRD [3]. This review displays the immense differences in response and remission rates between studies. These differences might be overcome by a more personalized approach. The authors underline the complexity of evaluating treatment effects in this patient group. Important inroads are also being made in the understanding of DBS working mechanisms in the treatment of TRD using preclinical studies. Animal studies show distant stimulation effects in the limbic network and neuroplasticity, as well as modifications at the molecular level.

In contrast to major depressive disorder, DBS for obsessive compulsive disorder (OCD) has the approval of the FDA as a humanitarian device exemption. The individual outcome of DBS, however, varies between patients. Generally, several pharmaceutical, as well as non-pharmaceutical, behavioral therapies are offered to patients before DBS surgery. The potential amplifying effect of these therapies in combination with DBS has insufficient attention. The review by Görmezoğlu et al. highlights the need to better investigate the synergetic effects of cognitive behavioral therapy (CBT) and DBS in patients suffering from OCD [4].

Chronic pain is a debilitating neurological symptom which is difficult to treat. Its inherently chronic nature has a huge impact on the quality of life of the individual affected, as well as societal costs. From a pathophysiological perspective, it is not surprising that many efforts have been made to treat patients using DBS. Yet, clinical studies thus far are not very promising. Caston et al. provide a complete overview on the cerebral pain network and potential targets for DBS [5]. The authors put forward a novel avenue to define potential DBS targets. They postulate combining electrocorticography or stereo-EEG (sEEG) with the thermal grill illusion method to map the cerebral pain network to depict possible targets. An interesting approach suggested by Shirvalkar and colleagues is to use sEEG [6]. They propose a trial period in which the electrodes are initially externalized. The effect of stimulation can then first be evaluated before a complete DBS system is implanted. Moreover, this strategy gives the opportunity to obtain neural signals, which might be used as biomarkers of stimulation-induced pain relief.

The most widely used indications for DBS remain Parkinson's disease (PD) and essential tremor (ET). DBS is considered a standard treatment for these disorders. Still, there is plenty of room for improvement. In this prospect, Bogdan and colleagues propose a novel individualized approach to optimize DBS settings for patients with ET [7]. Optimal tremor control can be achieved in patients who do not respond to conventional DBS settings or show habituation. Therefore, commercial DBS parties need to provide access for clinicians to stimulation options beyond the standard set of stimulation settings.

Traditionally, DBS electrodes are implanted whilst using local analgesia on the patient. A trend is to conduct DBS surgeries under general anesthesia [8]. Park and colleagues argue that the classical view, that DBS surgeries for PD patients are best performed in an awake condition to conduct micro-electrode recordings (MER) and macrostimulation, is ready for a change. Their literature review forms the basis to initiate non-inferiority studies to confirm the safety and efficacy of DBS surgeries under general anesthesia. In our electrophysiology study, we studied the effects of procedural sedation and analgesia (PSA) on MER [9]. One of our main findings was that dexmedetomidine reduces the power of the multi-unit activity (MUA) in a dose-dependent matter. The power of the MUA is a parameter which is commonly used to identify the subthalamic nucleus (STN). To what extent the use of anesthetics alters the MER signal that hampers accurate identification of the STN needs further study. Of utmost importance to achieve an optimal lead placement is the quality of the planning based on magnetic resonance imaging (MRI). Our imaging group provided a critical viewpoint on the optimization of pre-operative imaging at the level of acquisition, data-processing and planning software [10]. The individual success of DBS relates considerably to psychological aspects. Baertschi et al. show that illness representations and coping strategies in PD patients are not changed by DBS. However, psychological variances between PD patients should be considered in the acceptation process of life with DBS [11]. Finally, we are challenged by Artusi and colleagues to advance our decision making in the selection process for DBS in PD patients. The current clinical assessment could well benefit from decision support systems, including well-defined phenotypic as well as genetic aspects [12].

The novel concepts to optimize DBS have been developed in a fascinating rally over recent decades. Imaging techniques, using high-field MRI, have evolved considerably. New generations of DBS systems offer more programming options, thereby expanding the therapeutic window. The failure of randomized controlled DBS trials for several different disorders is reflected by the critical reviews presented in this Special Issue. A trend towards a different scientific policy using a more individualized approach for each patient will open new avenues in the field of DBS, while further neurotechnical advances may, in the future, allow DBS or alternatives to DBS to be offered to a broader group of patients. To conclude, we endorse a mechanism-based approach using translational research programs involving diverse experts ranging from basic neuroscientist, engineers, ethicists and clinicians to advance the field of DBS.

Funding: This research received no external funding.

Conflicts of Interest: The authors declare no conflict of interest.

References

1. Hitti, F.L.; Yang, A.I.; Cristancho, M.A.; Baltuch, G.H. Deep brain stimulation is effective for treatment-resistant depression: A meta-analysis and meta-regression. *J. Clin. Med.* **2020**, *9*, 2796. [CrossRef] [PubMed]
2. Roet, M.; Boonstra, J.; Sahin, E.; Mulders, A.E.; Leentjens, A.F.; Jahanshahi, A. Deep brain stimulation for treatment-resistant depression: Towards a more personalized treatment approach. *J. Clin. Med.* **2020**, *9*, 2729. [CrossRef] [PubMed]
3. Khairuddin, S.; Ngo, F.Y.; Lim, W.L.; Aquili, L.; Khan, N.A.; Fung, M.-L.; Chan, Y.; Temel, Y.; Lim, L.W. A decade of progress in deep brain stimulation of the subcallosal cingulate for the treatment of depression. *J. Clin. Med.* **2020**, *9*, 3260. [CrossRef] [PubMed]
4. Görmezoğlu, M.; Van Der Vlis, T.A.M.B.; Schruers, K.R.J.; Ackermans, L.; Polosan, M.; Leentjens, A.F. Effectiveness, timing and procedural aspects of cognitive behavioral therapy after deep brain stimulation for therapy-resistant obsessive compulsive disorder: A systematic review. *J. Clin. Med.* **2020**, *9*, 2383. [CrossRef] [PubMed]
5. Caston, R.M.; Smith, E.H.; Davis, T.; Rolston, J.D. the cerebral localization of pain: Anatomical and functional considerations for targeted electrical therapies. *J. Clin. Med.* **2020**, *9*, 1945. [CrossRef] [PubMed]
6. Shirvalkar, P.; Sellers, K.K.; Schmitgen, A.; Prosky, J.; Joseph, I.; Starr, P.A.; Chang, E.F. A deep brain stimulation trial period for treating chronic pain. *J. Clin. Med.* **2020**, *9*, 3155. [CrossRef] [PubMed]
7. Bogdan, I.D.; Laar, T.; Oterdoom, D.M.; Drost, G.; Van Dijk, J.M.C.; Beudel, M. Optimal parameters of deep brain stimulation in essential tremor: A meta-analysis and novel programming strategy. *J. Clin. Med.* **2020**, *9*, 1855. [CrossRef] [PubMed]
8. Park, H.-R.; Lim, Y.H.; Song, E.J.; Lee, J.M.; Park, K.; Park, K.H.; Lee, W.-W.; Kim, H.-J.; Jeon, B.; Paek, S.H. Bilateral subthalamic nucleus deep brain stimulation under general anesthesia: Literature review and single center experience. *J. Clin. Med.* **2020**, *9*, 3044. [CrossRef]
9. Bos, M.J.; Sanchez, A.M.A.; Bancone, R.; Temel, Y.; De Greef, B.T.A.; Absalom, A.R.; Gommer, E.D.; Van Kranen-Mastenbroek, V.H.; Buhre, W.F.; Roberts, M.; et al. Influence of anesthesia and clinical variables on the firing rate, coefficient of variation and multi-unit activity of the subthalamic nucleus in patients with parkinson's disease. *J. Clin. Med.* **2020**, *9*, 1229. [CrossRef]
10. Isaacs, B.R.; Keuken, M.C.; Alkemade, A.; Temel, Y.; Bazin, P.-L.; Forstmann, B.U. Methodological considerations for neuroimaging in deep brain stimulation of the subthalamic nucleus in Parkinson's disease patients. *J. Clin. Med.* **2020**, *9*, 3124. [CrossRef]
11. Baertschi, M.; Favez, N.; Dos Santos, J.F.A.; Radomska, M.; Herrmann, F.; Burkhard, P.R.; Canuto, A.; Weber, K.; Ghisletta, P. Illness representations and coping strategies in patients treated with deep brain stimulation for parkinson's disease. *J. Clin. Med.* **2020**, *9*, 1186. [CrossRef] [PubMed]
12. Artusi, C.A.; Lopiano, L.; Morgante, F. Deep brain stimulation selection criteria for Parkinson's disease: Time to go beyond CAPSIT-PD. *J. Clin. Med.* **2020**, *9*, 3931. [CrossRef]

Publisher's Note: MDPI stays neutral with regard to jurisdictional claims in published maps and institutional affiliations.

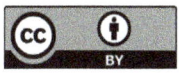

© 2021 by the authors. Licensee MDPI, Basel, Switzerland. This article is an open access article distributed under the terms and conditions of the Creative Commons Attribution (CC BY) license (http://creativecommons.org/licenses/by/4.0/).

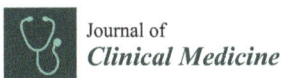

Article

Deep Brain Stimulation Is Effective for Treatment-Resistant Depression: A Meta-Analysis and Meta-Regression

Frederick L. Hitti [1,*], Andrew I. Yang [1], Mario A. Cristancho [2] and Gordon H. Baltuch [1]

1. Department of Neurosurgery, Pennsylvania Hospital, University of Pennsylvania, 800 Spruce St, Philadelphia, PA 19107, USA; andrew.yang@pennmedicine.upenn.edu (A.I.Y.); gordon.baltuch@pennmedicine.upenn.edu (G.H.B.)
2. Department of Psychiatry, University of Pennsylvania, 3535 Market Street, Philadelphia, PA 19104, USA; marioc@pennmedicine.upenn.edu
* Correspondence: Frederick.Hitti@uphs.upenn.edu; Tel.: +1-215-834-0444

Received: 21 July 2020; Accepted: 27 August 2020; Published: 30 August 2020

Abstract: Major depressive disorder (MDD) is a leading cause of disability and a significant cause of mortality worldwide. Approximately 30–40% of patients fail to achieve clinical remission with available pharmacological treatments, a clinical course termed treatment-resistant depression (TRD). Numerous studies have investigated deep brain stimulation (DBS) as a therapy for TRD. We performed a meta-analysis to determine efficacy and a meta-regression to compare stimulation targets. We identified and screened 1397 studies. We included 125 citations in the qualitative review and considered 26 for quantitative analysis. Only blinded studies that compared active DBS to sham stimulation (k = 12) were included in the meta-analysis. The random-effects model supported the efficacy of DBS for TRD (standardized mean difference = −0.75, <0 favors active stimulation; $p = 0.0001$). The meta-regression did not demonstrate a statistically significant difference between stimulation targets ($p = 0.45$). While enthusiasm for DBS treatment of TRD has been tempered by recent randomized trials, this meta-analysis reveals a significant effect of DBS for the treatment of TRD. Additionally, the majority of trials have demonstrated the safety and efficacy of DBS for this indication. Further trials are required to determine the optimal stimulation parameters and patient populations for which DBS would be effective. Particular attention to factors including electrode placement technique, patient selection, and long-term follow-up is essential for future trial design.

Keywords: deep brain stimulation; treatment-resistant depression; depression; meta-analysis; meta-regression; subcallosal cingulate gyrus; medial forebrain bundle; inferior thalamic peduncle; ventral capsule; ventral striatum

1. Introduction

Major depressive disorder (MDD) is one of the most common psychiatric diseases, and while a number of therapies are available, many patients remain symptomatic despite treatment [1,2]. Well-established treatment modalities for MDD include psychotherapy, medication, and electroconvulsive therapy (ECT) [3–9]. While ECT is efficacious for many patients resistant to medication and therapy, there are significant adverse effects associated with ECT, including cognitive and memory dysfunction [3]. Furthermore, there are patients who are refractory to multiple available therapies, including ECT. Patients who fail to improve following treatment with two or more therapies are considered to have treatment-resistant depression (TRD) [5,8,10–12]. Due to the considerable number of treatment non-remitters (30–40% of patients with MDD), developing novel therapies for TRD represents a major unmet need.

Deep brain stimulation (DBS) is a technique that uses implanted intracranial electrodes to modulate neural activity. It is currently a well-established, FDA-approved treatment for movement disorders such as Parkinson's disease (PD) and essential tremor (ET) [13,14]. In addition to movement disorders, DBS has been explored as a treatment modality for psychiatric conditions. Multiple human trials have explored the efficacy of DBS for TRD. Anatomic targets have included the ventral anterior limb of the internal capsule (vALIC) [15], ventral capsule/ventral striatum (VC/VS) [16], subcallosal cingulate (SCC) [17–22], inferior thalamic peduncle (ITP) [23], medial forebrain bundle (MFB) [24,25], and lateral habenula [26]. Reports regarding the efficacy of DBS for TRD have been mixed, with some studies demonstrating encouraging results, while others have shown a lack of efficacy relative to sham stimulation. To leverage all of the available data, we performed a meta-analysis to determine the efficacy of DBS for TRD. We then performed a meta-regression to compare stimulation targets. While prior meta-analyses have been undertaken [27–29], here we included only studies that compared active to sham stimulation in a blinded fashion. Furthermore, our analysis includes more recent studies.

2. Methods

2.1. Search Strategy

We used the PubMed database to identify studies investigating DBS for MDD and screened all studies for inclusion. We used the following search terms to identify relevant studies: ("deep brain stimulation"[MeSH Terms] OR ("deep"[All Fields] AND "brain"[All Fields] AND "stimulation"[All Fields]) OR "deep brain stimulation"[All Fields] OR "DBS"[All Fields]) AND ("depressive disorder"[MeSH Terms] OR ("depressive"[All Fields] AND "disorder"[All Fields]) OR "depressive disorder"[All Fields] OR "depression"[All Fields] OR "depression"[MeSH Terms]). All studies were considered, including studies written in other languages. The search was conducted on 10/16/2019, and the analysis followed the Preferred Reporting Items for Systematic reviews and Meta-Analyses (PRISMA) guidelines.

2.2. Study Inclusion and Exclusion Criteria

Only studies that investigated the efficacy of DBS for MDD were included. We excluded studies that utilized other therapies to treat MDD (e.g., ECT, epidural stimulation, vagal nerve stimulation, transcranial magnetic stimulation, or tDCS). We also excluded studies that investigated comorbid depression in the context of other disorders, such as epilepsy, dystonia, Tourette syndrome, anorexia nervosa, obsessive–compulsive disorder, schizophrenia, headache, ET, and PD. We excluded all non-human studies. Of the studies relevant to DBS as a treatment for MDD, we excluded case reports, non-systematic reviews, perspectives, commentaries, editorials, and opinions. We included the remainder of the studies for our qualitative review. For the quantitative meta-analysis, we only included studies in which sham stimulation was compared to active stimulation in a blinded fashion (either single- or double-blind). The clinical trial designs were varied and included both crossover and parallel studies.

2.3. Data Extraction and Outcome Measures

Our primary outcome was the efficacy of DBS as a treatment for depression as assessed by changes in the Hamilton Depression Rating Scale (HDRS) or Montgomery–Åsberg Depression Rating Scale (MADRS) scores. We compared sham stimulation scores to active stimulation scores. The data were extracted from tables when provided. If tables with the raw data were not provided, the WebPlotDigitizer tool was used to extract data from published graphs. We also extracted the number of patients, stimulation target, side effects of treatment, adverse events, study design, and depression rating scale used.

2.4. Statistical Methods

Statistical analysis was conducted in R using the meta, metaphor, and dmetar packages. We followed the guide published by Harrer et al. to conduct the analysis [30]. A random-effects model was employed for the meta-analysis to account for differences in study populations. We used the DerSimonian–Laird estimator for τ^2 (variance of true effect magnitude distributions), as it is the most widely used estimator. The studies included in the quantitative analysis used different depression rating scales. Therefore, we computed standardized mean differences so that the studies could be compared. We also calculated heterogeneity (I^2) of the studies in R. The differential efficacies of the various stimulation targets were compared with mixed-effects meta-regression. R was used to generate funnel plots and conduct Egger's test. Means are presented with their corresponding standard deviations. A p-value < 0.05 was considered statistically significant.

3. Results

We used fairly broad search terms (see Section 2) to ensure the inclusion of all studies relevant to the use of DBS as a therapy for depression. Our search identified 1397 studies, and all were screened for inclusion (Figure 1). We excluded 964 studies at the abstract/title level because these studies either did not use DBS as the therapeutic modality, examined depressive symptomatology in the context of other diseases, or were non-human animal studies. Of the remaining relevant studies, 308 were excluded because they were case reports, non-systematic reviews, perspectives, commentaries, editorials, or opinions. The remaining 125 studies were included in our qualitative review. We then screened these studies for inclusion in our quantitative meta-analysis. Twenty-six studies were candidates for inclusion at the abstract level. Thirteen studies were excluded because they did not compare active to sham stimulation [31–43], and one study was excluded as it included only three patients [44]. Therefore, 12 studies [15–25] (186 unique patients) were included in the meta-analysis and meta-regression (Table 1). The Raymaekers et al. study was analyzed as two separate studies, because this study included two anatomically distinct stimulation targets, and both targets were evaluated with blinded stimulation periods.

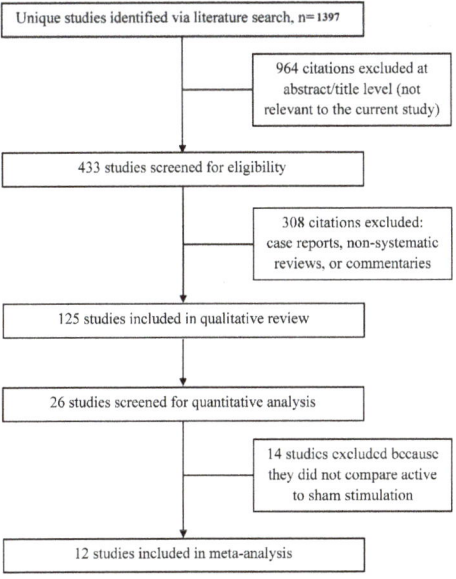

Figure 1. Flowchart of studies selected for inclusion in the qualitative review and quantitative meta-analysis.

Table 1. Studies included in meta-analysis and meta-regression.

Study	Location	N	Blinded Crossover
Bergfeld et al. 2016	vALIC	16	Yes
Coenen et al. 2019	MFB	16	No
Dougherty et al. 2015	VC/VS	29	No
Fenoy et al. 2018	MFB	6	Yes
Holtzheimer et al. 2012	SCC	10	Yes
Holtzheimer et al. 2017	SCC	85	No
Merkl et al. 2013	SCC	6	Yes
Merkl et al. 2018	SCC	4	Yes *
Puigdemont et al. 2015	SCC	5	Yes
Ramasubbu et al. 2013	SCC	4	Yes
Raymaekers et al. 2017	IC/BST	5	Yes
Raymaekers et al. 2017	ITP	5	Yes

* Only half of the patients crossed over. IC/BST: internal capsule/bed nucleus of the stria terminalis; ITP: inferior thalamic peduncle; MFB: medial forebrain bundle; SCC: subcallosal cingulate; vALIC: ventral anterior limb of the internal capsule; VC/VS: ventral capsule/ventral striatum.

The studies included in the meta-analysis had varied trial designs (Table 1). Due to our inclusion criteria, all studies contained a period of blinded sham stimulation and blinded active stimulation. The duration of the active and sham stimulation periods, however, was heterogeneous. The average blinded stimulation duration was 7.5 ± 6.6 weeks. All studies contained an open-label period of long-term active stimulation following the blinded phases. These long-term data were not included in the meta-analysis, since the goal of the present study was to compare blinded active stimulation to blinded sham stimulation. The majority of the trials (75%) were done in a crossover fashion (Table 1). Thus, all of the patients in these studies received both active and sham stimulation in a blinded fashion. Importantly, these study designs allow for within-subject comparisons and may enhance statistical power.

Using a random-effects model, our meta-analysis revealed that active stimulation results in a greater decline in HDRS/MADRS scores relative to sham stimulation (standardized mean difference (SMD) = −0.75; −1.13 to −0.36, 95% confidence interval (CI); p-value = 0.0001; Figure 2). There was moderate heterogeneity across studies (I^2 = 59%).

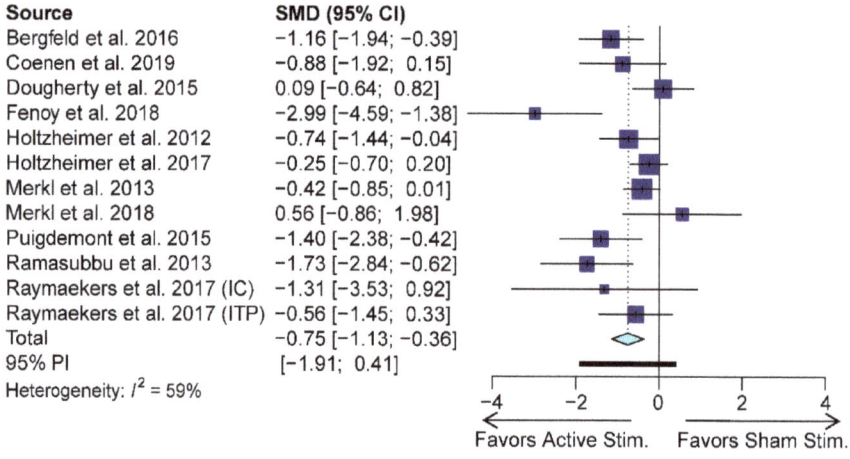

Figure 2. Meta-analysis forest plot depicting changes in HDRS/MADRS scores with active stimulation compared to sham stimulation. CI: confidence interval; IC: internal capsule; ITP: inferior thalamic peduncle; SMD: standardized mean difference; PI: prediction interval.

In addition to differences in study design, the studies also investigated the efficacy of DBS for TRD using different stimulation targets (Table 1). The most common target was the SCC (50% of studies), followed by the internal capsule (IC, 25%), MFB (17%), and ITP (8%). While there were a limited number of studies, we utilized meta-regression to determine if the available data would reveal an optimal stimulation target. The meta-regression, however, did not demonstrate a statistically significant difference ($p = 0.45$) between stimulation targets (Figure 3).

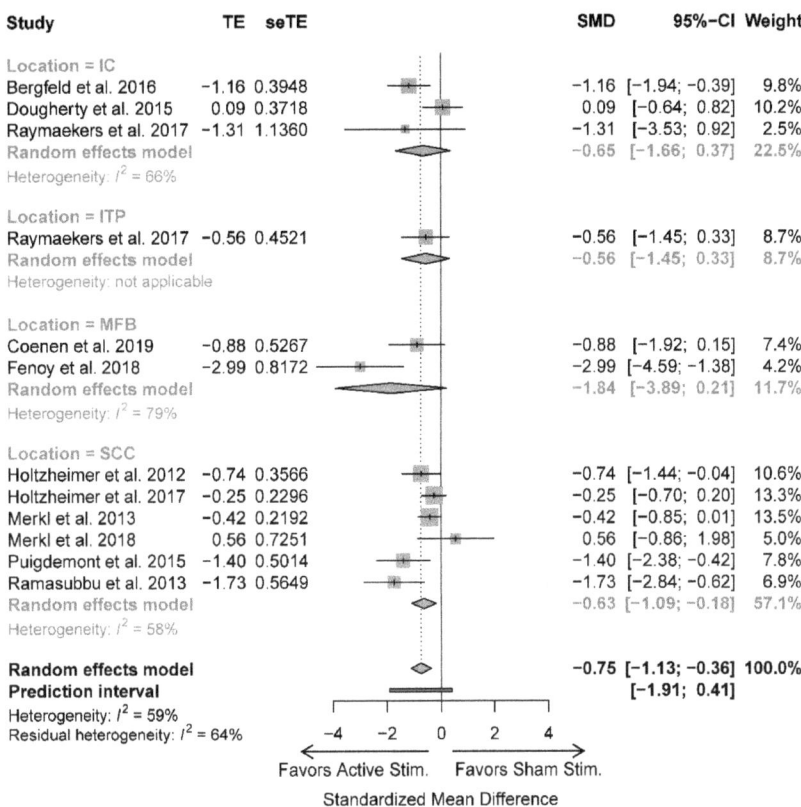

Figure 3. Meta-regression forest plot comparing various stimulation targets. CI: confidence interval; IC: internal capsule; ITP: inferior thalamic peduncle; MFB: medial forebrain bundle; SCC: subcallosal cingulate; SMD: standardized mean difference; TE: treatment effect; seTE: standard error of treatment effect.

Since the duration of stimulation during the blinded phase varied between studies, we performed another meta-regression to determine if there was an association between the duration of active stimulation and SMD. Our analysis did not reveal a significant effect of stimulation duration on SMD outcomes ($p = 0.20$).

Publication bias is an important concern when conducting a meta-analysis. We investigated for possible publication bias by first generating a funnel plot (Figure 4). We then tested for asymmetry of the funnel plot with Egger's test. The test revealed that there was no statistically significant asymmetry in the plot (intercept -1.9; 95% CI -3.864–0.056; $p = 0.07$), thus arguing against publication bias. Given the strong trend of Egger's test and the fact that one study (Fenoy et al. 2018) was a clear outlier, as depicted in the funnel plot, we re-analyzed the data with this outlier study excluded. Using a random-effects model, a meta-analysis of the pared data confirmed that active stimulation results in a greater decline in HDRS/MADRS scores relative to sham stimulation (SMD = −0.62; 95% CI −0.95 to −0.30; p = 0.0002). Removing the outlier study decreased study heterogeneity (I^2 = 45%) and decreased the likelihood of publication bias as estimated by Egger's test (intercept −1.3; 95% CI −3.26–0.66; p = 0.21).

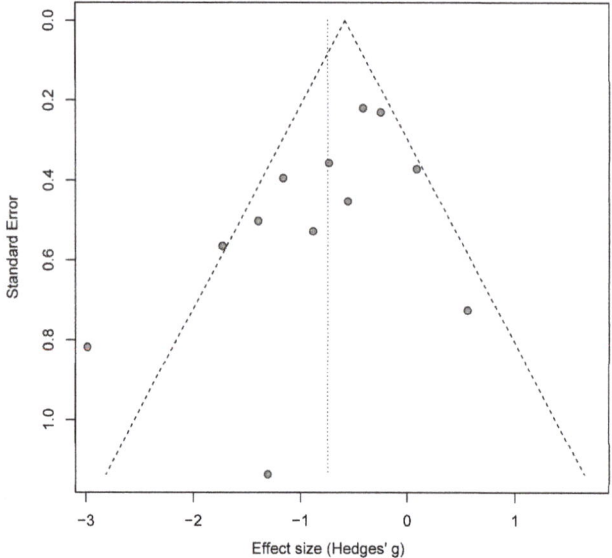

Figure 4. Funnel plot of studies included in the quantitative analysis.

We examined and compiled the adverse events reported in the studies included in the quantitative meta-analysis. The adverse events occurring in greater than 1% of patients are listed in Table 2, and the full list of adverse events in each study is detailed in Supplementary Table S1. The most common complaint was headache (26% of patients), followed by visual disturbances (21%), worsening depression (16%), sleep disturbances (16%), and anxiety (14%). All other adverse events were only seen in less than 10% of patients (Table 2). The authors of the original studies reported that the vast majority of adverse events were transient and were often resolved by stimulation parameter adjustment. The headaches were often postoperative and resolved a few days after surgery. A significant number of patients (n = 16, 8%) expressed suicidal ideation, and a similar number of patients (n = 15, 8%) attempted suicide. Completed suicides were rare. In two studies, one patient from each study who had no response to DBS committed suicide [15,16]. In one large study, there were two deaths by suicide in the control group during the open-label phase [17]. Finally, in another study, two patients committed suicide [23]. These suicides were deemed to be unrelated to DBS, because both patients had a history of suicide attempts and DBS did not appear to increase impulsivity [23].

Table 2. Adverse events.

Adverse Event	Patients (N)	Patients (%)
Headache	50	26
Blurred Vision/Diplopia	41	21
Worsening depression	31	16
Sleep Disturbances	30	16
Anxiety	26	14
Pain Around Neurostimulator	17	9
Nausea	16	8
Suicidal Ideation	16	8
Pain Around Incisions	16	8
Post-operative discomfort	16	8
Suicide Attempt	15	8
Device Infection	15	8
Balance/Gait Problems	13	7
Non-Specific Somatic Complaints	12	6
Pain/pulling sensation around Extension Wires	11	6
Other infections	10	5
Agitation	9	5
Paresthesias	9	5
Restlessness	8	4
Disinhibition/Impulsivity	8	4
Hypomania	8	4
Confusion/Cognitive impairment	8	4
Swollen Eyes	6	3
Excessive Sweating	6	3
Memory Disturbance	6	3
Weight Gain/hyperphagia	6	3
Lethargy	6	3
Abnormal Body Temperature	5	3
Hypertension	5	3
Postoperative Delirium	4	2
Constipation	4	2
Speech difficulties	4	2
Panic attack	4	2
Diarrhea	4	2
Irritability	4	2
Libido decrease/increase	4	2
Increase in drug side effects	4	2
Skin Disorder	4	2
Neuralgia	4	2
Drowsiness	4	2
Palpations Around Neurostimulator	3	2
Neck Pain	3	2
Mania	3	2
Hallucinations	3	2
Palpitations	3	2
Weakness	3	2
Mood swings	3	2
Difficulty voiding/urinary retention	3	2
Back pain	3	2
Electrode revision	3	2
Elective hospitalization	3	2

4. Discussion

MDD is a very prevalent neuropsychiatric condition. Although there are a number of existing treatment modalities, many patients remain symptomatic despite adequate treatment protocols. There is an urgent need for additional treatment options for TRD, since it is a significant source of morbidity and mortality.

Pathological neural activity (either hyperactivity or hypoactivity) may lead to neurological or psychiatric disease, and non-pharmacological neuromodulatory techniques may be used to ameliorate these conditions. DBS is a neuromodulatory approach that is an FDA-approved treatment for movement disorders, so multiple investigators have trialed DBS as a therapy for TRD. Initial open-label reports regarding the efficacy of DBS for TRD were encouraging [36,45], and subsequently, multiple randomized trials were initiated and completed [16,17]. The large-scale trials, however, did not reveal a significant difference between the control and treatment groups. A number of reasons have been posited to explain these negative results, including choice of stimulation target, electrode placement technique, patient selection, and short-term follow-up of patients [43,46–52].

Due to the discrepancy between earlier reports and larger trials, we undertook a meta-analysis to investigate the efficacy of DBS for TRD. In agreement with prior analyses [27–29], we found a significant effect of DBS on TRD. Specifically, active stimulation was associated with an improvement in depression scores relative to sham stimulation. The effect size of this treatment is medium to large, as indicated by the SMD of −0.75 [53]. This effect size is much larger than the small effect sizes (~0.3) seen with pharmacologic antidepressant treatment of patients with MDD [54]. Our findings extend those of prior analyses by including all currently available studies and by only including blinded studies that utilized a trial design in which active stimulation was compared to sham stimulation. Importantly, analyzing the data in this manner allows for the control of placebo effects. While some patients are able to detect active stimulation due to side effects such as visual disturbances, these effects are largely absent with a stimulation parameter adjustment [24,25]. With most studies including an optimization phase prior to the blinded assessments, it is reasonable to propose that comparing active stimulation to sham stimulation controls for placebo effects.

We conducted a meta-regression to determine if the data would reveal an optimal stimulation target. Due to the limited number of available studies, our analysis did not demonstrate an optimal target. With further research, the answer to this question may be elucidated in the future; however, a significant limitation is the heterogeneous nature of MDD neurobiology (i.e., symptoms of depression as a common manifestation of multiple brain functional abnormalities). It may be that instead of one optimal stimulation target for all patients, the optimal stimulation target varies across individuals [46,55–58].

As with any therapy, there is a risk of publication bias since studies with positive results and large effect sizes are more likely to be published than studies with small effect sizes or negative results [59]. To investigate publication bias in DBS for depression, we plotted the studies in a funnel plot and used Egger's test to assess for asymmetry. We did not find evidence of publication bias in this series of studies.

DBS is a well-tolerated treatment for movement disorders, but it is important to critically evaluate potential side effects of DBS for depression. The thoroughness of adverse event reporting varied between the studies. Nonetheless, the majority of adverse events were transient. Furthermore, many side effects were relieved by a stimulation parameter adjustment, as is seen with DBS for movement disorders. Patients with MDD are at significant risk for suicide, and patients with TRD have an even higher risk of suicide [60,61]. Currently available data do not demonstrate an increased risk of suicide with DBS, since suicide was rare in these studies and occurred at a lower rate than in patients with severe MDD not receiving DBS [62]. Moreover, the completed suicides occurred in non-responders or were deemed unrelated to DBS. As an invasive therapy, DBS may be perceived by patients as a "last resort" for recovery. Therefore, non-responders may represent a particularly high-risk group for suicide. Psychoeducation and adequate discussion of post DBS treatment options to reframe those perceptions may decrease the risk of suicide. In summary, published trials have demonstrated the safety of DBS for TRD.

While the results of this meta-analysis are encouraging, additional large-scale clinical trials demonstrating the efficacy of DBS for TRD are essential. Crucial to these efforts will be careful consideration of future trial design [24,63]. The large-scale clinical trials of DBS for TRD conducted to date have utilized a parallel trial design, whereas many of the smaller trials employed a crossover design (Table 1). Given the negative outcomes of the large-scale trials, a crossover design may be optimal to investigate the efficacy of DBS for TRD. As a therapy, DBS is unique in that sham stimulation and active stimulation may be compared within individuals, thereby facilitating crossover trial design. Crossover studies require fewer patients to achieve significance, so this design optimizes statistical power [64]. Some studies have used customized trial designs with a variable optimization period [15,65]. Ensuring proper optimization prior to randomization may be necessary to determine the efficacy of DBS for TRD. Another important factor in trial design is the length of time that the patient undergoes therapy. Long-term open-label studies have demonstrated that the efficacy of DBS for TRD improves over time, so longer trials may be necessary [17,18,38,66,67]. Finally, depression severity waxes and wanes throughout a patient's disease course. Therefore, trial designs that compare groups at specific time points may not be optimal. Integrating scores over predefined time periods may enhance outcome assessment.

In addition to trial design, proper electrode targeting is important for the efficacy of DBS for the treatment of depression. Instead of targeting brain nuclei, as is routinely done, targeting fiber tracts using patient-specific tractography may be important for therapeutic efficacy [49–52,58,68]. Furthermore, stereotactic accuracy of electrode placement is essential. For example, intraoperative phenomena, such as brain shift, should be accounted for [48]. Patient selection is also a critical consideration for future studies. The available data have demonstrated that there is a subgroup of patients that respond to this therapy and a subgroup that does not. Determining patient-specific factors (e.g., anatomical or symptom-based) that predict response to DBS for TRD may enable targeted selection of patients for whom DBS would be therapeutic [43,69–75]. These patient-specific factors could then be used as study inclusion criteria to enhance the probability of study success.

5. Conclusions

While enthusiasm for DBS as a therapy for TRD has been tempered by recent randomized trials, this meta-analysis reveals that active stimulation significantly ameliorates depression in patients with TRD. The meta-regression did not reveal an optimal stimulation target to treat depression due to the small size and number of available studies, and also likely due to the heterogeneous nature of this condition's neurobiology. Additional trials are needed to determine optimal stimulation targets. Further studies are also required to establish the patient populations for whom DBS would be effective. Particular attention to factors that include electrode placement technique, patient selection, and long-term observation is essential for future trial design.

Supplementary Materials: The following are available online at http://www.mdpi.com/2077-0383/9/9/2796/s1, Table S1: Complete list of adverse events.

Author Contributions: Conceptualization, F.L.H. and G.H.B.; methodology, F.L.H.; validation, F.L.H., A.I.Y., M.A.C., G.H.B.; formal analysis, F.L.H and A.I.Y; investigation, F.L.H.; data curation, F.L.H.; writing—Original draft preparation, F.L.H. and A.I.Y.; writing—Review and editing, F.L.H., A.I.Y., M.A.C., G.H.B.; visualization, F.L.H.; supervision, G.H.B.; project administration, G.H.B. All authors have read and agreed to the published version of the manuscript.

Funding: This research received no external funding.

Conflicts of Interest: The authors declare no conflict of interest.

References

1. Ferrari, A.J.; Charlson, F.J.; Norman, R.E.; Patten, S.B.; Freedman, G.; Murray, C.J.L.; Vos, T.; Whiteford, H.A. Burden of Depressive Disorders by Country, Sex, Age, and Year: Findings from the Global Burden of Disease Study 2010. *PLoS Med.* **2013**, *10*, e1001547. [CrossRef] [PubMed]
2. Steel, Z.; Marnane, C.; Iranpour, C.; Chey, T.; Jackson, J.W.; Patel, V.; Silove, D. The global prevalence of common mental disorders: A systematic review and meta-analysis 1980–2013. *Int. J. Epidemiol.* **2014**, *43*, 476–493. [CrossRef] [PubMed]
3. Bailine, S.H.; Rifkin, A.; Kayne, E.; Selzer, J.A.; Vital-Herne, J.; Blieka, M.; Pollack, S. Comparison of Bifrontal and Bitemporal ECT for Major Depression. *Am. J. Psychiatry* **2000**, *157*, 121–123. [CrossRef] [PubMed]
4. Fava, M.; Rush, A.J.; Wisniewski, S.R.; Nierenberg, A.A.; Alpert, J.E.; McGrath, P.J.; Thase, M.E.; Warden, D.; Biggs, M.; Luther, J.F.; et al. A comparison of mirtazapine and nortriptyline following two consecutive failed medication treatments for depressed outpatients: A STAR*D report. *Am. J. Psychiatry* **2006**, *163*, 1161–1172. [CrossRef]
5. Hollon, S.D.; Jarrett, R.B.; Nierenberg, A.A.; Thase, M.E.; Trivedi, M.; Rush, A.J. Psychotherapy and Medication in the Treatment of Adult and Geriatric Depression: Which Monotherapy or Combined Treatment? *J. Clin. Psychiatry* **2005**, *66*, 455–468. [CrossRef]
6. Nierenberg, A.A.; Fava, M.; Trivedi, M.H.; Wisniewski, S.R.; Thase, M.E.; McGrath, P.J.; Alpert, J.E.; Warden, D.; Luther, J.F.; Niederehe, G.; et al. A Comparison of Lithium and T 3 Augmentation Following Two Failed Medication Treatments for Depression: A STAR*D Report. *Am. J. Psychiatry* **2006**, *163*, 1519–1530. [CrossRef]
7. Rush, A.J.; Trivedi, M.H.; Wisniewski, S.R.; Stewart, J.W.; Nierenberg, A.A.; Thase, M.E.; Ritz, L.; Biggs, M.M.; Warden, D.; Luther, J.F.; et al. Bupropion-SR, sertraline, or venlafaxine-XR after failure of SSRIs for depression. *N. Engl. J. Med.* **2006**, *354*, 1231–1242. [CrossRef]
8. Thase, M.E.; Friedman, E.S.; Biggs, M.M.; Wisniewski, S.R.; Trivedi, M.H.; Luther, J.F.; Fava, M.; Nierenberg, A.A.; McGrath, P.J.; Warden, D.; et al. Cognitive Therapy Versus Medication in Augmentation and Switch Strategies as Second-Step Treatments: A STAR*D Report. *Am. J. Psychiatry* **2007**, *164*, 739–752. [CrossRef]
9. Trivedi, M.H.; Rush, A.J.; Wisniewski, S.R.; Nierenberg, A.A.; Warden, D.; Ritz, L.; Norquist, G.; Howland, R.H.; Lebowitz, B.; McGrath, P.J.; et al. Evaluation of Outcomes With Citalopram for Depression Using Measurement-Based Care in STAR*D: Implications for Clinical Practice. *Am. J. Psychiatry* **2006**, *163*, 28–40. [CrossRef]
10. Souery, D.; Papakostas, G.I.; Trivedi, M.H. Treatment-resistant depression. *J. Clin. Psychiatry* **2006**, *67* (Suppl. 6), 16–22.
11. Greden, J.F. The burden of disease for treatment-resistant depression. *J. Clin. Psychiatry* **2001**, *62* (Suppl. 16), 26–31.
12. Taipale, H.; Reutfors, J.; Tanskanen, A.; Brandt, L.; Tiihonen, J.; DiBernardo, A.; Mittendorfer-Rutz, E.; Brenner, P. Risk and risk factors for disability pension among patients with treatment resistant depression- a matched cohort study. *BMC Psychiatry* **2020**, *20*, 232. [CrossRef] [PubMed]
13. Hitti, F.L.; Ramayya, A.G.; McShane, B.J.; Yang, A.I.; Vaughan, K.A.; Baltuch, G.H. Long-term outcomes following deep brain stimulation for Parkinson's disease. *J. Neurosurg.* **2019**. [CrossRef] [PubMed]
14. Miocinovic, S.; Somayajula, S.; Chitnis, S.; Vitek, J.L. History, Applications, and Mechanisms of Deep Brain Stimulation. *JAMA Neurol.* **2013**, *70*, 163–171. [CrossRef] [PubMed]
15. Bergfeld, I.O.; Mantione, M.; Hoogendoorn, M.L.C.; Ruhe, H.G.; Notten, P.; van Laarhoven, J.; Visser, I.; Figee, M.; de Kwaasteniet, B.P.; Horst, F.; et al. Deep Brain Stimulation of the Ventral Anterior Limb of the Internal Capsule for Treatment-Resistant Depression: A Randomized Clinical Trial. *JAMA Psychiatry* **2016**, *73*, 456–464. [CrossRef] [PubMed]
16. Dougherty, D.D.; Rezai, A.R.; Carpenter, L.L.; Howland, R.H.; Bhati, M.T.; O'Reardon, J.P.; Eskandar, E.N.; Baltuch, G.H.; Machado, A.D.; Kondziolka, D.; et al. A Randomized Sham-Controlled Trial of Deep Brain Stimulation of the Ventral Capsule/Ventral Striatum for Chronic Treatment-Resistant Depression. *Biol. Psychiatry* **2015**, *78*, 240–248. [CrossRef]

17. Holtzheimer, P.E.; Husain, M.M.; Lisanby, S.H.; Taylor, S.F.; Whitworth, L.A.; McClintock, S.; Slavin, K.V.; Berman, J.; McKhann, G.M.; Patil, P.G.; et al. Subcallosal cingulate deep brain stimulation for treatment-resistant depression: A multisite, randomised, sham-controlled trial. *Lancet Psychiatry* **2017**, *4*, 839–849. [CrossRef]
18. Holtzheimer, P.E.; Kelley, M.E.; Gross, R.E.; Filkowski, M.M.; Garlow, S.J.; Barrocas, A.; Wint, D.; Craighead, M.C.; Kozarsky, J.; Chismar, R.; et al. Subcallosal cingulate deep brain stimulation for treatment-resistant unipolar and bipolar depression. *Arch. Gen. Psychiatry* **2012**, *69*, 150–158. [CrossRef]
19. Merkl, A.; Schneider, G.-H.; Schonecker, T.; Aust, S.; Kuhl, K.-P.; Kupsch, A.; Kuhn, A.A.; Bajbouj, M. Antidepressant effects after short-term and chronic stimulation of the subgenual cingulate gyrus in treatment-resistant depression. *Exp. Neurol.* **2013**, *249*, 160–168. [CrossRef]
20. Merkl, A.; Aust, S.; Schneider, G.-H.; Visser-Vandewalle, V.; Horn, A.; Kuhn, A.A.; Kuhn, J.; Bajbouj, M. Deep brain stimulation of the subcallosal cingulate gyrus in patients with treatment-resistant depression: A double-blinded randomized controlled study and long-term follow-up in eight patients. *J. Affect. Disord.* **2018**, *227*, 521–529. [CrossRef]
21. Puigdemont, D.; Portella, M.; Perez-Egea, R.; Molet, J.; Gironell, A.; de Diego-Adelino, J.; Martin, A.; Rodriguez, R.; Alvarez, E.; Artigas, F.; et al. A randomized double-blind crossover trial of deep brain stimulation of the subcallosal cingulate gyrus in patients with treatment-resistant depression: A pilot study of relapse prevention. *J. Psychiatry Neurosci. JPN* **2015**, *40*, 224–231. [CrossRef] [PubMed]
22. Ramasubbu, R.; Anderson, S.; Haffenden, A.; Chavda, S.; Kiss, Z.H.T. Double-blind optimization of subcallosal cingulate deep brain stimulation for treatment-resistant depression: A pilot study. *J. Psychiatry Neurosci. JPN* **2013**, *38*, 325–332. [CrossRef] [PubMed]
23. Raymaekers, S.; Luyten, L.; Bervoets, C.; Gabriels, L.; Nuttin, B. Deep brain stimulation for treatment-resistant major depressive disorder: A comparison of two targets and long-term follow-up. *Transl. Psychiatry* **2017**, *7*, e1251. [CrossRef] [PubMed]
24. Coenen, V.A.; Bewernick, B.H.; Kayser, S.; Kilian, H.; Bostrom, J.; Greschus, S.; Hurlemann, R.; Klein, M.E.; Spanier, S.; Sajonz, B.; et al. Superolateral medial forebrain bundle deep brain stimulation in major depression: A gateway trial. *Neuropsychopharmacol. Off. Publ. Am. Coll. Neuropsychopharmacol.* **2019**, *44*, 1224–1232. [CrossRef]
25. Fenoy, A.J.; Schulz, P.E.; Selvaraj, S.; Burrows, C.L.; Zunta-Soares, G.; Durkin, K.; Zanotti-Fregonara, P.; Quevedo, J.; Soares, J.C. A longitudinal study on deep brain stimulation of the medial forebrain bundle for treatment-resistant depression. *Transl. Psychiatry* **2018**, *8*, 111. [CrossRef] [PubMed]
26. Sartorius, A.; Kiening, K.L.; Kirsch, P.; von Gall, C.C.; Haberkorn, U.; Unterberg, A.W.; Henn, F.A.; Meyer-Lindenberg, A. Remission of Major Depression Under Deep Brain Stimulation of the Lateral Habenula in a Therapy-Refractory Patient. *Biol. Psychiatry* **2010**, *67*, e9–e11. [CrossRef]
27. Zhou, C.; Zhang, H.; Qin, Y.; Tian, T.; Xu, B.; Chen, J.; Zhou, X.; Zeng, L.; Fang, L.; Qi, X.; et al. A systematic review and meta-analysis of deep brain stimulation in treatment-resistant depression. *Prog. Neuropsychopharmacol. Biol. Psychiatry* **2018**, *82*, 224–232. [CrossRef]
28. Kisely, S.; Li, A.; Warren, N.; Siskind, D. A systematic review and meta-analysis of deep brain stimulation for depression. *Depress. Anxiety* **2018**, *35*, 468–480. [CrossRef]
29. Berlim, M.T.; McGirr, A.; Van den Eynde, F.; Fleck, M.P.A.; Giacobbe, P. Effectiveness and acceptability of deep brain stimulation (DBS) of the subgenual cingulate cortex for treatment-resistant depression: A systematic review and exploratory meta-analysis. *J. Affect. Disord.* **2014**, *159*, 31–38. [CrossRef]
30. Harrer, M.; Cuijpers, P.; Furukawa, T.; Ebert, D. Doing Meta-Analysis in R: A Hands-on Guide. Available online: https://bookdown.org/MathiasHarrer/Doing_Meta_Analysis_in_R/ (accessed on 26 June 2020).
31. Lozano, A.M.; Mayberg, H.S.; Giacobbe, P.; Hamani, C.; Craddock, R.C.; Kennedy, S.H. Subcallosal cingulate gyrus deep brain stimulation for treatment-resistant depression. *Biol. Psychiatry* **2008**, *64*, 461–467. [CrossRef]
32. Lozano, A.M.; Giacobbe, P.; Hamani, C.; Rizvi, S.J.; Kennedy, S.H.; Kolivakis, T.T.; Debonnel, G.; Sadikot, A.F.; Lam, R.W.; Howard, A.K.; et al. A multicenter pilot study of subcallosal cingulate area deep brain stimulation for treatment-resistant depression. *J. Neurosurg.* **2012**, *116*, 315–322. [CrossRef] [PubMed]
33. Puigdemont, D.; Perez-Egea, R.; Portella, M.J.; Molet, J.; de Diego-Adelino, J.; Gironell, A.; Radua, J.; Gomez-Anson, B.; Rodriguez, R.; Serra, M.; et al. Deep brain stimulation of the subcallosal cingulate gyrus: Further evidence in treatment-resistant major depression. *Int. J. Neuropsychopharmacol.* **2012**, *15*, 121–133. [CrossRef] [PubMed]

34. Bewernick, B.H.; Hurlemann, R.; Matusch, A.; Kayser, S.; Grubert, C.; Hadrysiewicz, B.; Axmacher, N.; Lemke, M.; Cooper-Mahkorn, D.; Cohen, M.X.; et al. Nucleus accumbens deep brain stimulation decreases ratings of depression and anxiety in treatment-resistant depression. *Biol. Psychiatry* **2010**, *67*, 110–116. [CrossRef] [PubMed]
35. Millet, B.; Jaafari, N.; Polosan, M.; Baup, N.; Giordana, B.; Haegelen, C.; Chabardes, S.; Fontaine, D.; Devaux, B.; Yelnik, J.; et al. Limbic versus cognitive target for deep brain stimulation in treatment-resistant depression: Accumbens more promising than caudate. *Eur. Neuropsychopharmacol. J. Eur. Coll. Neuropsychopharmacol.* **2014**, *24*, 1229–1239. [CrossRef]
36. Malone, D.A.J.; Dougherty, D.D.; Rezai, A.R.; Carpenter, L.L.; Friehs, G.M.; Eskandar, E.N.; Rauch, S.L.; Rasmussen, S.A.; Machado, A.G.; Kubu, C.S.; et al. Deep brain stimulation of the ventral capsule/ventral striatum for treatment-resistant depression. *Biol. Psychiatry* **2009**, *65*, 267–275. [CrossRef]
37. Bewernick, B.H.; Kayser, S.; Gippert, S.M.; Switala, C.; Coenen, V.A.; Schlaepfer, T.E. Deep brain stimulation to the medial forebrain bundle for depression- long-term outcomes and a novel data analysis strategy. *Brain Stimulat.* **2017**, *10*, 664–671. [CrossRef]
38. Crowell, A.L.; Riva-Posse, P.; Holtzheimer, P.E.; Garlow, S.J.; Kelley, M.E.; Gross, R.E.; Denison, L.; Quinn, S.; Mayberg, H.S. Long-Term Outcomes of Subcallosal Cingulate Deep Brain Stimulation for Treatment-Resistant Depression. *Am. J. Psychiatry* **2019**. [CrossRef]
39. Schlaepfer, T.E.; Bewernick, B.H.; Kayser, S.; Madler, B.; Coenen, V.A. Rapid effects of deep brain stimulation for treatment-resistant major depression. *Biol. Psychiatry* **2013**, *73*, 1204–1212. [CrossRef]
40. Bewernick, B.H.; Kayser, S.; Sturm, V.; Schlaepfer, T.E. Long-term effects of nucleus accumbens deep brain stimulation in treatment-resistant depression: Evidence for sustained efficacy. *Neuropsychopharmacol. Off. Publ. Am. Coll. Neuropsychopharmacol.* **2012**, *37*, 1975–1985. [CrossRef]
41. Eitan, R.; Fontaine, D.; Benoit, M.; Giordana, C.; Darmon, N.; Israel, Z.; Linesky, E.; Arkadir, D.; Ben-Naim, S.; Iserlles, M.; et al. One year double blind study of high vs low frequency subcallosal cingulate stimulation for depression. *J. Psychiatr. Res.* **2018**, *96*, 124–134. [CrossRef]
42. Accolla, E.A.; Aust, S.; Merkl, A.; Schneider, G.-H.; Kuhn, A.A.; Bajbouj, M.; Draganski, B. Deep brain stimulation of the posterior gyrus rectus region for treatment resistant depression. *J. Affect. Disord.* **2016**, *194*, 33–37. [CrossRef] [PubMed]
43. Sankar, T.; Chakravarty, M.M.; Jawa, N.; Li, S.X.; Giacobbe, P.; Kennedy, S.H.; Rizvi, S.J.; Mayberg, H.S.; Hamani, C.; Lozano, A.M. Neuroanatomical predictors of response to subcallosal cingulate deep brain stimulation for treatment-resistant depression. *J. Psychiatry Neurosci. JPN* **2019**, *44*, 1–10. [CrossRef] [PubMed]
44. Schlaepfer, T.E.; Cohen, M.X.; Frick, C.; Kosel, M.; Brodesser, D.; Axmacher, N.; Joe, A.Y.; Kreft, M.; Lenartz, D.; Sturm, V. Deep Brain Stimulation to Reward Circuitry Alleviates Anhedonia in Refractory Major Depression. *Neuropsychopharmacology* **2008**, *33*, 368–377. [CrossRef] [PubMed]
45. Mayberg, H.S.; Lozano, A.M.; Voon, V.; McNeely, H.E.; Seminowicz, D.; Hamani, C.; Schwalb, J.M.; Kennedy, S.H. Deep brain stimulation for treatment-resistant depression. *Neuron* **2005**, *45*, 651–660. [CrossRef]
46. Dandekar, M.P.; Fenoy, A.J.; Carvalho, A.F.; Soares, J.C.; Quevedo, J. Deep brain stimulation for treatment-resistant depression: An integrative review of preclinical and clinical findings and translational implications. *Mol. Psychiatry* **2018**, *23*, 1094–1112. [CrossRef]
47. Fins, J.J.; Kubu, C.S.; Mayberg, H.S.; Merkel, R.; Nuttin, B.; Schlaepfer, T.E. Being open minded about neuromodulation trials: Finding success in our "failures". *Brain Stimulat.* **2017**, *10*, 181–186. [CrossRef]
48. Choi, K.S.; Noecker, A.M.; Riva-Posse, P.; Rajendra, J.K.; Gross, R.E.; Mayberg, H.S.; McIntyre, C.C. Impact of brain shift on subcallosal cingulate deep brain stimulation. *Brain Stimulat.* **2018**, *11*, 445–453. [CrossRef]
49. Noecker, A.M.; Choi, K.S.; Riva-Posse, P.; Gross, R.E.; Mayberg, H.S.; McIntyre, C.C. StimVision Software: Examples and Applications in Subcallosal Cingulate Deep Brain Stimulation for Depression. *Neuromodulation J. Int. Neuromodulation Soc.* **2018**, *21*, 191–196. [CrossRef]
50. Riva-Posse, P.; Choi, K.S.; Holtzheimer, P.E.; Crowell, A.L.; Garlow, S.J.; Rajendra, J.K.; McIntyre, C.C.; Gross, R.E.; Mayberg, H.S. A connectomic approach for subcallosal cingulate deep brain stimulation surgery: Prospective targeting in treatment-resistant depression. *Mol. Psychiatry* **2018**, *23*, 843–849. [CrossRef]
51. Tsolaki, E.; Espinoza, R.; Pouratian, N. Using probabilistic tractography to target the subcallosal cingulate cortex in patients with treatment resistant depression. *Psychiatry Res. Neuroimaging* **2017**, *261*, 72–74. [CrossRef]

52. Coenen, V.A.; Sajonz, B.; Reisert, M.; Bostroem, J.; Bewernick, B.; Urbach, H.; Jenkner, C.; Reinacher, P.C.; Schlaepfer, T.E.; Madler, B. Tractography-assisted deep brain stimulation of the superolateral branch of the medial forebrain bundle (slMFB DBS) in major depression. *NeuroImage Clin.* **2018**, *20*, 580–593. [CrossRef] [PubMed]
53. Faraone, S.V. Interpreting Estimates of Treatment Effects. *Pharm. Ther.* **2008**, *33*, 700–711.
54. Locher, C.; Koechlin, H.; Zion, S.R.; Werner, C.; Pine, D.S.; Kirsch, I.; Kessler, R.C.; Kossowsky, J. Efficacy and Safety of Selective Serotonin Reuptake Inhibitors, Serotonin-Norepinephrine Reuptake Inhibitors, and Placebo for Common Psychiatric Disorders Among Children and Adolescents. *JAMA Psychiatry* **2017**, *74*, 1011–1020. [CrossRef] [PubMed]
55. Drobisz, D.; Damborska, A. Deep brain stimulation targets for treating depression. *Behav. Brain Res.* **2019**, *359*, 266–273. [CrossRef]
56. Guo, C.C.; Hyett, M.P.; Nguyen, V.T.; Parker, G.B.; Breakspear, M.J. Distinct neurobiological signatures of brain connectivity in depression subtypes during natural viewing of emotionally salient films. *Psychol. Med.* **2016**, *46*, 1535–1545. [CrossRef]
57. Williams, N.R.; Okun, M.S. Deep brain stimulation (DBS) at the interface of neurology and psychiatry. *J. Clin. Investig.* **2013**, *123*, 4546–4556. [CrossRef]
58. Coenen, V.A.; Schlaepfer, T.E.; Reinacher, P.C.; Mast, H.; Urbach, H.; Reisert, M. Machine learning-aided personalized DTI tractographic planning for deep brain stimulation of the superolateral medial forebrain bundle using HAMLET. *Acta Neurochir. (Wien)* **2019**, *161*, 1559–1569. [CrossRef]
59. van Aert, R.C.M.; Wicherts, J.M.; van Assen, M.A.L.M. Publication bias examined in meta-analyses from psychology and medicine: A meta-meta-analysis. *PLoS ONE* **2019**, *14*, e0215052. [CrossRef]
60. Bergfeld, I.O.; Mantione, M.; Figee, M.; Schuurman, P.R.; Lok, A.; Denys, D. Treatment-resistant depression and suicidality. *J. Affect. Disord.* **2018**, *235*, 362–367. [CrossRef]
61. Seo, H.-J.; Jung, Y.-E.; Jeong, S.; Kim, J.-B.; Lee, M.-S.; Kim, J.-M.; Yim, H.W.; Jun, T.-Y. Persistence and resolution of suicidal ideation during treatment of depression in patients with significant suicidality at the beginning of treatment: The CRESCEND study. *J. Affect. Disord.* **2014**, *155*, 208–215. [CrossRef]
62. Wulsin, L.R.; Vaillant, G.E.; Wells, V.E. A systematic review of the mortality of depression. *Psychosom. Med.* **1999**, *61*, 6–17. [CrossRef] [PubMed]
63. Bari, A.A.; Mikell, C.B.; Abosch, A.; Ben-Haim, S.; Buchanan, R.J.; Burton, A.W.; Carcieri, S.; Cosgrove, G.R.; D'Haese, P.-F.; Daskalakis, Z.J.; et al. Charting the road forward in psychiatric neurosurgery: Proceedings of the 2016 American Society for Stereotactic and Functional Neurosurgery workshop on neuromodulation for psychiatric disorders. *J. Neurol. Neurosurg. Psychiatry* **2018**, *89*, 886–896. [CrossRef] [PubMed]
64. Jones, B.; Lewis, J.A. The case for cross-over trials in phase III. *Stat. Med.* **1995**, *14*, 1025–1038. [CrossRef] [PubMed]
65. Mayberg, H.S.; Riva-Posse, P.; Crowell, A.L. Deep Brain Stimulation for Depression: Keeping an Eye on a Moving Target. *JAMA Psychiatry* **2016**, *73*, 439–440. [CrossRef]
66. Kennedy, S.H.; Giacobbe, P.; Rizvi, S.J.; Placenza, F.M.; Nishikawa, Y.; Mayberg, H.S.; Lozano, A.M. Deep brain stimulation for treatment-resistant depression: Follow-up after 3 to 6 years. *Am. J. Psychiatry* **2011**, *168*, 502–510. [CrossRef]
67. van der Wal, J.M.; Bergfeld, I.O.; Lok, A.; Mantione, M.; Figee, M.; Notten, P.; Beute, G.; Horst, F.; van den Munckhof, P.; Schuurman, P.R.; et al. Long-term deep brain stimulation of the ventral anterior limb of the internal capsule for treatment-resistant depression. *J. Neurol. Neurosurg. Psychiatry* **2020**, *91*, 189–195. [CrossRef]
68. Bhatia, K.D.; Henderson, L.; Ramsey-Stewart, G.; May, J. Diffusion tensor imaging to aid subgenual cingulum target selection for deep brain stimulation in depression. *Stereotact. Funct. Neurosurg.* **2012**, *90*, 225–232. [CrossRef]
69. Coenen, V.A.; Schlaepfer, T.E.; Bewernick, B.; Kilian, H.; Kaller, C.P.; Urbach, H.; Li, M.; Reisert, M. Frontal white matter architecture predicts efficacy of deep brain stimulation in major depression. *Transl. Psychiatry* **2019**, *9*, 197. [CrossRef]
70. Riva-Posse, P.; Choi, K.S.; Holtzheimer, P.E.; McIntyre, C.C.; Gross, R.E.; Chaturvedi, A.; Crowell, A.L.; Garlow, S.J.; Rajendra, J.K.; Mayberg, H.S. Defining critical white matter pathways mediating successful subcallosal cingulate deep brain stimulation for treatment-resistant depression. *Biol. Psychiatry* **2014**, *76*, 963–969. [CrossRef]

71. Howell, B.; Choi, K.S.; Gunalan, K.; Rajendra, J.; Mayberg, H.S.; McIntyre, C.C. Quantifying the axonal pathways directly stimulated in therapeutic subcallosal cingulate deep brain stimulation. *Hum. Brain Mapp.* **2019**, *40*, 889–903. [CrossRef]
72. McInerney, S.J.; McNeely, H.E.; Geraci, J.; Giacobbe, P.; Rizvi, S.J.; Ceniti, A.K.; Cyriac, A.; Mayberg, H.S.; Lozano, A.M.; Kennedy, S.H. Neurocognitive Predictors of Response in Treatment Resistant Depression to Subcallosal Cingulate Gyrus Deep Brain Stimulation. *Front. Hum. Neurosci.* **2017**, *11*, 74. [CrossRef] [PubMed]
73. Quraan, M.A.; Protzner, A.B.; Daskalakis, Z.J.; Giacobbe, P.; Tang, C.W.; Kennedy, S.H.; Lozano, A.M.; McAndrews, M.P. EEG power asymmetry and functional connectivity as a marker of treatment effectiveness in DBS surgery for depression. *Neuropsychopharmacol. Off. Publ. Am. Coll. Neuropsychopharmacol.* **2014**, *39*, 1270–1281. [CrossRef] [PubMed]
74. Broadway, J.M.; Holtzheimer, P.E.; Hilimire, M.R.; Parks, N.A.; Devylder, J.E.; Mayberg, H.S.; Corballis, P.M. Frontal theta cordance predicts 6-month antidepressant response to subcallosal cingulate deep brain stimulation for treatment-resistant depression: A pilot study. *Neuropsychopharmacol. Off. Publ. Am. Coll. Neuropsychopharmacol.* **2012**, *37*, 1764–1772. [CrossRef]
75. Lujan, J.L.; Chaturvedi, A.; Malone, D.A.; Rezai, A.R.; Machado, A.G.; McIntyre, C.C. Axonal pathways linked to therapeutic and nontherapeutic outcomes during psychiatric deep brain stimulation. *Hum. Brain Mapp.* **2012**, *33*, 958–968. [CrossRef] [PubMed]

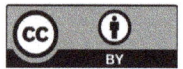

© 2020 by the authors. Licensee MDPI, Basel, Switzerland. This article is an open access article distributed under the terms and conditions of the Creative Commons Attribution (CC BY) license (http://creativecommons.org/licenses/by/4.0/).

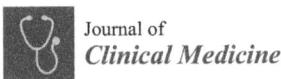

Review

Deep Brain Stimulation for Treatment-Resistant Depression: Towards a More Personalized Treatment Approach

Milaine Roet [1,2], Jackson Boonstra [1,2], Erdi Sahin [3], Anne E.P. Mulders [1,2,4], Albert F.G. Leentjens [2,4] and Ali Jahanshahi [1,2,*]

1. Department of Neurosurgery, Maastricht University Medical Center, P. Debyelaan 25, 6202 AZ Maastricht, The Netherlands; m.roet@maastrichtuniversity.nl (M.R.); j.boonstra@maastrichtuniversity.nl (J.B.); a.mulders@maastrichtuniversity.nl (A.E.P.M.)
2. European Graduate School of Neuroscience (EURON); 6229 ER Maastricht, The Netherlands; a.leentjens@maastrichtuniversity.nl
3. Department of Neurology, Istanbul Faculty of Medicine, Istanbul University Capa, Istanbul 34093, Turkey; erdisahin@gmail.com
4. Department of Psychiatry and Psychology, Maastricht University Medical Center, P. Debyelaan 25, 6202 AZ Maastricht, The Netherlands
* Correspondence: a.jahanshahi@maastrichtuniversity.nl; Tel.: +31-43-388-4124; Fax: +31-43-387-6038

Received: 23 July 2020; Accepted: 19 August 2020; Published: 24 August 2020

Abstract: Major depressive disorder (MDD) affects approximately 4.4% of the world's population. One third of MDD patients do not respond to routine psychotherapeutic and pharmacotherapeutic treatment and are said to suffer from treatment-resistant depression (TRD). Deep brain stimulation (DBS) is increasingly being investigated as a treatment modality for TRD. Although early case studies showed promising results of DBS, open-label trials and placebo-controlled studies have reported inconsistent outcomes. This has raised discussion about the correct interpretation of trial results as well as the criteria for patient selection, the choice of stimulation target, and the optimal stimulation parameters. In this narrative review, we summarize recent studies of the effectiveness of DBS in TRD and address the relation between the targeted brain structures and clinical outcomes. Elaborating upon that, we hypothesize that the effectiveness of DBS in TRD can be increased by a more personalized and symptom-based approach. This may be achieved by using resting-state connectivity mapping for neurophysiological subtyping of TRD, by using individualized tractography to help decisions about stimulation target and electrode placement, and by using a more detailed registration of symptomatic improvements during DBS, for instance by using 'experience sampling' methods.

Keywords: major depressive disorder; treatment resistant depression; deep brain stimulation; neuropsychological subtypes; personalized treatment approach

1. Introduction

Major depressive disorder (MDD) is a common mood disorder that affects one's feelings, thoughts, and behavior. According to the DSM-5, for a diagnosis of MDD, five of the following symptoms need to be present for at least two weeks: depressed mood, reduced interest or pleasure, weight loss or reduced appetite, insomnia or hypersomnia, psychomotor agitation or retardation, fatigue or loss of energy, worthlessness or excessive guilt, impaired concentration or indecisiveness, and recurrent thoughts of death or suicidal ideation or attempts. Either 'depressed mood' or 'loss of interest or pleasure' is essential for a diagnosis [1]. The total number of people suffering from MDD worldwide was estimated to be 322 million in 2015 and its prevalence increased by 18.4% between 2005 and 2015 [2]. Therefore, effective treatment of MDD merits intense consideration.

Whereas psychotherapy and antidepressant medication are effective in the majority of patients, approximately one third of patients do not respond to these therapies. In the Sequenced Treatment Alternatives to Relieve Depression (STAR*D) trial, the cumulative remission rate of MDD patients after four successive treatments was 67% [3]. In line with this, a meta-analysis of 92 studies of the effectiveness of psychotherapy showed that 62% of patients no longer met the criteria of depression after treatment [4]. Failure to respond to a treatment algorithm of several steps is commonly referred to as treatment resistance, although there is still discussion about the exact definition of treatment refractoriness [5]. Treatment-resistant depression (TRD) is associated with more (comorbid) mental health disorders, a higher number of hospitalizations, and more suicide attempts, leading to higher treatment costs compared to non-TRD [6]. In addition, patients with TRD show a higher demand of healthcare resources and costs of health care compared to non-TRD patients [7]. Various alternative treatment options for TRD are currently being investigated, including vagal nerve stimulation [8], repetitive transcranial magnetic stimulation (rTMS) [9], and deep brain stimulation (DBS) [10].

The aim of this narrative review is to provide an overview of recent studies of the effectiveness of DBS in TRD with a special focus on the relationship between the targeted brain structures and clinical outcomes. Based on these findings, we discuss the importance of distinguishing between different clinical phenotypes of depression that would allow for more personalized symptom-based treatment approaches, which may be a key factor in improving treatment outcomes.

2. Recent Insights on the Pathophysiology of Depression

It is hypothesized that in depression, there is an imbalance in the limbic cortico-striatal-thalamo-cortical (CSTC) mood circuits [11,12], yet many aspects of circuitopathy in MDD remain largely unknown. Based on different models [11,12], three main components of the CSTC mood circuits have been proposed (Figure 1). First, the ventral component is essential for recognizing emotions and initiating an adequate emotional and behavioral response. In this circuit, the amygdala, ventral striatum, ventral part of the anterior cingulate cortex, orbitofrontal cortex, ventrolateral prefrontal cortex, and downstream structures such as the hypothalamus and locus coeruleus are involved. Second, the dorsal component that regulates the emotional responses and requires cognitive processing. Here, the dorsolateral and dorsomedial prefrontal cortex, the dorsal part of the anterior cingulate cortex, and the hippocampus are involved. Third, a modulating region is present, although no consensus has been made about its precise anatomical organization and function. Some have suggested that this component consists of the thalamus and the rostral part of the anterior cingulate cortex [11–13]. As implied by Mayberg et al., the model of depression indicates that depression is associated with a decreased activity in dorsal limbic and neocortical regions and a relative increase in ventral paralimbic regions. Treatment of depression therefore requires the inhibition of the overactive ventral regions, resulting in the disinhibition of the underactive dorsal regions. To mediate this process, proper functioning of the rostral cingulate cortex is required [12]. These mood circuits overlap with the circuitry involved in compulsive traits; DBS of the ventral capsule/ventral striatum (VC/VS) in treatment resistant obsessive-compulsive disorder (OCD) patients has led to improvements in mood which prompted studying the application of DBS in TRD patients [14,15].

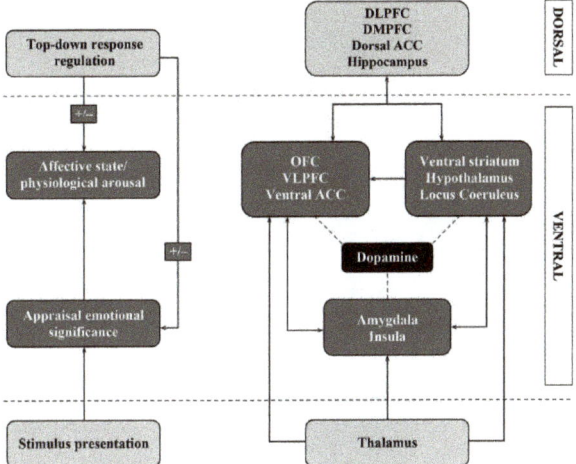

Figure 1. Schematic representation of emotional processing and its neurobiological base. Figure from Moonen et al. (2017) [16] with permission.

Expanding the Cortico-Striatal-Thalamo-Cortical Mood Circuits

One region that is not included in the CSTC mood circuits and yet has been a region of interest for DBS targeting in depression for over a decade is the subgenual cingulate gyrus/cortex (SCG/SCC) [10]. This region has shown hyperactivity in untreated depressed patients [17], is part of the ventral component, and has projections to the amygdala, hippocampus, superior and medial temporal gyri, ventral striatum, mid- and posterior cingulate cortex, thalamus, hypothalamus, periaqueductal gray, and lateral habenula [18,19]. Furthermore, in recent years, it has become known that several other brain areas all belonging to the ventral component play a role in the pathophysiology of depression. Among these are the thalamic peduncles (THp) that interconnects with the prefrontal cortex including the orbitofrontal cortex (OFC) [20], the medial forebrain bundle (MFB) that projects to the frontal cortex, the NAcc and ventral striatum [21], and the ventral part of the anterior limb of the internal capsule (vALIC) which forms a homeostatic system with the MFB and the bed nucleus of the stria terminalis (BNST) [22] (Figure 2).

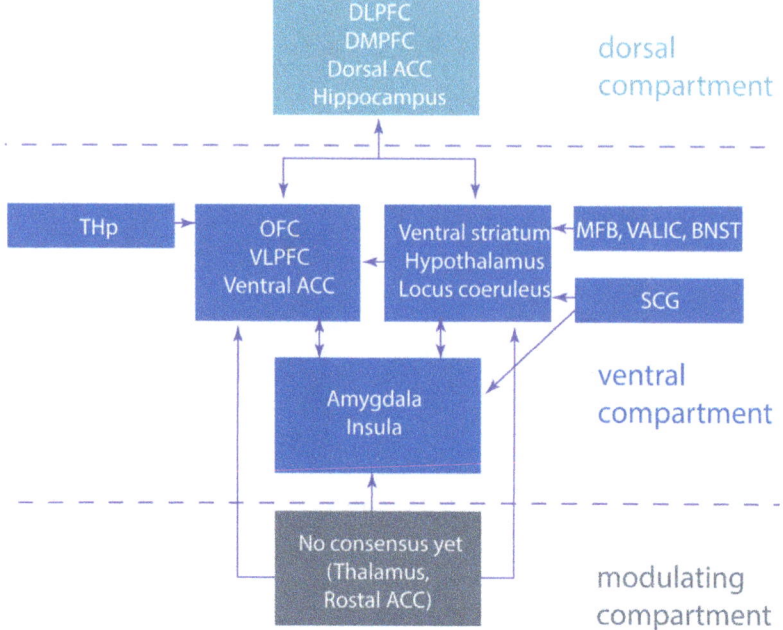

Figure 2. Cortico-striatal-thalamic-cortico mood circuits divided in a dorsal, ventral, and modulating compartment based on Alexander et al. [11], Mayberg et al. [12], and Moonen et al. [16] expanded with regions researched with deep brain stimulation (DBS) for treatment-resistant depression (TRD). DLPFC; dorsolateral prefrontal cortex, DMPFC; dorsomedial prefrontal cortex, ACC; anterior cingulate cortex, THp; thalamic peduncles, OFC; orbitofrontal cortex, VLPFC; ventrolateral prefrontal cortex, MFB; medial forebrain bundle, vALIC, ventral part of the anterior limb of the internal capsule, BNST; bed nucleus of the stria terminalis, SCG; subgenual cingulate gyrus, HPA axis; hypothalamic pituitary adrenal axis.

3. Deep Brain Stimulation for Treatment-Resistant Depression

DBS is an invasive neuromodulation technique that is effective in managing clinical symptoms of neurological and psychiatric disorders, such as Parkinson's disease (PD) [23,24] and OCD [25]. At stimulation settings commonly used in clinical practice, DBS decreases the spontaneous firing of neuronal populations and activates axonal projections near the electrode [26]. This modulates pathological activity and replaces it with regular patterns of discharge with intervals of burst activity [27,28]. More recent theories suggest that DBS destabilizes abnormal synchronous oscillatory activity within the basal ganglia circuitry improving hyperkinetic symptomology [24]. However, the exact mechanism(s) by which DBS normalizes electrical activity in the basal ganglia and exerts beneficial effects on PD symptoms remain unknown. In DBS for TRD, target selection has mostly been based on either neuroimaging studies or clinical observations of mood improvement following DBS in OCD [10,15,29]. For these reasons, the underlying mechanisms of action are poorly studied. DBS studies for TRD (Table 1) and the outcomes for selected brain targets (Table 2) are described below.

Table 1. DBS in treatment-resistant depression (TRD); published open-label and randomized clinical trials.

Region (DBS)	Study	Open-Labeled, RCT or Case-Report	N	Follow-Up	Age (Mean)	Length of Current Depressive Episode, Years (Mean)	Response Rate (%) in HDRS or MADRS Scores	Remission Rate (%)	Serious Adverse Events (N)
SCG	Mayberg et al., 2005	Open-label	6	6 months	46	5.58	33.3 (1 month), # 83 (2 months), # 66.6 (6 months), #	0 (1 month) 33.3 (3 months) 33.3 (6 months)	Suicidal ideation: 2 Syncope: 1 Lead problem: 1
	Lozano et al., 2008	Open-label	20	12 months	47.4	6.9	60 (6 months), # 55 (12 months), #	35 (6 months) 35 (12 months)	Seizure: 1 Lead problem: 3
	Kennedy et al., 2011	Open-label	20	1, 2 and 3 years, last follow-up (3–6 years)	47.4	6.9	62.5 (1 year), # 46.2 (2 years), # 75 (3 years), # 64.3 (last follow-up), #	18.8 (1 year) 15.4 (2 years) 50 (3 years)	Worsening depression:3 Suicidal ideation:3
	Puigdemont et al., 2012	Open-label	8	12 months	47.4	6.3	87.5 (1 week), # 37.5 (1 month), # 87.5 (6 months), # 62.5 (12 months), #	50 (1 week) 37.5 (6 months) 50 (12 months)	Suicide attempt: 1
	Lozano et al., 2012	Open-label	21	12 months	47.3	5.0	57 (1 month), # 48 (6 months), # 29 (12 months), #	-	Suicide: 1 Suicide attempt: 1
	Holtzheimer et al., 2012	Open-label	17	24 months	42	5.34	41 (6 months), # 36 (12 months), # 92 (24 months), #	18 (6 months) 36 (12 months) 58 (24 months)	Suicidal ideation: 1 Suicide attempt: 2
	Merkl et al., 2013	Open-label	6	24 h Last follow up (24–36 weeks)	50.66	2.13	33.33 (36 weeks), #	33.33 (36 weeks)	Headaches: 6 Tenseness in neck region: 1
	Holtzheimer et al., 2017	RCT	60 (52)	6 months (24 months)	50.53	12.62	22 (6 months), ‡ 54 (12 months), ‡ 48 (24 months), ‡	10 (6 months) 17 (12 months) 25 (24 months)	Suicide attempt: 2 Suicidal ideation: 2 Seizure: 2
	Eitan et al., 2018	RCT HF vs. LF DBS	9	13 months	46	-	44.44 (13 months), ‡		-

Table 1. *Cont.*

Region (DBS)	Study	Open-Labeled, RCT or Case-Report	N	Follow-Up	Age (Mean)	Length of Current Depressive Episode, Years (Mean)	Response Rate (%) in HDRS or MADRS Scores	Remission Rate (%)	Serious Adverse Events (N)
	Merkl et al., 2018	RCT	8	28 months (n = 6) 4 years (n = 2)	48.25	2	37.5 (6 months), # 43.0 (12 months), # 23.0 (28 months), #	12.5 (6 months) 14.2 (12 months) 33.0 (24 months) 33.3 (28 months)	Manic episode: 1
	Crowell et al., 2019	Open-label	28	4 (n = 14) 8 (n = 11) years	44.9 (45.9)	45.1 (46.6)	18 #	21	Suicide attempt: 6 Suicidal ideation: 8 Anxiety: 6 Worsening depression: 2
PGR	Accolla et al., 2016	Open-label	5 (1)	6 months (24 months)	45.20	-	-	-	-
NAcc	Schlaepfer et al., 2008	Open-label	3	6–24 weeks	46.7	7.2	-	-	None
	Bewernick et al., 2010	Open-label	10	10 months	48.6	10.8	50 (1 month), # 50 (6 months), # 50 (12 months), #	30 (1 month)	Suicide: 1 Suicide attempt: 1
	Bewernick et al., 2012	Open-label	11	12 months 24 months Last follow up (max 4 years)	48.36	9.26	45 (12 months), #	9.1 (24 months)	Pain: 4 Seizure: 1 Agitation: 3 Suicide:1 Suicide attempt: 1
VC/VS	Malone et al., 2009	Open-label	15	6 months (n = 15) 12 months (n = 11)	46.3	21	20 (1 month), # 40 (6 months), # 53.3 (last follow-up) #	20 (6 months) 40 (last follow-up)	Suicidal ideation: 2 Syncope: 1 Lead problem: 1
	Dougherty et al., 2015	RCT	30	24 months	47.7	11.4	20 (16 weeks), ¥ 20 (12 months), ¥ 23.3 (24 months), ¥	13 (12 months) 20 (24 months)	Suicide: 1 (stimulation off) Suicide attempt: 4 Suicidal ideation: 5 Lead revision: 3

Table 1. Cont.

Region (DBS)	Study	Open-Labeled, RCT or Case-Report	N	Follow-Up	Age (Mean)	Length of Current Depressive Episode, Years (Mean)	Response Rate (%) in HDRS or MADRS Scores	Remission Rate (%)	Serious Adverse Events (N)
vALIC	Van der Wal et al., 2020 (follow-up of the RCT Bergfeld et al. 2016)	Open-label	25	2 years	52.5	7.42	32.0 (2 years, ITT) #	20.0 (2 years, ITT)	Pain: 1 Agitation: 3 Suicidal ideation: 6 Fatigue: 4
	Bergfeld et al., 2016	RCT	25	52 weeks	53.2	6.98	40 (after optimization of DBS settings (T_2)) #	20 (T_2)	Suicide attempt: 4 Suicidal ideation: 3 Automutilation: 1
LHb	Sartorius et al., 2009	Case-report	1	60 weeks	64.0	9.0	-	-	-
MFB	Schlaepfer et al., 2013	Open-label	7	12–33 weeks	42.6	7.6	86, ¥	57	Cranial bleeding: 1
	Fenoy et al., 2016 (interim analysis)	Open-label	4	52 weeks	-	-	75 (7 days) ¥ 66 (26 weeks, OC) ¥	-	-

"-": has not been mentioned in this article, RCT: response criteria; #: 50% or greater reduction in Hamilton Depression Rating Scale (HDRS) (17 or 28) scores, ¥: 50% or greater reduction in MADRS scores, ‡: 40% or greater reduction in MADRS scores, RCT: randomized controlled trial, ITT: intention to treat, OC: observed case.

Table 2. Targets for DBS in treatment resistant depression (TRD), functions, pathophysiology and the effect of DBS.

Brain Region	Function	Pathological Activity in MDD	HF-DBS Effect
SCG	Contains three white matter bundles; forceps minor + uncinate fasciculus connecting to the medial frontal cortex, cingulum connecting to the rostral and dorsal ACC and fronto-striatal fibers connecting to the NAcc, CN, Pt and anterior Th. Connects higher 'top-down' cortical regions with subcortical modulatory regions. Involvement in brain DMN [30]	Increased activity [31] Reduced volume in familial depression [32] Projections to: (1) NAcc may play a role in lack of interest, disruption in reward and underlie anhedonia (2) Hth and brainstem may play a role in circadian and sleep disturbances, problems with appetite and an abnormal stress responds and cortisol metabolism [31].	Disruption of pathological activity Modulation of multiple regions connected to the SCG [31]
NAcc	Receives projections from VTA, AG, OFC, mPFC, dCN, GP and Hip and projects to Cg25, mPFC, VP, Th, AG and Hth. Transmits information from emotion centers to motor control regions, causing motivational behavior to obtain rewards [33]. Processes reward and pleasure information	In severe anhedonia; smaller size and less activation to reward [34]	Acute: Increase in exploratory motivation Chronic: reduction in anhedonia PET Imaging: ↑ activity in VS, bilateral dlPFC and dmPFC, cingulate cortex and bilateral AG. ↓ activity in vmPFC and vlPFC, dCN and Th [33]
VC/VS	Contains fibers connecting the dPFC, dACC, OFC and vmPFC with THAL, AG, Hth and brainstem (SN, VTA, RN and DMN) [35]	Increased activity [36] Activation of the connection from left vs. to left caudate has been associated with anhedonia Increased connectivity of vs. to DMN is positively correlated to higher depression scores in the CES-D score [37]	-
vALIC	Contains two fiber bundles: the anterior thalamic radiation and the supero-lateral branch of the MFB connecting the PFC to different subcortical structures such as the Th, NAcc, VTA and VS. Decreased integrity of the right vALIC in depressed patients [38]	-	Decreased metabolism in OFC, subgenual ACC and right DLPFC in patients with OCD [39]
LHb	Activity corresponds negatively to anticipation and reception of a reward [40]	Increased activity [41] Possible down regulation of serotonergic, noradrenergic and dopaminergic systems [42], volume reduction [43]	Localized metabolic increase in one patient with FDG-PET, presumably due to functional inhibition [44]
ITP	Interconnects the intralaminar nucleus and TRN with the OFC [30,45]	Hyperactivation in both TRN and OFC [46]	Cortical desynchronization Disruption of adrenergic and serotonergic malfunction [46]

Table 2. Cont.

Brain Region	Function	Pathological Activity in MDD	HF-DBS Effect
MFB	Interconnects the Nacc, VTA, vmHth, lHth and AG ventromedial and lateral nuclei of the Hth and AG with convergence onto the PFC [47,48] Plays a crucial role in the reward pathway;	Dysfunctional reward system. Responders showed a strong connectivity between the active electrode contact and the mPFC pre-operatively using individual DTI [49]	Insignificant changes in metabolism in 3 patients with PET measurements pre-operatively, 6 and 12 months post-operatively [49]
BNST	Mayor output pathway of the AG Regulates stress response Integrates information from multiple brain areas to perform 'valence surveillance' [22,30]	Oscillatory activity with high α-power [50]	-

"-": not investigated; (d) ACC; (dorsal) anterior cingulate cortex, AG; amygdala, CES-D score; center for epidemiologic studies depression score, (d) CN; (dorsal) caudate nucleus, DMN; default mode network, DTI; deterministic diffusion tensor imaging, GP; globus pallidus, Hip; hippocampus, Hth; hypothalamus, MFB; medial forebrain bundle, OFC; Orbitofrontal cortex, (m/dl/dm/vm/vl) PFC (medial/dorsolateral/dorsomedial/ventromedial/ventrolateral) Prefrontal cortex, PGR; posterior gyrus rectus, PTN; pedunculopontine tegmental nucleus, Pt: putamen, RN; raphe nuclei, SN; substantia nigra, Th; thalamus, TRN; thalamic reticular nucleus, VP; ventral pallidum, VS; ventral striatum, VTA; ventral tegmental area.

3.1. Subgenual Cingulate Gyrus/Cortex

The first clinical trial of DBS of the SCG for TRD was performed in 2005 and included six patients with MDD [10]. The severity of depression was measured using the Hamilton Depression Rating Scale (HDRS) and the Montgomory Asberg Depression Rating Scale (MADRS). The HDRS has been the gold standard for the assessment of depression for years [51]. A clinical response is commonly defined as a decrease in the HDRS score of more than 50% compared to baseline, and clinical remission is defined as a decrease in the HDRS score to eight or less. After one month, two out of six patients met the criteria for response. At the end of the sixth month, a response was seen in four out of six patients, with three of the patients reaching remission or near remission. Preliminary observations with positron emission tomography (PET) showed a metabolic hyperactive SCG (Brodmann area 25, Cg 25) during depressive states. It was speculated that DBS would reduce this hyperactivity [17] (Table 2). The improvement in depression scores after DBS was thought to be due to effectively disrupting focal pathological activity in limbic-cortical circuits. After 3 months of stimulation of the subgenual cingulate region (CG25) in patients suffering from TRD, local cerebral blood flow (CBF) was decreased in CG25 and the adjacent orbitofrontal cortex (Brodmann area 11). Moreover, after three and six months of stimulation, CBF was decreased in the hypothalamus, anterior insula, and medial frontal cortex of long-term responders, while CBF increased in the dorsolateral prefrontal cortex (dlPFC), dorsal anterior, posterior cingulate, and premotor and parietal regions (Table 2) [10]. In the different open-label trials, response rates varied from 20 to 57% after 1 month, 33.3 to 87.5% after 6 months, and 29 to 62.5% after 12 months (Table 1) [10,33,49,52–61]. In a long term follow-up, Kennedy et al. (2011) reported response rates at 1, 2, and 3 years after DBS implantation in the SCC of TRD patients of 62.5%, 46,2%, and 75%, respectively [52] (Table 1). In a case series of DBS of the SCG in five TRD patients, a decrease in the score of the depression rating scale was only found in one of the five TRD patients. This patient turned out to be stimulated in the posterior gyrus rectus (PGR) based on single subject tractography results rather than the initially targeted CG25 [62]. A recent exploratory meta-analysis of four observational studies investigating DBS for TRD (Holtzheimer et al. 2012, Lozano et al. 2012, Puigdemont et al. 2012, and Kennedy et al. 2011) reported relatively large response and remission rates following DBS treatment: the twelve-month response and remission rates were 39.9% (95% CI = 28.4% to 52.8%) and 26.3% (95% CI = 13% to 45.9%). The included studies reported a significant decrease in depression scores between 3 and 6 months (Hedges' g = −0.27, p = 0.003), while no additional decrease was found between 6 and 12 months, suggesting that maximal antidepressant effects occur mostly within the first 6 months of treatment [63]. However, adverse events can occur, including worsening of depression, suicidal ideation, and seizures (Table 1). A study consisting of a double-blind active vs. sham stimulation phase of four weeks, followed by an open-label stimulation for up to 24 months, reported no significant differences between the active and sham stimulation of the SCG and no reduction in HDRS scores in the first four weeks. In the open-label phase, response rates were 37.5%, 43% and 23% after 6, 12 and 28 months, respectively. Remission rates were 12.5% and 14.2% at 6 and 12 months, respectively, and 33.3% at 24 and 28 months [64].

A randomized controlled trial (RCT) investigating DBS of the subcallosal cingulate, known as the BROADEN trial, was aborted prematurely. The study lasted six months, during which all patients should have received SCC implantation surgery. After six months, blinding would have been uncovered and both groups would have been offered open-label DBS for another six months. At the end of the first six months, responses of the treatment group and control group were predicted to be 40% and 18.5%, respectively. In this trial, the response rate was defined as more than or equal to a 40% decrease in MADRS scores from baseline. However, after six months, only 20% of patients (n = 12) in the treatment group showed a response versus 17% of patients (n = 5) in the control group. At that time, a futility analysis predicted the probability of a successful study outcome to be 17% or less leading to the funding for DBS electrodes for this study to be discontinued. The actual study was never published, but results were published and mentioned in Morishita et al. (2014) [65,66]. It has been postulated that the patients enrolled in the BROADEN trial had extreme and chronic depression with a mean duration of the current depressive episode of 12 years, nearly twice that of previous open-label studies. Therefore, these patients could have required a longer treatment period before significant results emerge. Long-term outcomes of SCG DBS in TRD patients for up to 8 years show that most patients have a sustained antidepressant response [60]. However, these results need to be interpreted carefully as the patient group consisted of both MDD and bipolar type-II disorder patients. Further comparison between high- and low frequency DBS in the SCG in TRD showed no significant difference in effectiveness between the two groups and a 44.44% response rate at 13 months of stimulation [67].

3.2. Nucleus Accumbens

Another brain region involved in MDD is the nucleus accumbens (NAcc), part of the mesolimbic dopaminergic circuit involved in different cognitive functions such as motivation and reward [33] (Table 2). DBS of the NAcc exerts immediate and long-term positive clinical effects in TRD and has been shown to significantly improve depression scores within one week [33]. Visualized with PET–computed tomography (PET-CT or PET/CT), NAcc-DBS increased metabolic activity in the ventral striatum, dlPFC, dorsomedial PFC (dmPFC), cingulate cortex, and the amygdala. Furthermore, metabolic activity in the vmPFC, ventrolateral prefrontal cortex (vlPFC), dorsal caudate nucleus, and part of the thalamus were decreased. Targeting the NAcc was essential for the effect of DBS on anhedonia (i.e., the inability to feel pleasure) in patients suffering from TRD. However, when Schlaepfer et al. (2008) looked at single items of depression rating scales, capturing aspects of anhedonia such as 'work and activities', 'apparent sadness', and the 'inability to feel', no significant improvements were found following NAcc-DBS. A follow-up study showed a 50% response rate in 10 patients suffering from TRD undergoing NAcc-DBS after 10 months [53]. In a more recent study reporting the long term effects of NAcc-DBS, 45% of TRD patients ($n = 11$) were classified as responders with a 50% reduction in HDRS scores after 12 months of stimulation, which remained until the last follow-up of 4 years [54] (Table 1). Several side effects were reported, such as seizure, agitation, and a transient increase in anxiety. In addition, one attempted suicide and one completed suicide were reported, for which the relation with the DBS treatment is uncertain.

3.3. Ventral Capsule/Ventral Striatum

The ventral capsule/ventral striatum (VC/VS) is thought to be hyperactive in MDD [36] (Table 2). Capsulotomy (i.e., lesioning) of the VC/VS improved not only OCD symptoms but also depressive symptoms, inspiring stimulation of the VC/VS for TRD [15]. In an open-label trial that stimulated the VC/VS in 15 TRD patients, responder rates at three months, six months, and 12 months were 53.3%, 46.7%, and 53.3%, respectively, using the MADRS as an outcome measure, and were 46.7%, 40%, and 53.3%, respectively, using the HDRS as an outcome measure [55]. Adverse events ranged from pain or discomfort at the incision site, to hypomania, mixed bipolar state, and increased depression due to battery depletion.

The first RCT of DBS of the VC/VS for TRD was performed by Dougherty et al. (2015) who stimulated 30 patients for 16 weeks. There were no significant differences in response rates between the intervention and sham group in the double-blind phase [68,69]. Another RCT of VC/VS DBS in eight TRD patients was discontinued after an interim futility analysis of active vs. sham stimulation showed no difference in effects between the two groups after 16 weeks. These results were never published but were discussed by Rezai et al. [70].

3.4. The Ventral Part of the Anterior Limb of the Internal Capsule

The anterior limb of the internal capsule (ALIC) is another brain region that was initially studied for DBS in OCD. One study aimed at stimulating the NAcc discovered that most treated OCD patients (9 out of 16) actually received DBS in the ventral part of the ALIC (vALIC), which improved obsessive compulsive scale scores, showed anti-depressive effects, and led to the clinical implementation of vALIC-DBS in TRD [29]. DBS of the vALIC has also been associated with a decreased metabolism in the OFC, subgenual anterior cingulate cortex, and right dlPFC [71–73] (Table 2).

The first RCT of DBS of the vALIC for TRD was conducted by Bergfeld et al. (2016), investigating 25 TRD patients during a 52 week open-label trial, which resulted in a significant decrease in HDRS scores in the whole group during the optimization phase, although overall HDRS scores were still in the depression range (22.2 at baseline vs. 15.9 after optimization phase). Ten of the 25 patients could be classified as responders, with a more than 50% decrease on the HDRS. After the optimization phase, a RCT with a cross-over design including nine responders and seven non-responders ensued and showed a significantly lower score in the active DBS phase compared with the sham DBS phase (mean HDRS score of 13.6 (95% CI; 9.8–17.4 vs. 23.1 (95% CI; 20.6–25.6)) (HDRS < 0.001). However, the scores on the HDRS in the active treatment group were still within the mild to moderate depression range [74]. Both crossover phases lasted approximately 21 and 18 days, respectively.

3.5. Lateral Habenula

The activity of the lateral habenula (LHb) is negatively associated with reward, meaning its neurons increase their firing rate in a non-reward situation or in the omission of a reward. LHb hyperactivity could therefore explain the lower reward-seeking behavior in TRD [75] (Table 2). Speculation that DBS of the LHb could lead to the inhibition of hyperactivity prompted the first case study of LHb-DBS in TRD, which notably led to full remission of the patients' depressive symptoms [44]. A clinical non-randomized study in six patients suffering from TRD is currently being held, investigating the safety, tolerability, and benefit of LHb DBS in TRD. Patients that respond at 12 months of stimulation will enter a randomized, staggered withdrawal phase. During this phase, a double-blind discontinuation will be attempted at month 12 or 13, decreasing the stimulation by 50% and then completely discontinuing it during the following two weeks. Evaluation will take place at 15 months, where, in the meantime, escape criteria are included, and if met, will stop the blinded phase in continuing with an open treatment [76].

3.6. Thalamic Peduncles

The inferior thalamic peduncle (ITP) is a bundle of fibers connecting the OFC to the thalamus. The OFC is thought to play a role in the non-reward tractor theory of depression, where the orbitofrontal non-reward system is more easily triggered in depression, causing negative emotional states [77] (Table 2). Stimulating the ITP could disrupt this enhanced triggering and lead to less depressive symptoms. ITP stimulation for OCD has already shown improvements of the score on the Yale-Brown Obsessive-Compulsive scale in five OCD patients [45]. A case study in one TRD patient reported that DBS of the ITP decreased depressive symptoms [78]. However, within this study, two brain regions were investigated, the second being the BNST.

3.7. Bed Nucleus of the Stria Terminalis

The BNST is involved in a range of behaviors, such as stress response, social behavior, and extended duration of fear states. This nucleus assesses sensory information from the environment, coupled together with the subjects current mood and arousal, integrating a proper response to environmental and social setting changes [22] (Table 2). Raymaekers et al. (2017) indicated that both BNST and ITP stimulation could alleviate depressive symptoms; however, due to a small sample size, no statistical analyses were conducted [78].

3.8. Medial Forebrain Bundle

The medial forebrain bundle (MFB) is a fiber tract connected to various parts of the limbic system thought to play a role in reward-seeking systems [21] (Table 2). In one trial, DBS of the superolateral branch of the MFB resulted in more than a 50% decrease in depressive symptoms in six out of seven TRD patients within seven days [47]. An additional interim analysis of MFB-DBS in TRD confirmed these findings, showing more than a 50% decrease in depressive symptoms in three out of four patients within seven days of stimulation. At 26 weeks follow-up, two patients showed more than an 80% decrease in depression rating scales [49] (Table 1).

Taken together, the results of the aforementioned studies of DBS for TRD imply that stimulation at a number of different brain areas can alleviate depressive symptoms, which is in line with the view that MDD is a circuitopathy involving various brain regions and networks mainly within the limbic CSTC mood circuits [12,79]. However, how DBS of those targets improves the depressive symptoms is not completely clear. Moreover, stimulation parameters vary between studies due to a need to adjust and balance therapeutic effects to side effects.

MDD is a circuitopathy that involves a wide range of brain structures and exhibits diverse clinical manifestations. Therefore, a one-size-fits-all approach to the DBS targeting may not be beneficial in all patients, whereas a patient-centric selection based on individually disrupted neurocircuits could improve therapeutic outcomes. In evaluating the effects of DBS, one needs to focus on overall improvement on depression rating scales as well as individual scores and symptom-specific improvements. This will enhance the understanding of the effects of DBS and eventually contribute to the development of more personalized treatment approaches. Seemingly, this also applies in other psychiatric disorders such as OCD, where personalized approaches with content-specific DBS targets have already proven to be beneficial [80].

4. Towards a More Personalized DBS Treatment Approach for Treatment-Resistant Depression

Since open-label trials and RCT data on DBS in TRD show inconsistent results, this gives rise to discussion about the chosen study designs, the correct interpretation of results, and the best target(s) for neuromodulation. Depression entails different clinical subtypes and looking at homogenous subgroups of depressed patients may lead to a personalized DBS approach. This would be superior to looking at primary outcomes across all participants. Importantly, a prerequisite to this approach is the ability to determine pathoanatomical substrates of specific subtypes. How to implement such a more personalized approach to DBS treatment for TRD is discussed below.

4.1. Clinical and Neurophysiological Subtypes of Depression

Most response rates in depression treatments to date have been measured with changes in average levels among all patients treated. However, depressive symptomatology varies highly among individuals, making the standardization of positive outcomes challenging. Mood, sleep rhythm, concentration, psychomotor, and cognitive domains can all be disturbed in depression, while treating one selected brain structure within the mood circuit may not have an effect on all aforementioned symptoms nor have an effect on the main symptomatology of all depressed patients.

Subdividing TRD into different subtypes, involving distinct clinical symptoms as well as distinct patterns of dysfunctional connectivity in limbic and frontal striatal networks, may reveal different subtype-related outcomes for each investigated brain region, and if so, patient selection for a given brain target could enhance treatment effectiveness [81]. Analysis of resting-state connectivity biomarkers previously revealed four connectivity-based biotypes of depression characterized by either anxiety, increased anhedonia, psychomotor retardation, and/or increased anergia and fatigue. Moreover, patients could not be differentiated into a particular subtype based on clinical features alone and clustering them based on functional connectivity was needed [82]. Therefore, imaging procedures as well as featured symptoms should be taken into account when treating TRD with DBS. It is conceivable that subdividing TRD patients according to connectivity-based biotypes will shed new light on the interpretation of previous DBS study results, and that the integration of functional connectivity in future DBS studies will reveal clinically relevant subgroups that might respond to DBS of a specific target within the mood circuit. Altogether, it can be suggested that better assessment of therapeutic outcomes at symptom level might be accomplished when TRD patients with dominant anergia/fatigue symptoms (biotype 2) are stimulated within the CG 25; and patients characterized by more anxiety (biotype 4) are stimulated within the thalamic region, as suggested by Drysdale and coworkers [82]. Likewise, SCG stimulation could alleviate sleep disturbances and NAcc stimulation could improve anhedonia (Table 2).

4.2. Individual Tractography

Another way in which DBS efficiency can be improved is to ameliorate the implantation of electrodes with the usage of individualized, patient-specific, deterministic tractography targeting. Riva-Posse et al. (2018) used individualized patient-specific tractography targeting for SCC-DBS surgeries in TRD patients, aiming at the convergence of the four white matter bundles: the forceps minor, uncinate fasciculus, cingulum, and fronto-striatal fibers. This resulted in a response rate of 81.8% and a remission rate of 54% after a one year trial period, which proved greater than the previous open-label trials [83]. In a recent study, diffusion tensor imaging (DTI) tractography was used to target SCC-DBS more optimally, and the authors examined the impact of tract activation on clinical response at 6 and 12 months. Stimulation of vmPFC pathways by SCC-DBS was associated with a positive response and stimulation of the cingulum was associated with a 6 month, but not a 12 months DBS response. Monopolar stimulation of 130 Hz was applied with either pulse width (90–450 μs) or amplitude (4–8 V) progressively increased every month, based on response status. Patients were changed to bipolar settings if monopolar stimulation caused adverse effects. It was speculated that targeting more ventral, rather than the dorsal mPFC projections, might improve the response [84].

4.3. Combining Deep Brain Stimulation with Cognitive-Behavioral Therapy

It is plausible that better therapeutic outcomes could be achieved if DBS is applied in combination with concurrent treatments, such as pharmacotherapy with antidepressants or cognitive-behavioral therapy (CBT) in TRD. Studies focusing on the added effect of concurrent treatments to DBS have not been conducted in patients with TRD. The results from studies in OCD patients treated with DBS show that adding CBT to DBS has added beneficial effects [85]. Studies targeted at revealing the added effects of concomitant treatments after DBS for TRD would also provide information that may facilitate establishing a treatment algorithm to determine the place of these treatments in DBS patients.

4.4. Biomarkers

Biomarkers are quantifiable characteristics of biological processes, which could prove helpful in improving diagnostic objectivity of MDD and TRD as well as help in personalizing its treatment. For MDD, no specific biomarkers have yet been found, though several markers have been shown to be potential candidates, such as brain-derived neurotrophic factor (BDNF), interleukins (IL) 1 and 6, tumor necrosis factor (TNF), malondialdehyde (MDA), hypothalamic-pituitary-adrenal (HPA) activity, and cortisol responses [86,87]. Every biomarker as a standalone shows a low sensitivity and specificity, partly explained by the heterogeneity of MDD. To overcome this shortcoming, either examining a biological panel of several markers [88] or phenotyping MDD and TRD into distinct subtypes could be considered. However, a recent meta-analysis showed that only cortisol has a predictive effect on onset/relapse and recurrence of MDD making the integration of biomarkers for personalizing TRD treatment a futuristic milestone yet to be discovered [89].

4.5. Insights into Symptomatic Improvement after Deep Brain Stimulation

For TRD, different regions in the mood circuit can be stimulated with DBS (Table 2), although it is still unclear which depressive-symptoms respond to the stimulation of a specific target. More research into the mood circuit is needed to untangle which emotions arise from specific brain regions. This may vary from basic animal research, disentangling neuronal function per brain region, and ultra-high field MR studies in humans, all of which could shed light on the dysfunctional brain circuits in TRD. In contrast to the motor system that is studied thoroughly [90,91], emotional circuitry is far less understood. One reason for this is that animal research into mood circuitry remains complicated as there is considerable heterogeneity between species [92]. Modeling depression in animals is complex as there are several depressive-like behavior models, such as the chronic unpredictable stress paradigm (CUS), which give insight into depression pathology [93]. DBS is investigated within these models to unravel behavioral and cellular changes following DBS [94].

Alongside the standard clinical rating scales, the use of momentary assessment techniques, such as the experience sampling method (ESM), could enhance the documentation of the momentary mood states [95]. The ESM includes short repeated assessments of experiences and behaviors, as well as moment-to-moment changes in mental states in the context of daily life. Research has shown that depressed patients can improve their depressive symptomology while using weekly ESM for six weeks, and add-on ESM derived feedback resulted in a significant decrease in HDRS scores compared to controls ($p < 0.01$; −5.5 point reduction in HDRS at 6 months) [96]. In add-on-derived feedback, a psychologist or psychiatrist gives feedback on the association between the participants momentary affective states and specific daily life contexts [97]. ESM-derived feedback could further improve treatment by showing within-subject changes in a heterogeneous TRD population and contribute to clinical decision-making [97]. In the case of DBS, the use of ESM may reveal specific response patterns depending on the brain region that is stimulated, which can provide valuable information about emotional circuitry. This can be done using well-evaluated day-to-day scores, including questionnaires that go into detail on current mood and adaptive functioning.

5. Conclusions

More personalized treatment approaches hold the potential to increase the overall efficacy of DBS for TRD. Precise evaluations of symptoms, biomarkers, and resting-state connectivity patterns are essential when distinguishing clinical subtypes of TRD. Moreover, subtyping may provide more insight into the working mechanisms of DBS and help in selecting optimal targets in patients. Monitoring of biomarkers at multiple time points during treatment along with evaluation of ESM data, in parallel with clinical assessments of mood using standardized depression-rating scales, will lead to a better understanding of symptom changes when stimulating specific brain regions. Such considerations could further lead to optimal adjustments of stimulation parameters as long-term effects of DBS on mood occur.

Author Contributions: M.R. and E.S. prepared the first draft. J.B., A.E.P.M., A.F.G.L. and A.J. provided inputs and revised the manuscript. A.J. supervised the process. All authors have read and agreed to the published version of the manuscript.

Funding: This research received no external funding.

Conflicts of Interest: The authors declare no conflict of interest.

References

1. Uher, R.; Payne, J.L.; Pavlova, B.; Perlis, R.H. Major depressive disorder in DSM-5: Implications for clinical practice and research of changes from DSM-IV. *Depress. Anxiety* **2014**, *31*, 459–471. [CrossRef] [PubMed]
2. WHO. *Depression and Other Common Mental Disorders Global Health Estimates*; World Health Organization: Geneva, Switzerland, 2017.
3. Rush, A. Acute and Longer-Term Outcomes in Depressed Outpatients Requiring One or Several Treatment Steps: A STAR*D Report. *Am. J. Psychiatry* **2006**, *163*, 1905. [CrossRef] [PubMed]
4. Cuijpers, P.; Karyotaki, E.; Weitz, E.; Andersson, G.; Hollon, S.D.; van Straten, A. The effects of psychotherapies for major depression in adults on remission, recovery and improvement: A meta-analysis. *J. Affect. Disord.* **2014**, *159*, 118–126. [CrossRef] [PubMed]
5. Gaynes, B.N.; Asher, G.; Gartlehner, G.; Hoffman, V.; Green, J.; Boland, E.; Lux, L.; Weber, R.P.; Randolph, C.; Bann, C.; et al. *Definition of Treatment-Resistant Depression in the Medicare Population*; Agency for Healthcare Research and Quality: Rockville, MD, USA, 2018.
6. Amital, D.; Fostick, L.; Silberman, A.; Beckman, M.; Spivak, B. Serious life events among resistant and non-resistant MDD patients. *J. Affect. Disord.* **2008**, *110*, 260–264. [CrossRef]

7. Ivanova, J.I.; Birnbaum, H.G.; Kidolezi, Y.; Subramanian, G.; Khan, S.A.; Stensland, M.D. Direct and indirect costs of employees with treatment-resistant and non-treatment-resistant major depressive disorder. *Curr. Med. Res. Opin.* **2010**, *26*, 2475–2484. [CrossRef]
8. Johnson, R.L.; Wilson, C.G. A review of vagus nerve stimulation as a therapeutic intervention. *J. Inflamm. Res.* **2018**, *11*, 203–213. [CrossRef]
9. George, M.S.; Taylor, J.J.; Short, E.B. The expanding evidence base for rTMS treatment of depression. *Curr. Opin. Psychiatry* **2013**, *26*, 13–18. [CrossRef]
10. Mayberg, H.S.; Lozano, A.M.; Voon, V.; McNeely, H.E.; Seminowicz, D.; Hamani, C.; Schwalb, J.M.; Kennedy, S.H. Deep brain stimulation for treatment-resistant depression. *Neuron* **2005**, *45*, 651–660. [CrossRef]
11. Alexander, G.E.; DeLong, M.R.; Strick, P.L. Parallel organization of functionally segregated circuits linking basal ganglia and cortex. *Annu. Rev. Neurosci.* **1986**, *9*, 357–381. [CrossRef]
12. Mayberg, H.S. Limbic-cortical dysregulation: A proposed model of depression. *J. Neuropsychiatry Clin. Neurosci.* **1997**, *9*, 471–481.
13. Temel, Y.; Leentjens, A.F.G.; de Bie, R.M.A. *Handboek Diepe Hersenstimulatie Bij Neurologische En Psychiatrische Aandoeningen*; Bohn Stafleu van Loghum: Houten, The Netherlands, 2016; pp. 137–142.
14. Gabriels, L.; Cosyns, P.; Nuttin, B.; Demeulemeester, H.; Gybels, J. Deep brain stimulation for treatment-refractory obsessive-compulsive disorder: Psychopathological and neuropsychological outcome in three cases. *Acta Psychiatry Scand.* **2003**, *107*, 275–282. [CrossRef]
15. Greenberg, B.D.; Malone, D.A.; Friehs, G.M.; Rezai, A.R.; Kubu, C.S.; Malloy, P.F.; Salloway, S.P.; Okun, M.S.; Goodman, W.K.; Rasmussen, S.A. Three-year outcomes in deep brain stimulation for highly resistant obsessive-compulsive disorder. *Neuropsychopharmacology* **2006**, *31*, 2384–2393. [CrossRef] [PubMed]
16. Moonen, A.J.H.; Wijers, A.; Dujardin, K.; Leentjens, A.F.G. Neurobiological correlates of emotional processing in Parkinson's disease: A systematic review of experimental studies. *J. Psychosom. Res.* **2017**, *100*, 65–76. [CrossRef]
17. Mayberg, H.S.; Liotti, M.; Brannan, S.K.; McGinnis, S.; Mahurin, R.K.; Jerabek, P.A.; Silva, J.A.; Tekell, J.L.; Martin, C.C.; Lancaster, J.L.; et al. Reciprocal limbic-cortical function and negative mood: Converging PET findings in depression and normal sadness. *Am. J. Psychiatry* **1999**, *156*, 675–682. [PubMed]
18. Drevets, W.C.; Savitz, J.; Trimble, M. The subgenual anterior cingulate cortex in mood disorders. *CNS Spectr.* **2008**, *13*, 663–681. [CrossRef]
19. Ongur, D.; Ferry, A.T.; Price, J.L. Architectonic subdivision of the human orbital and medial prefrontal cortex. *J. Comp. Neurol.* **2003**, *460*, 425–449. [CrossRef]
20. Sun, C.; Wang, Y.; Cui, R.; Wu, C.; Li, X.; Bao, Y.; Wang, Y. Human Thalamic-Prefrontal Peduncle Connectivity Revealed by Diffusion Spectrum Imaging Fiber Tracking. *Front. Neuroanat.* **2018**, *12*, 24. [CrossRef]
21. Coenen, V.A.; Panksepp, J.; Hurwitz, T.A.; Urbach, H.; Madler, B. Human medial forebrain bundle (MFB) and anterior thalamic radiation (ATR): Imaging of two major subcortical pathways and the dynamic balance of opposite affects in understanding depression. *J. Neuropsychiatry Clin. Neurosci.* **2012**, *24*, 223–236. [CrossRef]
22. Lebow, M.A.; Chen, A. Overshadowed by the amygdala: The bed nucleus of the stria terminalis emerges as key to psychiatric disorders. *Mol. Psychiatry* **2016**, *21*, 450–463. [CrossRef]
23. Lozano, A.M.; Lipsman, N.; Bergman, H.; Brown, P.; Chabardes, S.; Chang, J.W.; Matthews, K.; McIntyre, C.C.; Schlaepfer, T.E.; Schulder, M.; et al. Deep brain stimulation: Current challenges and future directions. *Nat. Rev. Neurol.* **2019**, *15*, 148–160. [CrossRef]
24. Daneshzand, M.; Faezipour, M.; Barkana, B.D. Robust desynchronization of Parkinson's disease pathological oscillations by frequency modulation of delayed feedback deep brain stimulation. *PLoS ONE* **2018**, *13*, e0207761. [CrossRef] [PubMed]
25. Vicheva, P.; Butler, M.; Shotbolt, P. Deep brain stimulation for obsessive-compulsive disorder: A systematic review of randomised controlled trials. *Neurosci. Biobehav. Rev.* **2020**, *109*, 129–138. [CrossRef] [PubMed]
26. Agnesi, F.; Johnson, M.D.; Vitek, J.L. Deep brain stimulation: How does it work? *Handb. Clin. Neurol.* **2013**, *116*, 39–54. [PubMed]
27. Cheney, P.D.; Griffin, D.M.; Van Acker, G.M., III. Neural hijacking: Action of high-frequency electrical stimulation on cortical circuits. *Neuroscientist* **2013**, *19*, 434–441. [CrossRef]
28. Ashkan, K.; Rogers, P.; Bergman, H.; Ughratdar, I. Insights into the mechanisms of deep brain stimulation. *Nat. Rev. Neurol.* **2017**, *13*, 548–554. [CrossRef]

29. Van den Munckhof, P.; Bosch, D.A.; Mantione, M.H.; Figee, M.; Denys, D.A.; Schuurman, P.R. Active stimulation site of nucleus accumbens deep brain stimulation in obsessive-compulsive disorder is localized in the ventral internal capsule. *Acta Neurochir. Suppl.* **2013**, *117*, 53–59.
30. Drobisz, D.; Damborska, A. Deep brain stimulation targets for treating depression. *Behav. Brain Res.* **2019**, *359*, 266–273. [CrossRef]
31. Hamani, C.; Mayberg, H.; Stone, S.; Laxton, A.; Haber, S.; Lozano, A.M. The subcallosal cingulate gyrus in the context of major depression. *Biol. Psychiatry* **2011**, *69*, 301–308. [CrossRef]
32. Coryell, W.; Nopoulos, P.; Drevets, W.; Wilson, T.; Andreasen, N.C. Subgenual prefrontal cortex volumes in major depressive disorder and schizophrenia: Diagnostic specificity and prognostic implications. *Am. J. Psychiatry* **2005**, *162*, 1706–1712. [CrossRef]
33. Schlaepfer, T.E.; Cohen, M.X.; Frick, C.; Kosel, M.; Brodesser, D.; Axmacher, N.; Joe, A.Y.; Kreft, M.; Lenartz, D.; Sturm, V. Deep brain stimulation to reward circuitry alleviates anhedonia in refractory major depression. *Neuropsychopharmacology* **2008**, *33*, 368–377. [CrossRef]
34. Wacker, J.; Dillon, D.G.; Pizzagalli, D.A. The role of the nucleus accumbens and rostral anterior cingulate cortex in anhedonia: Integration of resting EEG, fMRI, and volumetric techniques. *Neuroimage* **2009**, *46*, 327–337. [CrossRef] [PubMed]
35. Makris, N.; Rathi, Y.; Mouradian, P.; Bonmassar, G.; Papadimitriou, G.; Ing, W.I.; Yeterian, E.H.; Kubicki, M.; Eskandar, E.N.; Wald, L.L.; et al. Variability and anatomical specificity of the orbitofrontothalamic fibers of passage in the ventral capsule/ventral striatum (VC/VS): Precision care for patient-specific tractography-guided targeting of deep brain stimulation (DBS) in obsessive compulsive disorder (OCD). *Brain Imaging Behav.* **2016**, *10*, 1054–1067.
36. Quevedo, K.; Ng, R.; Scott, H.; Kodavaganti, S.; Smyda, G.; Diwadkar, V.; Phillips, M. Ventral Striatum Functional Connectivity during Rewards and Losses and Symptomatology in Depressed Patients. *Biol. Psychol.* **2017**, *123*, 62–73. [CrossRef] [PubMed]
37. Hwang, J.W.; Xin, S.C.; Ou, Y.M.; Zhang, W.Y.; Liang, Y.L.; Chen, J.; Yang, X.Q.; Chen, X.Y.; Guo, T.W.; Yang, X.J.; et al. Enhanced default mode network connectivity with ventral striatum in subthreshold depression individuals. *J. Psychiatry Res.* **2016**, *76*, 111–120. [CrossRef] [PubMed]
38. Zhang, A.; Ajilore, O.; Zhan, L.; Gadelkarim, J.; Korthauer, L.; Yang, S.; Leow, A.; Kumar, A. White matter tract integrity of anterior limb of internal capsule in major depression and type 2 diabetes. *Neuropsychopharmacology* **2013**, *38*, 1451–1459. [CrossRef]
39. Alonso, P.; Cuadras, D.; Gabriels, L.; Denys, D.; Goodman, W.; Greenberg, B.D.; Jimenez-Ponce, F.; Kuhn, J.; Lenartz, D.; Mallet, L.; et al. Deep Brain Stimulation for Obsessive-Compulsive Disorder: A Meta-Analysis of Treatment Outcome and Predictors of Response. *PLoS ONE* **2015**, *10*, e0133591. [CrossRef]
40. Matsumoto, M.; Hikosaka, O. Lateral habenula as a source of negative reward signals in dopamine neurons. *Nature* **2007**, *447*, 1111–1115. [CrossRef]
41. Meng, H.; Wang, Y.; Huang, M.; Lin, W.; Wang, S.; Zhang, B. Chronic deep brain stimulation of the lateral habenula nucleus in a rat model of depression. *Brain Res.* **2011**, *1422*, 32–38. [CrossRef]
42. Sartorius, A.; Henn, F.A. Deep brain stimulation of the lateral habenula in treatment resistant major depression. *Med. Hypotheses* **2007**, *69*, 1305–1308. [CrossRef]
43. Ranft, K.; Dobrowolny, H.; Krell, D.; Bielau, H.; Bogerts, B.; Bernstein, H.G. Evidence for structural abnormalities of the human habenular complex in affective disorders but not in schizophrenia. *Psychol. Med.* **2010**, *40*, 557–567. [CrossRef]
44. Sartorius, A.; Kiening, K.L.; Kirsch, P.; von Gall, C.C.; Haberkorn, U.; Unterberg, A.W.; Henn, F.A.; Meyer-Lindenberg, A. Remission of major depression under deep brain stimulation of the lateral habenula in a therapy-refractory patient. *Biol. Psychiatry* **2010**, *67*, e9–e11. [CrossRef] [PubMed]
45. Lee, D.J.; Dallapiazza, R.F.; De Vloo, P.; Elias, G.J.B.; Fomenko, A.; Boutet, A.; Giacobbe, P.; Lozano, A.M. Inferior thalamic peduncle deep brain stimulation for treatment-refractory obsessive-compulsive disorder: A phase 1 pilot trial. *Brain Stimul.* **2019**, *12*, 344–352. [CrossRef] [PubMed]
46. Velasco, F.; Velasco, M.; Jimenez, F.; Velasco, A.L.; Salin-Pascual, R. Neurobiological background for performing surgical intervention in the inferior thalamic peduncle for treatment of major depression disorders. *Neurosurgery* **2005**, *57*, 439–448, Discussion 439–448. [CrossRef] [PubMed]
47. Schlaepfer, T.E.; Bewernick, B.H.; Kayser, S.; Madler, B.; Coenen, V.A. Rapid effects of deep brain stimulation for treatment-resistant major depression. *Biol. Psychiatry* **2013**, *73*, 1204–1212. [CrossRef]

48. Schoene-Bake, J.C.; Parpaley, Y.; Weber, B.; Panksepp, J.; Hurwitz, T.A.; Coenen, V.A. Tractographic analysis of historical lesion surgery for depression. *Neuropsychopharmacology* **2010**, *35*, 2553–2563. [CrossRef]
49. Fenoy, A.J.; Schulz, P.; Selvaraj, S.; Burrows, C.; Spiker, D.; Cao, B.; Zunta-Soares, G.; Gajwani, P.; Quevedo, J.; Soares, J. Deep brain stimulation of the medial forebrain bundle: Distinctive responses in resistant depression. *J. Affect. Disord.* **2016**, *203*, 143–151. [CrossRef]
50. Neumann, W.J.; Huebl, J.; Brucke, C.; Gabriels, L.; Bajbouj, M.; Merkl, A.; Schneider, G.H.; Nuttin, B.; Brown, P.; Kuhn, A.A. Different patterns of local field potentials from limbic DBS targets in patients with major depressive and obsessive compulsive disorder. *Mol. Psychiatry* **2014**, *19*, 1186–1192. [CrossRef]
51. Bagby, R.M.; Ryder, A.G.; Schuller, D.R.; Marshall, M.B. The Hamilton Depression Rating Scale: Has the gold standard become a lead weight? *Am. J. Psychiatry* **2004**, *161*, 2163–2177. [CrossRef]
52. Kennedy, S.H.; Giacobbe, P.; Rizvi, S.J.; Placenza, F.M.; Nishikawa, Y.; Mayberg, H.S.; Lozano, A.M. Deep brain stimulation for treatment-resistant depression: Follow-up after 3 to 6 years. *Am. J. Psychiatry* **2011**, *168*, 502–510. [CrossRef]
53. Bewernick, B.H.; Hurlemann, R.; Matusch, A.; Kayser, S.; Grubert, C.; Hadrysiewicz, B.; Axmacher, N.; Lemke, M.; Cooper-Mahkorn, D.; Cohen, M.X.; et al. Nucleus accumbens deep brain stimulation decreases ratings of depression and anxiety in treatment-resistant depression. *Biol. Psychiatry* **2010**, *67*, 110–116. [CrossRef]
54. Bewernick, B.H.; Kayser, S.; Sturm, V.; Schlaepfer, T.E. Long-term effects of nucleus accumbens deep brain stimulation in treatment-resistant depression: Evidence for sustained efficacy. *Neuropsychopharmacology* **2012**, *37*, 1975–1985. [CrossRef] [PubMed]
55. Malone, D.A., Jr.; Dougherty, D.D.; Rezai, A.R.; Carpenter, L.L.; Friehs, G.M.; Eskandar, E.N.; Rauch, S.L.; Rasmussen, S.A.; Machado, A.G.; Kubu, C.S.; et al. Deep brain stimulation of the ventral capsule/ventral striatum for treatment-resistant depression. *Biol. Psychiatry* **2009**, *65*, 267–275. [CrossRef] [PubMed]
56. Lozano, A.M.; Mayberg, H.S.; Giacobbe, P.; Hamani, C.; Craddock, R.C.; Kennedy, S.H. Subcallosal cingulate gyrus deep brain stimulation for treatment-resistant depression. *Biol. Psychiatry* **2008**, *64*, 461–467. [CrossRef] [PubMed]
57. Puigdemont, D.; Perez-Egea, R.; Portella, M.J.; Molet, J.; de Diego-Adelino, J.; Gironell, A.; Radua, J.; Gomez-Anson, B.; Rodriguez, R.; Serra, M.; et al. Deep brain stimulation of the subcallosal cingulate gyrus: Further evidence in treatment-resistant major depression. *Int. J. Neuropsychopharmacol.* **2012**, *15*, 121–133. [CrossRef]
58. Lozano, A.M.; Giacobbe, P.; Hamani, C.; Rizvi, S.J.; Kennedy, S.H.; Kolivakis, T.T.; Debonnel, G.; Sadikot, A.F.; Lam, R.W.; Howard, A.K.; et al. A multicenter pilot study of subcallosal cingulate area deep brain stimulation for treatment-resistant depression. *J. Neurosurg.* **2012**, *116*, 315–322. [CrossRef]
59. Holtzheimer, P.E.; Kelley, M.E.; Gross, R.E.; Filkowski, M.M.; Garlow, S.J.; Barrocas, A.; Wint, D.; Craighead, M.C.; Kozarsky, J.; Chismar, R.; et al. Subcallosal cingulate deep brain stimulation for treatment-resistant unipolar and bipolar depression. *Arch. Gen. Psychiatry* **2012**, *69*, 150–158. [CrossRef]
60. Crowell, A.L.; Riva-Posse, P.; Holtzheimer, P.E.; Garlow, S.J.; Kelley, M.E.; Gross, R.E.; Denison, L.; Quinn, S.; Mayberg, H.S. Long-Term Outcomes of Subcallosal Cingulate Deep Brain Stimulation for Treatment-Resistant Depression. *Am. J. Psychiatry* **2019**, *176*, 949–956. [CrossRef]
61. Merkl, A.; Schneider, G.H.; Schonecker, T.; Aust, S.; Kuhl, K.P.; Kupsch, A.; Kuhn, A.A.; Bajbouj, M. Antidepressant effects after short-term and chronic stimulation of the subgenual cingulate gyrus in treatment-resistant depression. *Exp. Neurol.* **2013**, *249*, 160–168. [CrossRef]
62. Accolla, E.A.; Aust, S.; Merkl, A.; Schneider, G.H.; Kuhn, A.A.; Bajbouj, M.; Draganski, B. Deep brain stimulation of the posterior gyrus rectus region for treatment resistant depression. *J. Affect. Disord.* **2016**, *194*, 33–37. [CrossRef]
63. Berlim, M.T.; McGirr, A.; Van den Eynde, F.; Fleck, M.P.; Giacobbe, P. Effectiveness and acceptability of deep brain stimulation (DBS) of the subgenual cingulate cortex for treatment-resistant depression: A systematic review and exploratory meta-analysis. *J. Affect. Disord.* **2014**, *159*, 31–38. [CrossRef]
64. Merkl, A.; Aust, S.; Schneider, G.H.; Visser-Vandewalle, V.; Horn, A.; Kuhn, A.A.; Kuhn, J.; Bajbouj, M. Deep brain stimulation of the subcallosal cingulate gyrus in patients with treatment-resistant depression: A double-blinded randomized controlled study and long-term follow-up in eight patients. *J. Affect. Disord.* **2018**, *227*, 521–529. [CrossRef] [PubMed]

65. Holtzheimer, P.E.; Husain, M.M.; Lisanby, S.H.; Taylor, S.F.; Whitworth, L.A.; McClintock, S.; Slavin, K.V.; Berman, J.; McKhann, G.M.; Patil, P.G.; et al. Subcallosal cingulate deep brain stimulation for treatment-resistant depression: A multisite, randomised, sham-controlled trial. *Lancet Psychiatry* **2017**, *4*, 839–849. [CrossRef]
66. Morishita, T.; Fayad, S.M.; Higuchi, M.A.; Nestor, K.A.; Foote, K.D. Deep brain stimulation for treatment-resistant depression: Systematic review of clinical outcomes. *Neurotherapeutics* **2014**, *11*, 475–484. [CrossRef] [PubMed]
67. Eitan, R.; Fontaine, D.; Benoit, M.; Giordana, C.; Darmon, N.; Israel, Z.; Linesky, E.; Arkadir, D.; Ben-Naim, S.; Iserlles, M.; et al. One year double blind study of high vs low frequency subcallosal cingulate stimulation for depression. *J. Psychiatry Res.* **2018**, *96*, 124–134. [CrossRef]
68. Dougherty, D.D.; Rezai, A.R.; Carpenter, L.L.; Howland, R.H.; Bhati, M.T.; O'Reardon, J.P.; Eskandar, E.N.; Baltuch, G.H.; Machado, A.D.; Kondziolka, D.; et al. A Randomized Sham-Controlled Trial of Deep Brain Stimulation of the Ventral Capsule/Ventral Striatum for Chronic Treatment-Resistant Depression. *Biol. Psychiatry* **2015**, *78*, 240–248. [CrossRef] [PubMed]
69. Peichel, D. A Clinical Evaluation of Different Device Parameters for the Management of Patients with Treatment Resistant Major Depressive Disorder, Single or Recurrent Episode, with Deep Brain Stimulation. Available online: https://clinicaltrials.gov/ct2/show/NCT01331330 (accessed on 24 August 2020).
70. Rezai, A. Feasibility, Safety and Efficacy of Deep Brain Stimulation of the Internal Capsule for Severe and Medically Refractory Major Depression. Available online: https://clinicaltrials.gov/ct2/show/NCT00555698 (accessed on 24 August 2020).
71. Nuttin, B.J.; Gabriels, L.A.; Cosyns, P.R.; Meyerson, B.A.; Andreewitch, S.; Sunaert, S.G.; Maes, A.F.; Dupont, P.J.; Gybels, J.M.; Gielen, F.; et al. Long-term electrical capsular stimulation in patients with obsessive-compulsive disorder. *Neurosurgery* **2003**, *52*, 1263–1272, Discussion 1264–1272. [CrossRef]
72. Abelson, J.L.; Curtis, G.C.; Sagher, O.; Albucher, R.C.; Harrigan, M.; Taylor, S.F.; Martis, B.; Giordani, B. Deep brain stimulation for refractory obsessive-compulsive disorder. *Biol. Psychiatry* **2005**, *57*, 510–516. [CrossRef]
73. Van Laere, K.; Nuttin, B.; Gabriels, L.; Dupont, P.; Rasmussen, S.; Greenberg, B.D.; Cosyns, P. Metabolic imaging of anterior capsular stimulation in refractory obsessive-compulsive disorder: A key role for the subgenual anterior cingulate and ventral striatum. *J. Nucl. Med.* **2006**, *47*, 740–747.
74. Bergfeld, I.O.; Mantione, M.; Hoogendoorn, M.L.; Ruhe, H.G.; Notten, P.; van Laarhoven, J.; Visser, I.; Figee, M.; de Kwaasteniet, B.P.; Horst, F.; et al. Deep Brain Stimulation of the Ventral Anterior Limb of the Internal Capsule for Treatment-Resistant Depression: A Randomized Clinical Trial. *JAMA Psychiatry* **2016**, *73*, 456–464. [CrossRef]
75. Loonen, A.J.; Ivanova, S.A. Circuits Regulating Pleasure and Happiness-Mechanisms of Depression. *Front. Hum. Neurosci.* **2016**, *10*, 571. [CrossRef]
76. Goodman, W. A Clinical Pilot Study Examining Bilateral Inhibition of the Lateral Habenula as a Target for Deep Brain Stimulation in Intractable Depression. Available online: https://clinicaltrials.gov/ct2/show/NCT01798407 (accessed on 24 August 2020).
77. Rolls, E.T. A non-reward attractor theory of depression. *Neurosci. Biobehav. Rev.* **2016**, *68*, 47–58. [CrossRef] [PubMed]
78. Raymaekers, S.; Luyten, L.; Bervoets, C.; Gabriels, L.; Nuttin, B. Deep brain stimulation for treatment-resistant major depressive disorder: A comparison of two targets and long-term follow-up. *Transl. Psychiatry* **2017**, *7*, e1251. [CrossRef] [PubMed]
79. Price, J.L.; Drevets, W.C. Neural circuits underlying the pathophysiology of mood disorders. *Trends Cogn. Sci.* **2012**, *16*, 61–71. [CrossRef]
80. Barcia, J.A.; Avecillas-Chasin, J.M.; Nombela, C.; Arza, R.; Garcia-Albea, J.; Pineda-Pardo, J.A.; Reneses, B.; Strange, B.A. Personalized striatal targets for deep brain stimulation in obsessive-compulsive disorder. *Brain Stimul.* **2019**, *12*, 724–734. [CrossRef] [PubMed]
81. Beijers, L.; Wardenaar, K.J.; van Loo, H.M.; Schoevers, R.A. Data-driven biological subtypes of depression: Systematic review of biological approaches to depression subtyping. *Mol. Psychiatry* **2019**, *24*, 888–900. [CrossRef]
82. Drysdale, A.T.; Grosenick, L.; Downar, J.; Dunlop, K.; Mansouri, F.; Meng, Y.; Fetcho, R.N.; Zebley, B.; Oathes, D.J.; Etkin, A.; et al. Resting-state connectivity biomarkers define neurophysiological subtypes of depression. *Nat. Med.* **2017**, *23*, 28–38. [CrossRef]

83. Riva-Posse, P.; Choi, K.S.; Holtzheimer, P.E.; Crowell, A.L.; Garlow, S.J.; Rajendra, J.K.; McIntyre, C.C.; Gross, R.E.; Mayberg, H.S. A connectomic approach for subcallosal cingulate deep brain stimulation surgery: Prospective targeting in treatment-resistant depression. *Mol. Psychiatry* **2018**, *23*, 843–849. [CrossRef]
84. Clark, D.L.; Johnson, K.A.; Butson, C.R.; Lebel, C.; Gobbi, D.; Ramasubbu, R.; Kiss, Z.H.T. Tract-based analysis of target engagement by subcallosal cingulate deep brain stimulation for treatment resistant depression. *Brain Stimul.* **2020**, *13*, 1094–1101. [CrossRef]
85. Gormezoglu, M.; van der Vlis, T.B.; Schruers, K.; Ackermans, L.; Polosan, M.; Leentjens, A.F.G. Effectiveness, Timing and Procedural Aspects of Cognitive Behavioral Therapy after Deep Brain Stimulation for Therapy-Resistant Obsessive Compulsive Disorder: A Systematic Review. *J. Clin. Med.* **2020**, *9*, 2383. [CrossRef]
86. Hacimusalar, Y.; Esel, E. Suggested Biomarkers for Major Depressive Disorder. *Noro Psikiyatr Ars* **2018**, *55*, 280–290. [CrossRef]
87. MacDonald, K.; Krishnan, A.; Cervenka, E.; Hu, G.; Guadagno, E.; Trakadis, Y. Biomarkers for major depressive and bipolar disorders using metabolomics: A systematic review. *Am. J. Med. Genet. B Neuropsychiatr. Genet.* **2019**, *180*, 122–137. [CrossRef] [PubMed]
88. Schmidt, H.D.; Shelton, R.C.; Duman, R.S. Functional biomarkers of depression: Diagnosis, treatment, and pathophysiology. *Neuropsychopharmacology* **2011**, *36*, 2375–2394. [CrossRef] [PubMed]
89. Kennis, M.; Gerritsen, L.; van Dalen, M.; Williams, A.; Cuijpers, P.; Bockting, C. Prospective biomarkers of major depressive disorder: A systematic review and meta-analysis. *Mol. Psychiatry* **2020**, *25*, 321–338. [CrossRef]
90. Rosin, B.; Nevet, A.; Elias, S.; Rivlin-Etzion, M.; Israel, Z.; Bergman, H. Physiology and pathophysiology of the basal ganglia-thalamo-cortical networks. *Parkinsonism Relat. Disord.* **2007**, *13* (Suppl. S3), S437–S439. [CrossRef]
91. Redgrave, P.; Rodriguez, M.; Smith, Y.; Rodriguez-Oroz, M.C.; Lehericy, S.; Bergman, H.; Agid, Y.; DeLong, M.R.; Obeso, J.A. Goal-directed and habitual control in the basal ganglia: Implications for Parkinson's disease. *Nat. Rev. Neurosci.* **2010**, *11*, 760–772. [CrossRef] [PubMed]
92. Panksepp, J. The basic emotional circuits of mammalian brains: Do animals have affective lives? *Neurosci. Biobehav. Rev.* **2011**, *35*, 1791–1804. [CrossRef] [PubMed]
93. Abelaira, H.M.; Reus, G.Z.; Quevedo, J. Animal models as tools to study the pathophysiology of depression. *Braz. J. Psychiatry* **2013**, *35* (Suppl. S2), S112–S120. [CrossRef] [PubMed]
94. Lim, L.W.; Prickaerts, J.; Huguet, G.; Kadar, E.; Hartung, H.; Sharp, T.; Temel, Y. Electrical stimulation alleviates depressive-like behaviors of rats: Investigation of brain targets and potential mechanisms. *Transl. Psychiatry* **2015**, *5*, e535. [CrossRef]
95. Verhagen, S.J.; Hasmi, L.; Drukker, M.; van Os, J.; Delespaul, P.A. Use of the experience sampling method in the context of clinical trials. *Evid. Based Ment. Health* **2016**, *19*, 86–89. [CrossRef]
96. Kramer, I.; Simons, C.J.; Hartmann, J.A.; Menne-Lothmann, C.; Viechtbauer, W.; Peeters, F.; Schruers, K.; van Bemmel, A.L.; Myin-Germeys, I.; Delespaul, P.; et al. A therapeutic application of the experience sampling method in the treatment of depression: A randomized controlled trial. *World Psychiatry* **2014**, *13*, 68–77. [CrossRef]
97. Davidson, K.W.; Peacock, J.; Kronish, I.M.; Edmondson, D. Personalizing Behavioral Interventions Through Single-Patient (N-of-1) Trials. *Soc. Pers. Psychol. Compass* **2014**, *8*, 408–421. [CrossRef] [PubMed]

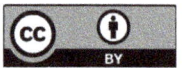 © 2020 by the authors. Licensee MDPI, Basel, Switzerland. This article is an open access article distributed under the terms and conditions of the Creative Commons Attribution (CC BY) license (http://creativecommons.org/licenses/by/4.0/).

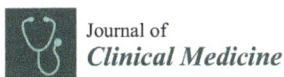

Review

A Decade of Progress in Deep Brain Stimulation of the Subcallosal Cingulate for the Treatment of Depression

Sharafuddin Khairuddin [1,†], Fung Yin Ngo [1,†], Wei Ling Lim [1,2], Luca Aquili [3], Naveed Ahmed Khan [4], Man-Lung Fung [1], Ying-Shing Chan [1], Yasin Temel [5] and Lee Wei Lim [1,2,*]

1. Neuromodulation Laboratory, School of Biomedical Sciences, Li Ka Shing Faculty of Medicine, The University of Hong Kong, L4 Laboratory Block, 21 Sassoon Road, Hong Kong, China; sharaf@hku.hk (S.K.); fyngo1@connect.hku.hk (F.Y.N.); weilingl@sunway.edu.my (W.L.L.); fungml@hku.hk (M.-L.F.); yschan@hku.hk (Y.-S.C.)
2. Department of Biological Sciences, School of Science and Technology, Sunway University, Bandar Sunway 47500, Malaysia
3. School of Psychological and Clinical Sciences, Charles Darwin University, NT0815 Darwin, Australia; luca.aquili@cdu.edu.au
4. Department of Biology, Chemistry and Environmental Sciences, College of Arts and Sciences, American University of Sharjah, Sharjah 26666, UAE; naveed5438@gmail.com
5. Departments of Neuroscience and Neurosurgery, Maastricht University, 6229ER Maastricht, The Netherlands; y.temel@maastrichtuniversity.nl
* Correspondence: drlimleewei@gmail.com
† These authors have joint first authorship.

Received: 14 August 2020; Accepted: 28 September 2020; Published: 12 October 2020

Abstract: Major depression contributes significantly to the global disability burden. Since the first clinical study of deep brain stimulation (DBS), over 446 patients with depression have now undergone this neuromodulation therapy, and 29 animal studies have investigated the efficacy of subgenual cingulate DBS for depression. In this review, we aim to provide a comprehensive overview of the progress of DBS of the subcallosal cingulate in humans and the medial prefrontal cortex, its rodent homolog. For preclinical animal studies, we discuss the various antidepressant-like behaviors induced by medial prefrontal cortex DBS and examine the possible mechanisms including neuroplasticity-dependent/independent cellular and molecular changes. Interestingly, the response rate of subcallosal cingulate Deep brain stimulation marks a milestone in the treatment of depression. DBS achieved response and remission rates of 64–76% and 37–63%, respectively, from clinical studies monitoring patients from 6–24 months. Although some studies showed its stimulation efficacy was limited, it still holds great promise as a therapy for patients with treatment-resistant depression. Overall, further research is still needed, including more credible clinical research, preclinical mechanistic studies, precise selection of patients, and customized electrical stimulation paradigms.

Keywords: deep brain stimulation; treatment-resistant depression; major depressive disorder; subcallosal cingulate; medial prefrontal cortex

1. Introduction

Major depressive disorder (MDD) contributes significantly to the global disability burden and social burden [1,2]. In the US from 2005 to 2010, the economic burden of patients with major depressive disorder increased by 21.5% to $210.5 billion [3]. The main symptoms of MDD include severe sadness, anxiety, cognitive deterioration, and suicidal thoughts [4]. Although its etiology is uncertain, genetic predisposition, developmental deficits, hormonal imbalance, and a stressful lifestyle may increase the risk for MDD [5–10].

Prior to the discovery of antidepressant medication, surgical ablation was used to effectively treat MDD in the US and Europe [11]. Pharmacological antidepressants first appeared in the late 20th century and these first-generation drugs became the first line treatment for depression [12]. However, newer generations of antidepressants were barely more effective than first-generation tricyclic antidepressants [13] and this has led to the emergence of treatment resistance. Treatment-resistant depression (TRD) is the failure to respond to the three different classes of treatment: antidepressants, psychotherapy, or electroconvulsive therapy given at a sufficient dose and time [14,15]. Approximately 20% to 30% of patients are refractory to pharmacotherapy and nearly 60% respond inadequately [16,17], which can result in worse clinical responses, leading to additional social burdens [18]. As the pathogenesis of MDD involves multiple structures, a broad-acting safe therapy needs to be developed [19,20].

With much progress in surgical techniques and advances in cardiac pacemakers, electrical stimulation has matured to become an adjustable stimulatory regimen [21]. Deep brain stimulation (DBS) is a procedure whereby deep brain structures are stimulated via precisely implanted electrodes. It was first used to alleviate movement disorders in patients with Parkinson's disease [22]. With advances in our understanding of the limbic circuitry, the focus has shifted to the antidepressant-like effects of DBS [23]. Some recent clinical studies have shown that DBS holds great promise in treating patients with TRD, and mechanistic studies in animals are currently in progress.

The use of DBS as a treatment for TRD was first proposed in a study by Kruger et al. on the differences in regional cerebral blood flow (rCBF) between remitted patients and bipolar depression (BD) patients [24]. They observed that rCBF in Brodmann Area 25 (BA25) was higher in remitted and BD patients compared to control patients and this was also seen in healthy patients with self-rated high negative affect [25]. Furthermore, Kruger et al. noted that mood provocation did not change the rCBF to this region in BD patients compared to MDD patients, indicating that dysfunction in the region was specific to depression [24]. Mayberg et al., who are pioneers of DBS as a treatment for depression, subsequently targeted BA25 after detecting metabolic abnormalities within the region that were consistent with those found in patients with TRD [19]. This landmark paper led to further developments in the application of DBS of this region as a treatment for depression.

Indeed, several research groups have used DBS to treat depression by targeting different brain regions in the limbic system. Jimenez et al. applied DBS to the inferior thalamic peduncle, whereas Schlaepfer et al. applied DBS in the nucleus accumbens core [26,27] and successfully performed DBS on the medial forebrain bundle [28]. With rapid developments in DBS as a treatment for TRD, research is now focusing on the subcallosal cingulate (SCC). This review aims to examine and consolidate clinical and preclinical research on the use of DBS as a treatment for depression, targeting the subcallosal cingulate in humans and the ventromedial prefrontal cortex, the anatomical correlate in rodents.

2. Outline of the Review

The online PubMed database was searched for research articles in English using a Boolean operation with keywords including "deep brain stimulation" AND "depression" AND "subcallosal cingulate" OR "rodent" AND "medial prefrontal cortex". Relevant articles cited in the reference lists of the identified publications were also included. PubMed was utilized due to its extensive collection of indexed peer-reviewed journals. This review highlights the development of DBS as a treatment for TRD and discusses the findings and limitations of preclinical and clinical studies published in the recent decade. The neuroplasticity-dependent and -independent aspects of the molecular and cellular changes due to DBS are also discussed. Lastly, some potential approaches that may improve the precision, safety, and efficacy of DBS are proposed.

3. The Development of Deep Brain Stimulation as a Treatment for Depression

Deep brain stimulation involves the stereotactic implantation of thin electrodes in deep brain structures that are used to deliver electrical stimulation generated by a subcutaneous pulse generator [29,30]. Stimulation is generally applied at either a low/moderate frequency (5–90 Hz) or high frequency (100–400 Hz). Since the inception of DBS, a number of studies have demonstrated that this modality has the ability to treat pain, obsessive-compulsive disorder, and Parkinson's disease [16,21,31]. Its efficacy has been verified in Parkinson's disease patients, in which high frequency stimulation (HFS) of specific brain region(s) in the basal ganglia was able to stop tremors [21,32]. The use of DBS has been given FDA approval for the management of obsessive-compulsive disorder since 2007, but it is only provided under a humanitarian device exemption [33,34].

The following sections summarize the clinical studies on deep brain stimulation in the subcallosal cingulate for treating patients with treatment-resistant depression and preclinical studies of deep brain stimulation in the medial prefrontal cortex (mPFC) of rodents.

4. Clinical and Preclinical Studies of SCC DBS for the Treatment of Depression

Clinical studies of depression utilize rating scales of depression that assess changes in depressive symptoms in patients. Some scales are completed by the researcher such as the Hamilton Depression Rating Scale (HDRS) and the Montgomery-Åsberg Depression Rating Scale (MADRS). These rating scales should allow more consistent assessment between patients, but can lack consensus in their interpretation among researchers, which could lead to misdiagnosis [35]. Another weakness of rating scales conducted in this manner is that the accuracy of the results is dependent on the communication skills of the patient, which might be hampered by the disease itself. Other scales are completed by patients such as the Beck Anxiety Inventory (BAI), Beck Depression Inventory (BDI), and Quick Inventory of Depressive Symptomatology (QIDS). These rating scales should allow for a more accurate reporting of depressive symptoms, although the number and/or depth of questions may vary across different tests.

4.1. Progress in the Development of SCC-DBS

Different papers have referred to the SCC and similar regions under different names, e.g., the subcallosal cingulate gyrus (SCG), the subgenual cingulate, as well as Brodmann areas. Different historical names allow for different historical context. The subgenual cortex is used more interchangeably with the term Brodmann Area 25, named after Korbinian Brodmann. The subgenual cortex is located in the cingulate region as a narrow band in the caudal portion of the subcallosal area adjacent to the paraterminal gyrus. By comparison, the SCG is comprised of Brodmann areas 25, 24, and 32 [36]; SCG circuits; and limbic structures. The SCG is pivotal in mood, learning, reward, and memory [37] and has been implicated as an aberrant region in MDD. As the SCC can be effectively targeted by antidepressants, this makes the SCG a potential target of DBS against TRD [38,39]. Tables 1 and 2 list 39 clinical studies on the treatment efficacy of SCC-DBS for TRD.

Table 1. A list of clinical studies on deep brain stimulation of the human subcallosal cingulate.

Authors	Main Inclusion Criteria	No. of Patients	Stimulation Target & DBS Design	Stimulation Parameters	Clinical Evaluation	Major Outcomes	Adverse Effects
Sankar et al. 2020 [40]	TRD MDE: Current MDE ≥ 12 months; HRSD-17 score ≥ 20; Non-responsive (NR) ≥ 4 antidepressant therapies; HRSD-17 score ≥ 20.	27	Target SCG	Implantation Bilateral Stimulation Monopolar Frequency 130 Hz Amplitude 3–6 V Pulse Width 90 μs	Volumetric analysis, Whole brain grey and white matter analysis	Left and average SCG volume significantly higher in responders compared to non-responders. Right and average amygdala volume significantly higher in responders compared to non-responders. Left, right, and average thalamus volume significantly higher in responders compared to non-responders. Brain grey matter volume significantly lower in responders compared to non-responders. Ratio of grey to white matter volume significantly higher in responders compared to non-responders.	N.A.
Riva-Posse et al. (2019) [41]	TRD MDE: Current MDE ≥ 12 months; HRSD-17 score ≥ 20; Non-responsive (NR) ≥ 4 antidepressant therapies; HRSD-17 score ≥ 20; GAF < 50.	9	Target SCC Study Design Intraoperative Sessions: 6 min session of 3 min stimulation ON and 3 min stimulation OFF. Number of sessions: 12 trials (one at each of the eight available contacts. Four per hemisphere, plus four sham trials). Sham-controlled, double-blinded trials (one case w/single blind trial)	Implantation Bilateral Stimulation Monopolar Frequency 130 Hz Amplitude 6 mA Pulse Width 90 μs	ECG, EDA, MRI Volume of Tissue Activated, Structural Connectivity Analysis	Autonomic changes with SCC-DBS correspond to salient behavioral responses. Distant effects of SCC-DBS in the midcingulate cortex. Increase in heart rate was only seen with left SCC-DBS. No significant relationship with skin conductance. These findings aid in the optimal selection of contacts and parameters in SCC-DBS surgery.	N.A.
Eitan et al. (2018) [42]	Both sexes, 21–70 years; Non-psychotic MDD; First MDE onset before 45 years old with current MDE ≥ 12 months; NR ≥ 4 antidepressant therapies; MADRS ≥ 22; GAF < 50; MMSE > 24; No changes in current antidepressant treatments ≥ 4 wks prior to study.	9	Target BA25 Study Design Double-blind, randomized. Two groups: High- OR low-frequency DBS for 12 months from 1 month after electrode implantation.	Implantation Bilateral Stimulation Monopolar Frequency 20 Hz or 130 Hz Amplitude 4–8 mA Pulse Width 91 μs	MADRS, HRSD-17, QIDS-SR, Q-LES-Q, GAF, HAM-A, CGI, PGI, CANTAB battery.	Four out of nine patients responded ° at the end of DBS (≥40% reduction in MADRS from baseline). The effect of DBS at 6-12 months was higher than DBS at 1–6 months. High-frequency DBS showed higher efficacy than low-frequency DBS. Non-responders crossed over after first 6 months of DBS.	Severe One patient overdosed on medication (dothiepin and valium).

Table 1. Cont.

Authors	Main Inclusion Criteria	No. of Patients	Stimulation Target & DBS Design	Stimulation Parameters	Clinical Evaluation	Major Outcomes	Adverse Effects
Merkl et al. (2018) [43]	Diagnosed MDD and disease lasted for >2 years; HAMD-24 score ≥ 20; ATHF Score ≥ 3; TRD: NR ≥ 2 antidepressant therapies; Failed to respond to antidepressants and ECT; No changes in current antidepressant treatments ≥6 wks prior to study.	8	Target SCC Study Design Randomized; Two groups: sham-DBS (delayed onset) OR non-delayed onset group for the first 8 weeks in a blinded manner. Open-label DBS afterwards for up to 28 months.	Implantation Bilateral Stimulation Monopolar Frequency 130 Hz Amplitude 5–7 V Pulse Width 90 μs	HAMD-24, BDI, MADRS.	Three out of eight patients responded ** after 6 months DBS; three out of seven with the same criteria after 12 months. Two out of six responded ** at the end of DBS, follow-up at 28 months. Two out of six patients reached remission □ at the end of DBS, follow-up at 28 months. This study showed a delayed response in patients; no significant antidepressant effects between sham and active stimulation compared to baseline.	Non-severe Headache; Pain; Scalp tingling; Dizziness; Light hypomania; Inconvenient movement; Severe NIL
Howell et al. (2018) [44]	Both sexes aged 18–70 years; current MDE ≥ 12 months; NR ≥ 4 antidepressant therapies; HRSD-17 score ≥ 20; GAF score ≤ 50.	6	Target SCC (Cingulum Bundle and Forceps Minor)	Implantation Bilateral Stimulation Monopolar Frequency 130 Hz Amplitude 4 V Pulse Width 90 μs	HDRS-17, MRI Field-cable modeling (non-VTA-based analysis)	All of the subjects responded. Left and right cingulum bundles as well as forceps minor are the most likely therapeutic targets. Right cingulum bundle activation beyond a threshold may protract recovery. Uncinate fasciculus and frontal pole were activated to a lesser extent, may not be necessary for anti-depressive effect of SCC-DBS. Time to a stable response (TSR) was 8–189 days, 1-year HDRS-17 was 2–11. Field cable modeling was more accurate than volume of activated tissue at approximating axonal activation. Overstimulation of CB-DBS can be detrimental to the recovery process.	N.A.
Waters et al. (2018) [45]	Both sexes aged 18–70 years; current MDE ≥ 12 months; NR ≥ 4 antidepressant therapies; HRSD-17 score ≥ 20; GAF score ≤ 50.	4	Target SCC Study Design Single-blinded, Session 3 min	Implantation Bilateral Stimulation Monopolar Frequency 130 Hz Amplitude 3–5 V Pulse Width 90 μs	HDRS-17, EEG	Symptom severity scores decreased. three out of four patients in remission (HDRS-17 ≤ 7). Test-retest reliability across four repeated measures over 14 months met or exceeded standards for valid test construction in three out of four patients for cortical-evoked responses studied.	N.A.

Table 1. Cont.

Authors	Main Inclusion Criteria	No. of Patients	Stimulation Target & DBS Design	Stimulation Parameters	Clinical Evaluation	Major Outcomes	Adverse Effects
Smart et al. (2018) [46]	TRD patients enrolled from two separate clinical trials for Deep Brain Stimulation. Trial 1 Both sexes aged 18–70 years; Diagnosis of a Major Depressive Episode or Bipolar Type II—current episode depressed, Current episode duration of at least 1 year, Non-responsive (NR) ≥ 4 antidepressant therapies. Trial 2 Both sexes aged 25–70 years; Current depressive episode of at least 2 years duration OR a history of more than four lifetime depressive episodes, Non-responsive (NR) ≥ 4 antidepressant therapies.	14	Target SCC Study Design Double-blinded. Intraoperative behavioral testing; Frequency: 130 Hz Pulse width: 90 μs Current: 6 mA Eight patients continued SCC local field potential.	Implantation Bilateral Stimulation Monopolar Frequency 130 Hz Amplitude 6–8 mA for St. Jude Medical devices, 3.5–5 V for Medtronic devices Pulse Width 90 μs	HDRS-17, MRI, LFP.	11 of 14 patients met the criteria for DBS antidepressant response by 6 months. Of the three 6 month non-responders, one responded after the 6 month study endpoint but without a contact change (Patient 2), one responded after a contact switch in the left hemisphere (Patient 7), and one remained a non-responder (Patient 6). Mean baseline HDRS-17 of 23.8 and SD of 2.8; HDRS-17 of 9.6 and SD of 4.5 at month 6; 19.9 weeks for stable response with SD of 20 weeks. Precision on the left may be more important than precision on the right, which is supported by theta decreases.	N.A.
Choi et al. (2018) [47]	Both sexes aged 18–70 years; current MDE ≥ 12 months; NR ≥ 4 antidepressant therapies; HRSD-17 score ≥ 20; GAF score ≤ 50.	15	Target SCC Study Design Patients went through SCC-DBS, followed by MRI scans.	Implantation Bilateral Stimulation Monopolar Frequency 130 Hz Amplitude 6 mA Pulse Width 90 μs	HDRS-17, MRI, DWI, Volume of Tissue Activated	Significant differences in the pathway activation changes over time between remitters and non-remitters. Non-remitters had significantly larger net changes in their pathway activation connection in both the near and long term relative to the initial plan.	N.A.
Conen et al. (2018) [48]	TRD (unipolar); NR ≥ 4 antidepressant therapies; MADRS Score ≥ 22.	7	Targets SCC followed by Ventral Anterior Capsule, nucleus accumbens (separately, unless patient in remission, and later combined, for non-responding patients). Study Design DBS was applied sequentially for 3 months per region, for a total period ranging from 16–45 months.	N.A.	MADRS, HAM-D 17, GAF.	Remitters had higher regional cerebral blood flow in the baseline prefrontal cortex and subsequent tests when compared to non-remitters and non-responders. Chronic DBS increased prefrontal cortex regional cerebral blood flow. Remitted patients had higher prefrontal cerebral blood flow at baseline.	N.A.

Table 1. *Cont.*

Authors	Main Inclusion Criteria	No. of Patients	Stimulation Target & DBS Design	Stimulation Parameters	Clinical Evaluation	Major Outcomes	Adverse Effects
Holtzheimer et al. (2017) [43]	Both sexes aged 21–70 years; Unipolar, non-psychotic MDD First MDE onset before 45 years old with current MDE ≥ 12 months; NR ≥ 4 antidepressant therapies, MADRS Score > 22; GAF < 50; MMSE > 24; No changes in current antidepressant treatments ≥ 4 wks prior to study.	60 (DBS) 30 (Sham)	Target SCG Study Design DBS or sham stimulation 2 weeks after implantation for 6 months in randomized and double-blind manner. Two groups: DBS or sham then both groups received open-label stimulation for 6 months or 2 years.	Implantation Bilateral Stimulation Monopolar Frequency 130 Hz Amplitude 4–8 mA Pulse Width 91 μs	MADRS, GAF HRSD-17, 30-item Inventory of Depressive Symptomatology, QIDS-SR, WSAS, PGI, CGI, QOL, HAM-A.	Insignificant difference in response * between sham and DBS at the end of the 6-month double-blind phase. 38 patients responded * and 20) remitted □ after 6 month DBS. In 2 years of open-label active DBS, 48% achieved antidepressant response and 25% achieved remission—clinically meaningful long-term outcomes.	Severe Eight of 40 events reported related to device or surgery: six infections (in five patients), one skin erosion over the extension wires, and one postoperative seizure.
McInerney et al. (2017) [44]	Current MDE ≥ 12 months; HRSD-17 Score ≥ 20; NR ≥ 4 antidepressant therapies.	20	Target SCG Study Design DBS for 12 months open-label	Implantation Bilateral Stimulation Monopolar Frequency 130 Hz Amplitude 3.5–5 V Pulse Width 90 μs	Wisconsin Card Sorting Task (WCST), Hopkins Verbal Learning Test, Controlled Oral Word Association Test (COWA), Finger Tap Test, Stroop Test, HRSD-17.	Significant reduction in HRSD-17 from baseline to experimental follow-up. Baseline scores differed significantly between responders and non-responders. 11 patients responded ** and nine were non-responders. WCST Test results indicated that the total errors were predictive of responsiveness to DBS. No significant deterioration in cognition and psychomotor speed. Improvements in verbal memory and verbal fluency.	N.A.
Riva-Posse et al. (2018) [49]	Both sexes aged 18–70 years; current MDE ≥ 12 months; NR ≥ 4 antidepressant therapies; HRSD-17 score ≥ 20; GAF score ≤ 50.	11	Target SCG Study Design DBS from 4 weeks after surgery and lasted for 6 months, open-label. Stimulation contacts were changed in non-responders and they were stimulated for 6 more months.	Implantation Bilateral Stimulation Monopolar Frequency 130 Hz Amplitude 6–8 mA Pulse Width 91 μs	HRSD-17	Eight out of 11 responded ** and six remitted □□ after 6 month DBS. Nine responded ** and six remitted □□ after 12 month DBS. Two did not respond throughout the study. Tractography-based surgery reduced variability in the effects of stimulation on patient-specific brain circuitry.	N.A.
Tsolaki et al. (2017) [50]	TRD	2	Target SCG	Implantation Bilateral Stimulation Monopolar Frequency 130 Hz Amplitude 8 mA Pulse Width 91 μs	MRI, DTI, CT, PSL Probabilistic tractography, Volume of Tissue Activated, MADRS.	One patient was a responder (81% change in MADRS score). Responder's contacts were closer to the Tractography-guided optimized target (TOT), unlike the non-responder.	N.A.

Table 1. Cont.

Authors	Main Inclusion Criteria	No. of Patients	Stimulation Target & DBS Design	Stimulation Parameters	Clinical Evaluation	Major Outcomes	Adverse Effects
Accolla et al. (2016) [51]	MDD; NR to treatments; Currently in a depressive episode as in DSM-IV Axis I disorders; HAMD-24 score of ≥ 20.	5	Target BA25 Study Design Double-blind. Each homologous electrode pair was activated separately on 5 consecutive days, then antidepressant effects was assessed 24 h later. Open-label DBS for up to 24 months. Pre- and post-DBS MRI images were taken.	Implantation N.A. Stimulation Monopolar Frequency 130 Hz Amplitude 5 V Pulse Width 90 µs	HAMD-24, BDI.	Four out of five patients did not show sustained response ** to DBS (also ≥50% reduction in DBI). One patient responded ** to DBS of the bilateral posterior gyrus rectus instead of the intended target (BA25).	N.A.
Richieri et al. (2016) [52]	Diagnosed MDD; Severe cognitive defects and relapsed after ECT.	1	Target BA25 Study Design DBS at Day 5 after electrode implantation.	Implantation Bilateral Stimulation Bipolar Frequency 130 Hz Amplitude 4.2 V Pulse Width 90 µs	QIDS SR-16	Remitted (QIDS SR-16 3/48) at 1 month after DBS and maintained at the end of DBS.	Seizure
Hilimire et al. (2015) [53]	Both sexes aged 18–70 years; Current MDE ≥ 12 months; Non-responsive (NR) ≥ 4 antidepressant therapies; HRSD-17 score ≥ 20, GAF score ≤ 50.	7	Target SCC Study Design DBS for 6 months, open-label. Behavioral testing and electrophysiological recording (i) before electrode implantation, (ii) after 1 month DBS and (iii) after 6 month DBS.	Implantation Bilateral Stimulation Monopolar Frequency 130 Hz Amplitude 4–8 mA Pulse Width 91 µs	HDRS-17, Emotional self-referential task, EEG recording.	Reduced proportion of negative self-descriptive words compared to baseline after 1 month and 6 month DBS. Significant reduction in P1 amplitude compared to baseline (for negative word self-description) after 1 month and 6 month DBS, and P3 amplitudes at 6 month DBS only. Reduced depression severity.	N.A.
Martin-Blanco et al. (2015) [54]	Both sexes aged 18–70 years; current MDE ≥ 12 months; NR ≥ 4 antidepressant therapies; HRSD-17 score ≥ 20; GAF score ≤ 50.	7	Target SCC Study Design Chronic DBS for 9 months on average for clinical stabilization. A PET scan was acquired (i) during active stimulation and (ii) after 48 h of inactive stimulation.	Implantation Bilateral Stimulation Monopolar Frequency 135 Hz Amplitude 3.5–5 V Pulse Width 120–210 µs	HAMD-17, PET	Decreased metabolism in BA24, BA6, caudate putamen after 48 h DBS. This study suggests metabolic changes spread after longer periods of no stimulation. No clinical changes were detected according to HAMD-17.	N.A.

Table 1. Cont.

Authors	Main Inclusion Criteria	No. of Patients	Stimulation Target & DBS Design	Stimulation Parameters	Clinical Evaluation	Major Outcomes	Adverse Effects
Puigdemont et al. (2015) [55]	Severe TRD; Both sexes aged 18–70 years; current MDE ≥ 12 months; NR ≥ 4 antidepressant therapies; HRSD-17 score ≥ 20; GAF score ≤ 50.	5	Target SCG Study Design Randomized, Double-blind. After stable clinical remission to DBS, patients were allocated to two groups, one with (i) 3 month DBS-ON, then (ii) 3 month sham stimulation (ON-OFF arm) or OFF-ON arm and the other, vice-versa.	Implantation Bilateral Stimulation Monopolar Frequency 130–135 Hz Amplitude 3.5–5 V Pulse Width 120–240 µs	Volume of Tissue Activated, HRSD-17	Active stimulation: four of five patients were remitted patients. Sham stimulation: Only two patients remained in remission, another two relapsed, and one showed a progressive worsening without reaching relapse criteria.	N.A.
Serra-Blasco et al. (2015) [56]	Treatment-Resistant Depression (TRD) Group Resistant to pharmacological treatment; min. stage IV of Thase-Rush scale; HDRS score ≥ 18. First Episode MDD (FE MDD) Group HDRS score ≥ 14; Newly diagnosed MDD.	16	Target SCG Study Design DBS began at 48 h postoperative and ended when each patient had stabilized response for at least three consecutive visits, tests conducted before surgery, and 12 months after DBS treatment.	Implantation Bilateral Stimulation Monopolar Frequency 135 Hz Amplitude 3.5–5 V Pulse Width 120–210 µs	Rey Auditory Verbal Learning Test, Trail Making Tests-A and -B, Wechsler Adult Intelligence Scale III, Tower of London Test, HDRS-17.	FE MDD and TRD saw significant improvements over time in memory. No significant difference was observed in both groups on executive functioning, language, and processing speed. DBS was well tolerated and had no adverse effect on neuropsychological and cognitive function.	N.A.
Choi et al. (2015) [57]	Both sexes aged 18–70 years; current MDE ≥ 12 months; NR ≥ 4 antidepressant therapies; HDRS-17 score ≥ 20; GAF score ≤ 50.	9	Target SCG Intraoperative Sessions: 6 min session of 3 min stimulation ON, and 3 min stimulation OFF. Number of sessions: 12 trials (one at each of the eight available contacts; four per hemisphere, plus four sham trials). Study Design Sham-controlled, Double-blind trials (one case w/single blind trial).	Acute Implantation Bilateral Stimulation Monopolar Frequency 130 Hz Amplitude 6 mA Pulse Width 90 µs	MRI with PSL analysis, Volume of Tissue Activated.	Behavioral switch was apparent to patients within the first minute of the initiation of stimulation and effects were sustained while stimulation remained on. Three common white matter bundles were affected by stimulation: (i) the uncinate fasciculus, (ii) the forceps minor, and (iii) the left cingulum bundle. Seven of nine patients with left hemispheric contact had a response to treatment at 6 months.	
Sun et al. (2015) [58]	NR ≥ 4 antidepressant therapies, Mean HRSD-17 score of 25 (3).	20	Target SCG Session: 100 min, w/15 min break EEG recording sessions/day Session 1: DBS On Session 2: DBS Random (On/Off) Session 3: DBS (Off)	Implantation Bilateral Stimulation Monopolar Frequency 130 Hz Amplitude 2–7.25 mA OR 2–6 V Pulse Width 90 µs	EEG, HDRS-17.	Suppression of gamma oscillations by DBS during working memory performance and the treatment efficacy of DBS for TRD may be associated with the improved GABAergic neurotransmission, previously shown to be deficient in MDD. The present study also suggests that modifying treatment parameters to achieve suppression of gamma oscillations and increased theta-gamma coupling may lead to optimized DBS efficacy for TRD.	N.A.

Table 1. Cont.

Authors	Main Inclusion Criteria	No. of Patients	Stimulation Target & DBS Design	Stimulation Parameters	Clinical Evaluation	Major Outcomes	Adverse Effects
Perez-Caballero et al. (2014) [59]	18–70 years old with MDE; Resistant to pharmacological treatment and at most, a partial response to ECT; HAMD-17 Score ≥ 18.	8	Target SCG Study Design All patients received chronic DBS within 48 h after implantation. Four patients took NSAIDs for up to 30 days postoperative, four patients did not.	Implantation Quadrupolar Stimulation 135 Hz Amplitude 3.5–5 V Pulse Width 120–210 µs	HDRS-17	At week 1 after surgery, all patients without NSAID prescription responded ** and two remitted □□□; three patients with NSAID responded **, and two remitted □□□. At week 4 after surgery, three patients without NSAID remitted □□□; no patients with NSAID responded **	N.A.
Merkl et al. (2013) [60]	MDD; NR to treatments; Currently in a depressive episode as in DSM-IV Axis I disorder; HAMD-24 score of ≥ 20; HDRS-24 score ≥ 24.	6	Target SCG Study Design DBS on 11–19 days after electrode implantation, 24 h acute stimulation followed by sham stimulation for each of the three electrode pairs. Up to 6 months of chronic stimulation.	Implantation Bilateral Stimulation Monopolar Frequency 130 Hz Amplitude 2.5–10 V Pulse Width 90 µs	HAMD-24, MADRS BDI, TMT-A, TMT-B, CVLT, TAP, Boston Naming Test, Stroop Test, Word Fluency Test.	Non-significant reduction in HAMD-24, BDI, and MADRS scores for acute DBS and sham stimulation. 0/4 contact pair locations showed significant BDI and MADRS improvements. Contact pair 3/7 for Patient 4 saw a 77% reduction in HAMD-24 score and 62% reduction of MADRS score. Reduced HDRS-24, BDI, and MADRS scores at the end of chronic stimulation. Two out of six remissions □ at the end of chronic stimulation.	Mild Headache; Pain; Scalp tingling; Dizziness; Sore throat; Hardware-related; Severe NIL
Ramasubbu et al. (2013) [61]	Aged between 20–60 years; Diagnosed MDD; HAMD-17 score ≥ 20; NR ≥ 4 antidepressant therapies. (Enrolled patients were among the most treatment resistant).	4	Target SCG Study Design Double-blind DBS optimization. Open-label continuous DBS for 6 months after optimization period. Varied parameters for each patient during optimization.	Implantation Bilateral Stimulation Monopolar Frequency 0/5/20/130/185 Hz Amplitude 0–10.5 V Pulse Width 0/90/150/ 270/450 µs	HAMD-17, MADRS, HAM-A, CGI.	Postoperative optimization: All four patients showed maximal response at longer pulse widths; three patients experienced a 50% reduction in HAMD-17 score. Longer pulse widths were correlated to short-term improvement. Longer pulse width also induced insomnia, confusion, and drowsiness; improved by turning off stimulation. Chronic stimulation: two patients responded ** at the end of open-label DBS, with longer pulse width. Electrode targets suggested to be individualized, as opposed to standard as in movement disorders, owing to the complexity of cortical gyral anatomy	Mild Anxiety; Drowsiness; Confusion; Insomnia.

Table 1. Cont.

Authors	Main Inclusion Criteria	No. of Patients	Stimulation Target & DBS Design	Stimulation Parameters	Clinical Evaluation	Major Outcomes	Adverse Effects
Torres et al. (2013) [62]	Type I bipolar depression; Poor response to ECT and pharmacotherapy.	1	Target SCC Study Design DBS from 15 days after implantation and follow-up for 9 months.	Implantation N.A. Stimulation Monopolar Frequency 130 Hz Amplitude 6 mA Pulse Width 91 μs	HDRS-17, BDI, MADRS, GAF, Young Mania Scale.	Scores improved across tests. Psychotic symptoms disappeared. Manic episodes reduced.	N.A.
Broadway et al. (2012) [63]	Both sexes aged 18–70 years; current MDE ≥ 12 months; NR ≥ 4 antidepressant therapies; HRSD-17 score ≥ 20; GAF score ≤ 50.	12	Target SCC Study Design DBS for up to 24 weeks.	Implantation N.A. Stimulation Monopolar Frequency 130 Hz Amplitude 6–8 mA Pulse Width 90 μs	HRSD-17, Frontal and posterior Theta cordance.	Reduced HDRS-17 scores between baseline and the end of DBS among all patients. Six patients had significantly reduced HRSD-17 scores ** at the end of DBS. Increased frontal theta cordance between baseline and week 4 in responders correlated with their decreased depressive state at later time points.	N.A.
Hamani et al. (2012) [64]	TRD; NR to respond to pharmacotherapy, psychotherapy, transcranial magnetic stimulation, ECT, vagus nerve stimulation. Relapsed after receiving 6 month SCC-DBS.	1	Target SCC Study Design Administered tranylcypromine before surgery. DBS for 6 months.	Implantation Bilateral Stimulation Monopolar Frequency 130 Hz Amplitude 2.5 V Pulse Width 90 μs	HAMD-17	Before relapse: SCC-DBS reduced HAMD-17 score from 22 to 9 after 4 month DBS. After relapse: MAOI supplementation restored the therapeutic effect of DBS; HAMD-17 score lowered from 22 to 16 (after 2 weeks), to 8 (after 2 months) and to 9 (after 4 months).	N.A.
Holtzheimer et al. (2012) [65]	Both sexes aged 18–70 years; current MDE ≥ 12 months; NR ≥ 4 antidepressant therapies; HRSD-17 score ≥ 20; GAF score ≤ 50.	17	Target SCC Study Design Intraoperative testing of electrode location for 12 or 17 patients. Stimulation: (i) 4 weeks of sham stimulation, followed by (ii) 24 weeks of open label DBS for 24 weeks, followed by (iii) single-blind discontinuation for 1 week and open label stimulation for up to 2 years.	Implantation Bilateral Stimulation Monopolar Frequency 130 Hz Amplitude 4–8 mA Pulse Width 91 μs	HRSD-17, BDI-II, GAF.	Reduced depression and increased function. 11 patients responded ** and seven further remitted ▢▢ after 2 year DBS. Efficacy was similar for patients with MDD and those with BP. A modest sham stimulation effect was found, likely due to a decrease in depression after the surgical intervention, but prior to entering the sham phase.	Anxiety; Worsened depression; Nausea; Headache; Infection; Suicide attempts.

49

Table 1. Cont.

Authors	Main Inclusion Criteria	No. of Patients	Stimulation Target & DBS Design	Stimulation Parameters	Clinical Evaluation	Major Outcomes	Adverse Effects
Lozano et al. (2012) [66]	Both sexes aged 30–60 years; First MDE before 35 years; HRSD-17 score ≥ 20; GAF < 50.	21	Target SCG Study Design DBS for 12 months, open label.	Implantation Bilateral Stimulation N.A. Frequency 110–140 Hz Amplitude 3.5–7 mA Pulse Width 65–182 μs	HRSD-17, CGI-S.	Improved global functioning and less severe depression. 13 patients responded ***, based on HRSD-17 scores.	Gastrointestinal problems; Skin problem; Suicide; Spasms; Weight gain; Insomnia.
Puigdemont et al. (2012) [67]	18–70 years old with MDE; Resistant to pharmacological treatment and at most, a partial response to ECT; HAMD-17 Score ≥ 18.	8	Target SCG Study Design Intraoperative feedback was provided during surgery for electrode placement. DBS began at 48 h postoperative and ended when each patient had stabilized their response for at least three consecutive visits.	Implantation Bilateral Stimulation Monopolar Frequency 135 Hz Amplitude 3.5–5 V Pulse Width 90 μs	HAMD-17, MADRS, CGI.	Seven patients responded ** and three remitted □□ after 6 month DBS. Five patients responded ** and four remitted □□ after 12 month DBS. Three out of four remitted patients after 12 month DBS had remitted after 3 month DBS.	Suicide ideation; Neck pain; Recurrence; Depression; Cephalalgia.
Kennedy et al. (2011) [18]	Current MDE ≥ 12 months; HRSD-17 score ≥ 20; NR ≥ 4 antidepressant therapies.	20	Target SCG DBS patients were monitored for 3–6 years.	Implantation Bilateral Stimulation Monopolar Frequency 124.7 Hz (average) Amplitude 4.3 V (average) Pulse Width 70.6 μs	HAMD-17 36-item Short-Form Healthy Survey Questionnaire.	64.3% patients responded ** at the last follow-up visit. 35% patients remitted □□ at the last follow-up visit. Scores at the last visit tended towards maintenance of therapeutic scores at 3 years.	Depression; Suicidal thoughts; Suicide (All determined to be unrelated to DBS).
Guinjoan et al. (2010) [68]	Chronic TRD; Family history of affective disorders; Poor response to antidepressants, ECT, and psychotherapy.	1	Target BA25 Study Design Positioning was aided by intraoperative feedback. Bilateral DBS was conducted for 12 months. Followed by unilateral-left, then right DBS, for 6 months	Implantation Bilateral Stimulation Monopolar Frequency 130 Hz Amplitude 3.5–5 V Pulse Width 90 μs	HAMD-17, BDI.	Patient's condition plateaued after 6 month bilateral DBS. Left unilateral DBS led to rapid worsening in mood. Right unilateral DBS reversed the symptoms and the patient made significant improvements over bilateral stimulation. Patient remitted at 18 months.	Orthostatic hypotension.

Table 1. Cont.

Authors	Main Inclusion Criteria	No. of Patients	Stimulation Target & DBS Design	Stimulation Parameters	Clinical Evaluation	Major Outcomes	Adverse Effects
Holtzheimer and Mayberg (2010) [69]	Showed signs and symptoms of MDD; Had suicidal ideation in current MDE; Did not improve in symptoms with pharmacotherapy, psychotherapy, and ECT HAM-D score was 25	1	Target SCC Study Design Positioning of electrodes was aided by intraoperative feedback 24 weeks of open-label DBS and chronic stimulation beyond the assessment	Implantation Bilateral Stimulation Monopolar Frequency 130 Hz Amplitude 6 mA Pulse Width 91 μs	HAMD-17	HAMD-17 score lowered to 9 at the end of DBS follow-up. Sustained antidepressant response up to 2 years after surgery	N.A.
Hamani et al. (2009) [70]	Diagnosed MDD; current MDE ≥ 12 months; HAMD-17 score >20; GAF ≤ 50; NR ≥ 4 antidepressant therapies.	20	Target SCG Study Design DBS began at 2 weeks after surgery and lasted for 12 months	Implantation Bilateral Stimulation Monopolar Frequency 130 Hz Amplitude 3–5 V Pulse Width 90 μs	HAMD-17	11 responded ** at the end of 6 month DBS follow-up. Electrodes in responders were positioned ventrally relative to the landmarks of the medial prefrontal lobe.	N.A.
Puigdemont et al. (2009) [71]	Suffered from MDD, with several MDE accompanied by psychotic symptoms; Responded poorly to pharmacotherapy and ECT; Relapse following SCG-DBS with different features; Psychotic as opposed to depressive from previous episodes.	1	Target SCG Study Design DBS for 4 months, then switched off because of relapse and administered ECT for 3 weeks Resumed DBS until 12 months from the beginning of DBS.	Implantation Bilateral Stimulation Monopolar Frequency 135 Hz Amplitude 3.6 V Pulse Width 90 μs	HAMD-17	Sustained response without the need of ECT before relapse. Maintained remission in DBS after ECT until the end of follow-up.	N.A.

Table 1. *Cont.*

Authors	Main Inclusion Criteria	No. of Patients	Stimulation Target & DBS Design	Stimulation Parameters	Clinical Evaluation	Major Outcomes	Adverse Effects
Lozano et al. (2008) [72]	Current MDE ≥ 12 months; HRSD-17 score ≥ 20; NR ≥ 4 antidepressant therapies.	20	Target SCG Study Design Blinded-DBS in between and after surgery, monitored for up to 1 year.	Implantation Bilateral Stimulation Monopolar Frequency 130 Hz Amplitude 3.5–5 V Pulse Width 90 µs	HRSD-17, Beck Anxiety Inventory, BDI, CGI-S, PET scans, Neuropsychological tests.	Mean HRSD-17 score lower than baseline at all time points. 12 patients responded ** to DBS, 7 remitted □□ after 6 month DBS. 11 patients responded ** to DBS, 7 were nearly remitted or remitted □□ after 12 month DBS. Eight responses maintained from 6 month to 12 month DBS. PET Scans: decreases in orbital, medial prefrontal cortex, and insula. Increases in lateral prefrontal cortex, parietal, anterior, and posterior cingulate by 6 months; increases in metabolic activity in regions adjacent to SCG.	Seven patients without adverse effects. Wound Infection; Headache; Pain; Seizure; Worsened mood; Irritability.
McNeely et al. (2008) [73]	Current MDE ≥ 12 months, HRSD-17 score ≥ 20, Non-responsive (NR) ≥ 4 antidepressant therapies,	6	Target BA25 Continuous DBS for 12 months.	Implantation Bilateral Stimulation Monopolar Frequency 130 Hz Amplitude 3–4.5 V Pulse Width 60 µs	HRSD-17 Object alternation Test Iowa gambling task Visual delayed recall memory Verbal delayed memory Verbal list learning Stroop color-word	6 months: four responded at the end of DBS.** General Neuropsychological Performance: Manual Motor Skills: Improved for dominant and non-dominant hand by 12 months. Verbal learning: Restored impairments in two patients at the end of 12 months. No significant correlations between change in mood and neuropsychological function at 6 and 12 months.	N.A.
Neimat et al. (2008) [74]	Family history of severe MDD. Failed to respond to antidepressants, adjuncts, and ECT. Relapsed after ablative cingulotomy	1	Target BA25 Study Design Started DBS on the day after electrode implantation and lasted for 30 months	Implantation Bilateral Stimulation Monopolar Frequency 130 Hz Amplitude 4.5 V Pulse Width 60 µs	HAMD-17	HAMD-17 score decreased from 19 before surgery to 8 at 6 months after DBS. Sustained remission until the end of DBS study (scored 7)	N.A.

Table 1. *Cont.*

Authors	Main Inclusion Criteria	No. of Patients	Stimulation Target & DBS Design	Stimulation Parameters	Clinical Evaluation	Major Outcomes	Adverse Effects
Mayberg, et al. (2005) [19]	Current MDE ≥ 12 months, HRSD-17 score ≥ 20, Non-responsive (NR) ≥ 4 antidepressant therapies.	6	Target BA25 Study Design 1–5 min on-off stimulation in acute DBS for 5 days postoperative. Chronic DBS for 6 months after pulse generator was implanted and optimized for 4 wks	Implantation Bilateral Stimulation Monopolar Acute: Frequency 10–130 Hz Amplitude 0.0–9.0V Pulse Width 30–250 μs Chronic: Frequency 130 Hz Amplitude 4 V Pulse Width 60 μs	HDRS-17, MADRS, CGI, Positive and Negative Affective Scale.	Acute effects: Sudden feeling of calmness Chronic effects: five patients responded ** after 2 month DBS. Response maintained in four patients at the end of 6 month DBS. Three patients achieved remission □□ or near remission at the end of 6 month DBS.	Mild Lightheadedness; Psychomotor slowing; Skin infection; Skin erosion.

* ≥40% reduction in MADRS and average GAF in months 4–6 not worse than baseline; ** ≥50% reduction in HRSD-17 (HAMD-17) score from baseline; *** ≥40% reduction in HRSD-17 score from baseline; ◊ ≥40% reduction in MADRS compared to mean baseline; □ HAMD-24 scores or MADRS scores ≤ 10 after DBS; □□ HRSD score < 8. □□□ HRSD score ≤ 8; Abbreviations: ATHF = Anti-depressant Treatment History Form, BA25 = Brodmann Area 25, BDI/-II = Beck Depression Inventory/-II, CGI, PGI, CANTAB = Clinician and Patient Global Impression of Severity and Improvement (CGI; PGI) and cognitive function (CANTAB); CVLT = California verbal learning test, DBS = deep brain stimulation, DWI = Diffusion-weighted imaging, ECG = electrocardiogram, ECT = electroconvulsive therapy, EDA = electrodermal activity, EEG = electroencephalography, GAF = Global assessment function, HAM-A = Hamilton Anxiety Rating Scale, HRSD-17/HDRS-17 = Hamilton Rating Scale for Depression/ Hamilton Depression Rating Scale, (f)MRI = (functional) magnetic resonance imaging, MADRS/MARDS = Montgomery-Åsberg Depression Rating Scale, MAOI = monoamine oxidase inhibitors, MDD = major depressive disorder, MDE = major depressive episodes, MMSE = Mini-Mental State Examination, NSAID = non-steroidal anti-inflammatory drug, NR = non-responsive, PET = positron emission tomography, QIDS/-SR = Quick Inventory of Depressive Symptomatology/-self report, Q-LES-Q = Quality of Life and Satisfaction Questionnaire, SCC = subcallosal cingulate, SCG = subcallosal cingulate gyrus, SCR = skin conductance response, QOL = Quality of Life Enjoyment and Satisfaction Questionnaire, TRD = treatment-resistant depression, WSAS = Work and Social Adjustment Scale.

Table 2. Summary of response and remission rates from clinical studies.

Authors	≤ 6 months		6–12 months		12–24 months		≥ 24 months	
	Response (%)	Remission (%)	Response (%)	Remission (%)	Response (%)	Remission (%)	Response (%)	Remission (%)
Sankar et al. 2020 [40]	NA	NA	NA	NA	NA	NA	NA	NA
Riva Posse et al. (2019) [41]	NA	NA	NA	NA	NA	NA	NA	NA
Eitan et al. (2018) [42]	NA	NA	NA	NA	44.4	NA	NA	NA
Merkl et al. (2018) [43]	37.5	12.5	43	14.2	33	33	33	NA
Howell et al. (2018) [44]	-	-	33.3	66.7	-	-	-	-
Waters et al. (2018) [45]	NA	NA	NA	NA	NA	NA	NA	NA
Smart et al. (2018) [46]	-	-	78.5	-	-	-	-	-
Choi et al. (2018) [47]	NA	NA	NA	NA	NA	NA	NA	NA
Conen et al. (2018) [48]	-	-	28.6	42.9	-	-	-	-
Holtzheimer et al. (2017) [15]	22 20 (sham)	10 7 (sham)	28 30 (sham)	12 7 (sham)	54 52 (sham)	17 20 (sham)	48 44 (sham)	25 12 (sham)
McInerney et al. (2017) [14]	-	-	55	-	-	-	-	-
Riva-Posse et al. (2018) [49]	72.7	54.5	81.8	54.5	-	-	-	-
Tsolaki et al. 2017 [50]	50	-	-	-	-	-	-	-
Accolla et al. (2016) [51]	-	-	-	-	79	20	-	-
Richieri et al. (2016) [52]	100 (Case Study)	-	-	-	-	-	-	-
Hilimire et al. (2015) [53]	NA	NA	NA	NA	NA	NA	NA	NA
Martin-Blanco et al. (2015) [54]	NA	NA	NA	NA	NA	NA	NA	NA
Puigdemont et al. (2015) [55]	-	80	-	-	-	-	-	-
Serra-Blasco et al. (2015) [56]	-	-	-	-	75 (F.E.) 87 (TRD)	-	-	-
Choi et al. 2015 [57]	NA	NA	NA	NA	NA	NA	NA	NA
Sun et al. 2015 [58]	NA	NA	NA	NA	NA	NA	NA	NA
Perez-Caballero et al. (2014) [59]	50	-	-	-	-	-	-	-
Merkl et al. (2013) [60]	-	-	-	30	-	-	-	-
Ramasubbu et al. (2013) [61]	50	-	-	-	-	-	-	-
Torres et al. (2013) [62]	100 (2 Case Studies)	-	100 (2 Case Studies)	-	100 (2 Case Studies)	-	100 (2 Case Studies)	-
Broadway et al. (2012) [63]	50	-	-	-	-	-	-	-
Hamani et al. (2012) [64]	-	100 (Case Study)	100 (Case Study)	-	-	-	-	-
Holtzheimer et al. (2012) [65]	18	41	36	36	58	92	-	-
Lozano et al. (2012) [66]	57	-	48	-	62	-	-	-
Puigdemont et al. (2012) [67]	37.5	37.5	87.5	37.5	62.5	50	-	-
Kennedy et al. (2011) [18]	-	-	62.5	-	46.2	-	75	-
Guinjoan et al. (2010) [68]	100 (Case Study)	-	100 (Case Study)	-	100 (Case Study)	-	-	100 (Case Study)
Holtzheimer and Mayberg (2010) [69]	100 (Case Study)	-	100 (Case Study)	-	100 (Case Study)	-	100 (Case Study)	-
Hamani et al. (2009) [70]	-	-	55	-	-	-	-	-
Puigdemont et al. (2009) [71]	100 (Case Study)	-	100 (Case Study)	-	-	-	-	-
Lozano et al. (2008) [72]	35	10	60	35	-	-	-	-
McNeely et al. (2008) [73]	66	NA	-	-	-	-	-	-
Neimat et al. (2008) [74]	100 (Case Study)	NA	-	-	-	-	100 (Case Study)	-
Mayberg et al. (2005) [19]	66	50	-	-	-	-	-	-
Average	63.8%	43.9%	66.5%	36.5%	69.3%	42.4%	76%	62.5%
Range	18–100	10–100	28.6–100	12–66.7	33–100	17–92	33–100	12–100

The first evidence-based clinical study on SCC-DBS was published by Mayberg et al. in 2005 [19]. Among six patients with an average of 5.6 years of major depressive episode (MDE), four responded to the treatment, but three remitted or nearly remitted during the stimulation, even without changing medications. The authors found that the metabolic activity in the SCC normalized from a hyperactive state and was accompanied by reduced local blood flow as detected by Positron Emission Tomography (PET) [19]. In a study from 2003 to 2006 by Lozano et al. on chronic DBS in 20 patients with an average of 6.9 years of current MDE, 11 patients responded, but seven remitted [72], which was similar to the response and remission rates of Mayberg et al. In a 3.5-year follow-up study, the response rate was consistent across time points, but the remission rate increased from 18.8% to 42.9% at the last visit [18]. Both studies reported changes in structures distal to SCC after DBS, which explains the persistent response throughout the DBS treatments [18,72].

In a case report by Neimat et al., a 55-year-old female TRD patient who relapsed after a subgenual cingulotomy, achieved sustained remission for up to 30 months with SCC-DBS treatment [74]. In a case reported by Guinjoan et al. in 2010, a 60-year-old male TRD patient responded to unilateral SCC-DBS in the right hemisphere, but unilateral stimulation in the left hemisphere worsened his mood. This is in line with the asymmetrical response to antidepressants in the SCC region. However, the authors noted a further study was needed with more patients to validate the effects of unilateral stimulation on mood enhancement [68].

Similarly, in a preliminary study in 2012 by Puigdemont et al. on eight patients with an average of 6.3 years of current MDE, they found that five patients responded at the end of the 12-month DBS, but three out of four final remitters remitted after 3 months of DBS [67]. Their cognitive functions were not exacerbated and their memory functions were actually improved in cognitive assessments in 2015 [56]. Concurrently, a clinical study conducted in three different medical centers also reported similar efficacies of SCC-DBS, suggesting that DBS has reliable stimulation effects. Among 21 patients with an average of 5 years of current MDE, 13 responded to the treatment and the rest performed better than at baseline by the end of the study, although one patient committing suicide by medication overdose [66].

4.2. Remission Rates

Some previous studies reported higher initial response and/or remission rates compared to more recent studies [19,67,72]. In the study by Perez-Caballero et al., they suggested that electrode insertion-induced inflammation could affect response and remission rates. Four of the eight recruited patients took non-steroidal anti-inflammatory drugs (NSAIDs), which resulted in a diminished antidepressant response toward DBS, whereas the other four not taking NSAIDs gradually responded and remitted. The authors also analyzed the role of inflammation in the early DBS response in rats [59], which is discussed in a later section of this review. A later study in 2015 by Puigdemont et al. reported that remission was maintained in four out of five remitted patients in the 3-month active stimulation group, whereas only two patients remitted in the sham stimulation group. They concluded that continuous active stimulation was important in maintaining the therapeutic effect [55]. This was supported by an earlier case of a 27-year-old patient on DBS for 2 years whose symptoms worsened due to battery depletion, but improved again upon battery replacement [69].

Table 2 reflects the different response and remission rates, at 6-month intervals, across the duration of the studies in Table 1. This reporting allows for a cursory longitudinal tracking in understanding how response and remission may change with time. Among the reviewed studies on DBS, the response rate ranged from 18% to 87.5% and remission rate ranged from 10% to 92% (excluding all case studies) across the different time points (see Table 2), which were comparable to earlier clinical studies [19,72]. However, large-scale controlled trials are needed to further validate the efficacy of DBS in patients with TRD. Some predictive markers discovered in these studies could facilitate the selection of more responsive patients and increase the safety of DBS. A noteworthy study by Holtzheimer and Mayberg demonstrated some changes in the response and remission rates with DBS [69]. The authors noted that several months after a response and/or remission in their depressive symptoms, worsening of symptoms was temporarily observed at 16 weeks. They attributed the temporary worsening of symptoms to the difficulty of some patients reintegrating into society. In an earlier study by Lozano et al. in 2008, they also observed a similar occurrence at 4 months. These findings highlight the complexity of treating neuropsychiatric diseases, as the recovery periods are not always consistent and can be affected by different factors.

4.3. Significant Challenges in the Development of SCC-DBS

A larger study that aimed to recruit 201 patients was conducted by Holtzheimer et al. in 2017 to further validate the therapeutic effects of DBS [15]. A futility analysis conducted after 90 patients had been recruited showed no significant differences between the DBS and sham groups, leading to the early termination of the study. During a 6-month double-blind trial, no significant differences were found in the response of the DBS group compared to the sham group. However, among 77 patients that received subsequent open-label DBS for up to 2 years, 38 responded and 20 remitted. Holtzheimer et al. offered several explanations for the observed result. First, the patients selected for the study had an average current episode duration of around 12 years, whereas most studies recruited patients with an average current depressive episode of about 3–5 years. Holtzheimer also posited the possibility of suboptimal contact during the first 12 months, further affecting the results. This landmark paper was initially thought to be the death knell for DBS as a treatment for TRD. However, a summit of key academics within the field determined that DBS protocols required further modification and patient recruitment needed refining to better assess the therapeutic effects of DBS for TRD [75]. Considering that multiple other studies showed the efficacy and effectiveness of DBS for TRD, the conference considered several possibilities for the discrepancies in the findings, some conclusions were that DBS was initiated too early before optimal targeting was secured, a lack of specificity and standardization in the improvement of symptoms, high placebo effects typically seen in the treatment of psychiatric disorders, and study design. The heterogeneity of the symptoms of the disease was also emphasized, which suggested that different circuitry might be involved in different individuals. The key conclusions from the summit included that patient selection should be better and more refined, study designs should be either fast to fail or fast to succeed, registries should be established for better subject tracking, and longitudinal data should be collected. The paper stressed that the complexities of the disease were real and better experimental designs were needed to truly reflect the effects of DBS as a treatment for TRD for a better response and remission rate and to allow the elucidation of the mechanistic role of DBS.

4.4. Adverse Effects

The safety of SCC-DBS was subsequently assessed following the initial results of the efficacy of DBS in treating TRD. In 2008, McNeely et al. conducted a trial on six patients with an average of 5.6 years of current MDE. They found that mood was significantly improved during the 1-year DBS treatment without serious cognitive deterioration [73]. Moreines et al. found that DBS treatment in both unipolar and bipolar TRD patients with at least 2 years of current MDE improved executive functions and stabilized their memory [76]. Similarly, SCC-DBS for 6 months followed by depression treatment in patients with MDD, who had increased negative emotional processing and/or reduced positive emotions, resulted in reduced negative emotional bias [53]. Martín-Blanco et al. reported that a 52-year-old female had a seizure after 5 weeks of DBS. As severe MDD may predispose patients to seizures, the authors recommended that patients should be evaluated for seizures before administering DBS and parameters might need to be adjusted to within safe ranges [52]. In a study in 2017 by McInerney et al. on 20 unipolar TRD patients with an average of 6.9 years of MDE, they reported that 11 patients responded at the end of the 12-month DBS without further deterioration of cognitive functions. They also found a correlation between verbal fluency and mood improvement, which could be predictive of the DBS response [14]. The side effects reported in this review range from mild symptoms, such as headaches, dizziness and gastrointestinal irritation [43,66], to more severe effects including suicidal ideation and device malfunction [15,67]. This reporting should not discourage the development of therapies. Indeed, many treatments including serotonin-selective reuptake inhibitors have severe side effects, including increased fractures and suicidal ideations [77,78]. In the study of therapies, it is important to report these side effects and to note that these therapies are administered by a professional, whose role is to detect and modulate the therapies accordingly.

4.5. Stimulation Parameters

Several studies have attempted to optimize the parameters of DBS for treating mood disorders. As previously mentioned, Eitan et al. reported that high-frequency stimulation (HFS) was more effective at lowering MADRS scores compared with low frequency stimulation [42]. Indeed, the most commonly used stimulation frequency was in the high frequency range of 130–135 Hz, although some studies have tested frequencies between 5 and 185 Hz [19,61] (see Table 1). The pulse width used in DBS also varied greatly across studies. In a study by Ramasubbu et al., they found that a long pulse width of 180–270 μs was effective [61]. However, this study also reported that DBS with a long pulse width caused patients to experience stimulation-induced insomnia, anxiety, confusion, and drowsiness. Previous studies by Lozano et al. and Holtzheimer et al. demonstrated that shorter pulse widths of 30–60 μs led to clinical improvements in depression symptoms without these side effects [66,72]. Indeed, Ramasubbu et al. suggested that longer pulse widths with lower amplitudes and shorter pulse widths with higher amplitudes could produce comparable therapeutic benefits. The amplitude of the stimulating current used in DBS to elicit a therapeutic response also tended to vary across studies. The amplitude is the first parameter to be adjusted when patients do not respond to the treatment. Among 38 clinical studies, the overall current range was 2–8 mA and voltage range was 2.5–10.5 V. The variability in the amplitude underscores the personalized nature of DBS, which requires specific adjustments to achieve individual therapeutic effects.

4.6. Electrode Implantation

Several clinical DBS studies have also tried to improve the accuracy of electrode implantation in order to precisely target regions of interest. The pioneering work by Mayberg et al. used PET scans of pathological glucose metabolism to guide the electrode implantation. Riva-Posse et al. used individualized tractography maps based on a group connectome blueprint of past responders to DBS to identify optimal target regions for electrode implantation [49]. Riva-Posse et al. used a four-bundle white matter blueprint, which resulted in good clinical outcomes in eight out of 11 patients, which suggests that the use of this method could improve the precision of implantation. Similarly, Tsolaki et al. investigated the use of FMRIB Software Library (FSL) probabilistic tractography in SCC-DBS [50]. Several studies have used other methods to try to specify the optimal stimulation points. Choi et al. investigated the best contact positions that elicited the best response during intraoperative testing [57]. They used diffusion-directed magnetic resonance imaging and patient-specific tractography maps to guide the implantation. They also used fiber tract probabilistic tractography to determine the putative fiber tract activation in patients, which was used to guide the electrode implantation for the best response, rather than the salient response. Contacts in the left hemisphere were found to produce the best consistent intraoperative response to DBS in seven out of nine patients at 6 months. Smart et al. validated this result in their study using local field potentials following unilateral HFS-DBS [46]. They found that left-sided stimulation evoked broadband effects, compared with right sided stimulation, which evoked only beta and gamma bands. Additionally, a decrease in theta bands was consistently accompanied by behavioral improvements. They concluded that the precision of electrodes in the left-hemisphere was more important and instructive than in the right hemisphere. In contrast, Guinjoan et al. and Howell et al. found that right hemisphere targets were critical for behavioral improvements [44,68]. Guinjoan et al. showed that right unilateral DBS could reverse and remit a patient's worsening mood induced by left unilateral DBS. Howell et al. showed that right cingulate bundle activation beyond a threshold could protract the recovery. Further research is needed to elucidate the differences in these studies.

4.7. Other Responses to DBS

With regard to other potential responses to DBS, recent studies have attempted to characterize non-behavioral evoked responses. Conen et al. identified higher rCBF in patients at baseline and during DBS therapy compared to non-remitters and non-responders [48]. Riva-Posse et al. observed autonomic changes in responders undergoing DBS [41]. In a study by Smart et al., assessing the efficacy of DBS, they found consistent changes in left theta local field potentials, which could provide another consistent parameter to monitor. Based on this finding, they proceeded to adjust the contacts for one non-responder, who was able to achieve a response by the end of the study. In a study by Sankar et al. on responders and non-responders who had previously undergone SCG-DBS, they found that both groups had significant volume differences in the left and average SCG; in the right and average amygdala; and in the left, right, and average thalamus (Sankar et al. 2020). Additionally, non-responders had significantly greater grey matter volume compared to responders and a greater grey to white matter ratio. This important information provides yet more criteria for assessing if a patient might respond to DBS. Expanding the breadth of data obtained during clinical trials has the potential to advise clinicians on the efficacy of DBS, and to help predict non-responders and adjust the stimulation parameters. This will improve patient welfare and allows for a more accurate examination of the mechanisms of DBS in improving depressive-like symptoms.

Furthermore, it would be prudent to use preclinical results to advise clinical cases. In a previous preclinical study, Hamani et al. reported that DBS supplemented with tranylcypromine increased the antidepressant-like response in animals by 20%–30% compared to either treatment alone. They later reported on a patient who relapsed after 4 years of remission following DBS treatment [64]. Based on their previous work, they administered tranylcypromine before the DBS treatment, which allowed the patient to enter remission again.

5. Preclinical Studies of Electrical Stimulation in the Medial Prefrontal Cortex in Rodents

Following the success of a number of preliminary clinical studies, several preclinical studies were conducted to investigate the antidepressant-like effects of DBS [79]. The mPFC in rats is widely regarded to be homologous to the SCC in humans. The mPFC together with the amygdala, hippocampus, and hypothalamus controls the stress response, autonomic functions, and cognition in rats [80–83]. Using PET imaging, glucose metabolism was observed to normalize in the mPFC from a hyperactive state following DBS, which was similarly observed in the SCC after 1 h of DBS [84]. However, the homology between subdivisions of mPFC and SCC is still under debate. The vmPFC can be further subdivided into the infralimbic (IL) and prelimbic (PrL) regions. Although there are overlaps, the IL and PrL innervate different regions to different extents, including the lateral hypothalamus, dorsal raphe nucleus, and amygdala, among efferent regions [85–87]. The PrL has been shown to innervate to important limbic regions associated with SCC projections [87]. Meanwhile, the infralimbic cortex (IL) is believed to be structurally homologous based on comparisons involving tractography analysis [88–90]. Some assert that the whole ventromedial prefrontal cortex (vmPFC) is homologous to the SCC [91,92]. Others assert that the vmPFC is functionally distinct from the dorsal medial prefrontal cortex [70,91]. Nevertheless, the vmPFC is generally regarded as homologous to BA25, although a thorough understanding of specific correlations remains to be seen. Table 3 lists 29 preclinical studies on the effects of vmPFC-DBS on animal behaviors.

5.1. vmPFC Stimulation

Hamani et al. published the first preclinical study of vmPFC-DBS in rats in 2010. They used the forced swim test (FST), which models "helplessness" in animals including anxiolytic-like and anti-anhedonic-like behavior. They found DBS reduced the immobility score in FST, indicating antidepressant-like effects. The authors attributed the behavioral changes to serotonergic function in the dorsal raphe nucleus (DRN) as lesions in this structure abolished the behavioral effects in FST [91]. Another animal study in 2012 found the optimal stimulation frequency and amplitude of vmPFC-DBS was 130 Hz and 200 µA that produced anti-anhedonic-like effects and produced a charge density similar to DBS in humans [93]. They found a lesion in the DRN abolished the higher sucrose consumption due to DBS, even with a normal hippocampal brain-derived neurotrophic factor (BDNF) profile. They postulated that an interaction between BDNF and neurochemical substances potentiated the antidepressant-like response [92]. The anti-anhedonic-like effects of DBS were also supported in studies by Rea et al. and Edemann-Callesen et al. They conducted an intracranial, self-stimulation paradigm in Flinders sensitive line and Flinders resistant line rats to assess reward-seeking behaviors, which demonstrated that the anti-anhedonic-like effect of vmPFC-DBS was independent of the dopaminergic reward system [94,95]. Bruchim-Samuel et al. reported that modulation of the ventral tegmental area could prolong the behavioral changes. They found that intermittent acute patterned stimulation administered to the ventral tegmental area of Flinders sensitive line rats resulted in antidepressant-like and anti-anhedonic-like behaviors [96]. Strikingly, a study by Bregman et al. in 2018 found that the antidepressant-like effect of DBS was serotonin transporter-independent. This could be of benefit to some patients with a mutated serotonin transporter-promoter gene (5-HTTLPR), which underlies the poor response to conventional selective serotonin re-uptake inhibitors that target serotonin transporters [97].

Beside changes in neurochemical and neurotrophin profiles, neuroplasticity changes induced by DBS have also been investigated. For instance, Bambico et al. reported increased hippocampal neurogenesis and BDNF levels after vmPFC-DBS, which led to anti-anhedonic-like behaviors, but was not sufficient for an overall antidepressant-like effect [98]. Correspondingly, Liu et al. found a correlation between vmPFC-HFS and hippocampal neurogenesis and improvements in short- and long-term memory in middle-aged rats. This suggests that DBS has therapeutic potential in age-dependent memory deficits [99].

5.2. Other Brain Targets

As preclinical studies have progressed, several brain targets of DBS have been established. Hamani et al. in 2014 demonstrated that DBS in the nucleus accumbens induced a similar antidepressant-like effect to DBS in the vmPFC, even though the stimulations modulated different circuits. This may contribute to more customized stimulation targeting based on the patient's symptoms [100]. Bregman et al. reported that the HFS of the medial forebrain bundle induced antidepressant-like behaviors in the FST [101]. Interestingly, this antidepressant effect was not mediated by increases in either serotonin or dopamine release in the nucleus accumbens. Lim et al. in 2015 emphasized that only HFS of the vmPFC led to anti-anhedonic-like effects and these pronounced antidepressant-like effects were induced by modulating the activity of serotonergic neurons in the DRN [102]. However, the authors did not investigate the effects of different stimulation parameters on depressive-like behaviors in various DBS targets. The study by Etiévant et al. supported the modulation of DRN by DBS and added that glial integrity was a prerequisite to the antidepressant-like outcome [103]. In another study, mice subjected to chronic social defeat stress were administered 7 days of 5-h vmPFC-DBS, which resulted in increased social interactive behavior accompanied by DRN modulation [104]. Interestingly, a recent study demonstrated that the potentiation of the anxiolytic response to vmPFC stimulation was associated with exposure to an enriched environment. This indicates that an enriched living environment can facilitate the beneficial effects of DBS intervention [105]. Creed et al. conducted DBS on the entopeduncular and the subthalamic nuclei to compare antidepressant-like effects [106]. Chronic Subthalamic nucleus DBS was reported to impair performance in the learned helplessness task, with no significant effects in anxiety tests. These results were associated with decreased hippocampal BDNF and TrkB mRNA. Interestingly, entopeduncular nucleus DBS did not increase depressive-like behavior in the learned helplessness task, indicating a superior target over the subthalamic nucleus for the treatment of depressive-like behaviors. Meng et al. reported reductions in depressive-like behaviors in animals stimulated in the lateral habenula; this observation was associated with elevations in dopamine, norepinephrine, and serotonin in both blood serum and in the hippocampus [107].

5.3. vmPFC-Linked Modulation of Other Structures

Other structures have been found to be modulated by vmPFC-DBS. For example, Lim et al. reported that activation of the medial subthalamic nucleus contributed to antidepressant-like behavior [108]. In a rat model of post-traumatic stress disorder, IL-DBS reduced firing in the basolateral amygdala, which attenuated fear and produced a slight anxiolytic-like effect [109]. A recent study showed that DBS resulted in elevated spontaneous firing of noradrenergic locus coeruleus neurons and strengthened the coherence between the prefrontal cortex and locus coeruleus. The latter was protective against stress and was responsible for the antidepressant-like effect seen in FST [110]. On the other hand, Insel et al. reported that there was reduced communication between IL and ventral hippocampus in rats after 10 days of 8-h IL-DBS and such coherence was higher in depressed subjects [111]. Jiménez-Sánchez et al. in 2016 reported two studies on acute IL-DBS in naive and olfactory bulbectomized rat models. In naive animals, IL-DBS induced antidepressant-like behaviors and increased prefrontal glutamate efflux, which activated the α-amino-3-hydroxy-5-methyl-4-isoxazolepropionic acid receptor (AMPAR) to modulate DRN output [81]. In olfactory bulbectomized rats, similar changes were noted in the prefrontal serotonergic and glutamatergic output with the activation of AMPAR and antidepressant-like behaviors [33].

5.4. Synergism with Other Treatments

Antidepressant-like effects in different DBS paradigms are leading to some advancements in the field. One such investigation by Laver et al. in 2014 examined the use of augmentation agents such as buspirone, risperidone, and pindolol to enhance DBS efficacy. However, these agents did not increase the antidepressant response of the rats receiving DBS treatment, when compared to those co-administered monoamine oxidase inhibitors in previous studies [64,112]. It is possible that a response may become evident in clinical trials. Perez-Caballero et al. in 2014 reported an interesting early response to stimulation, in which sham-treated rats had reduced immobility and increased swimming in FST at weeks 1 and 2, but not at week 6 post treatment. They reasoned that this was caused by insertion-induced inflammation as pretreatment by indomethacin reduced the expression of pro-inflammatory mediators (TNF-α, COX1, COX2) and reversed the antidepressant-like behaviors in sham-treated animals [59]. Rummel et al. in 2016 reported that chronic continuous HFS did not have more benefits than chronic intermittent stimulation in treatment-resistant rats with congenitally learned helplessness [113].

5.5. Other Biological Parameters Modulated

Similar to the research direction of clinical studies, preclinical studies have also attempted to characterize other biological parameters of DBS, including more precise electrode implantation. Lehto et al. characterized real-time fMRI responses in the brain following DBS, and found strong connectivity between the vmPFC and amygdala, which validated vmPFC as a target region [114]. Perez-Cabalerro et al. used PET scans to study the immediate effects of electrode implantation. They found that metabolism was decreased locally (vmPFC), but was increased in ventral regions, including dorsal and ventral hippocampus, piriform and insular cortex, nucleus accumbens, ventral tegmental area, ventral pallidum, hypothalamus, and the preoptic area [115]. This was in agreement with other studies on the effect of DBS on depressive-like behavior, but it is noteworthy to see these effects simply via electrode insertion.

Table 3. A list of preclinical studies on deep brain stimulation of the medial prefrontal cortex in rodents.

Authors	Target	Animal	Animal Models & DBS Design	Stimulation Parameters	Behavioral Tests	Outcomes
Jia et al. (2019) [116]	vmPFC	Sprague-Dawley rats, male.	CUS animal model. Open field test and forced swim test before DBS.	Unipolar High Frequency Frequency: 130 Hz Amplitude: 100 μA Pulse Width: 90 μs Low Frequency Frequency: 20 Hz Amplitude: 400 μA Pulse Width: 0.2 μs	Sucrose preference test	CUS rats had a lowered sucrose preference compared to control rats.
					Open field test	No significant difference in locomotion was recorded between CUS and control groups.
					Forced swim test	Both High- and Low-Frequency Stimulation reduced immobility compared to sham rats.
Papp et al. (2019) [117]	vmPFC	Wistar-Kyoto rats, male (DBS) Wistar rats, male [Venlafaxine(VFX)-treated]	CMS animal model. Two, 2-h DBS sessions were conducted, one on the preceding evening and the other on the following morning before each sucrose intake test and the NORT T1 session.	Frequency: 130 Hz Amplitude: 250 μA Pulse width: 90 μs	Sucrose intake test	During the first 2 wks of CMS, sucrose intake decreased >50% across groups. VFX treatment restored sucrose intake levels.
					Novel object recognition test	Wistar Kyoto rats: DBS rescued novel object recognition test across all groups. Wistar rats: VFX rescued novel object recognition test in CMS animals administered with D2 antagonist, but not in D2-administered CMS animals. VFX also did not rescue groups administered with D3 antagonist.
Bhaskar et al. (2018) [105]	vmPFC	Wistar rats, male.	Naïve animal model. DBS for 15 min prior to and throughout behavioral testing.	Bipolar Frequency: 100 Hz Amplitude: 200 μA Pulse Width: 100 μs	Home-cage emergence test	Enriched environment potentiated the efficacy of HFS on reduced escape latency time in the Naïve animal model.

Table 3. *Cont.*

Authors	Target	Animal	Animal Models & DBS Design	Stimulation Parameters	Behavioral Tests	Outcomes
Bregman et al. (2018) [97]	vmPFC	SERT homozygous knockout and wildtype mice, male.	Serotonin transporter (SERT) knockout model. DBS for 4 h before forced swim test and open field test.	Bilateral Monopolar Frequency: 130 Hz Amplitude: 100 μA Pulse Width: 90 μs	Elevated plus maze	HFS with an enriched environment reduced the anxiety index and increased head dips.
					Novel object recognition test	No significant difference.
					Forced swim test	Both wild-type and knockout-DBS mice had reduced immobility time compared to sham.
					Open field test	Knockout-DBS mice had lower locomotion counts than sham and wild-type mice.
Lehto et al. (2018) [114]	IL	Sprague-Dawley rats, male.	Naïve animal model. All stimulation paradigms consisted of three blocks of 60 s of rest and 18 s of stimulation, ending with an additional rest period, giving a total paradigm of 4 min 54 s.	Monopolar Frequency: 20/35/70/100/130/160/200 Hz tested in randomized order. Amplitude: 1.4–1.7 mA distributed equally among the three electrode channels Pulse Width: 180-μs	N.A.	fMRI conducted to characterize changes in the brain following DBS. IL-DBS at varying stimulation parameters significantly triggered the amygdala. Orientation selective stimulation was able to recruit neuronal pathways of distinct orientations relative to the position of the electrode.
Papp et al. (2018) [118]	vmPFC	Wistar rats, male.	CMS animal model. Two, 2-h DBS sessions were conducted, one on the previous evening and one the next morning 15 min before each behavioral test.	Bipolar Frequency: 130 Hz, Amplitude: 250 μA, Pulse Width: 90 μs	Sucrose intake test	DBS increased sucrose intake across all treatment groups, except for imipramine-treated animals.
					Elevated plus maze	DBS increased the anxiolytic open arm entries in all treatment groups.

Table 3. *Cont.*

Authors	Target	Animal	Animal Models & DBS Design	Stimulation Parameters	Behavioral Tests	Outcomes
					Novel object recognition test	DBS rescued the abolished novel object recognition in CMS sham-treated animals, across all treatment groups.
					Paw-pressure test	Ibuprofen, tramadol, and morphine significantly increased the paw withdrawal threshold in naive animals relative to respective vehicle alone, demonstrating a clear analgesic effect.
					Open field test	No analgesics altered the motor activity of rats.
Perez-Caballero et al. (2018) [115]	IL	Wistar rats, male.	Six independent sets of animals using naive (unoperated controls) and DBS-off animals.	N.A.	Modified forced swim test	Electrode implantation induced a significant reduction in the immobility scores of vehicle-treated animals. Ibuprofen abolished the antidepressant-like effect of electrode implantation in the modified forced swim test, increasing the DBS-off animal's immobility. Neither morphine nor tramadol counteracted the antidepressant-like effect of DBS-off animals.

Table 3. Cont.

Authors	Target	Animal	Animal Models & DBS Design	Stimulation Parameters	Behavioral Tests	Outcomes
Torres-Sanchez et al. (2018) [110]	vmPFC	Wistar rats, male.	Naive animal model. DBS for (i) 4 h at 24 h after surgery, then (ii) 2 h at 48 h after surgery	Bipolar Monophasic Frequency: 130 Hz Amplitude: 100 µA Pulse Width: 90 µs	Novelty suppressed feeding test	Electrode implantation reduced latency to feed compared to naive animals. Ibuprofen increased latency to feed relative to VEH-treated animals. Neither morphine nor tramadol reduced the latency to feed in electrode-implanted animals.
					Forced swim test	Reduced immobility time and increased climbing compared to control.
Volle et al. (2018) [119]	vmPFC	Sprague-Dawley rats, male.	Stimulation was delivered 1 week after surgery for either (i) a single day (acute stimulation; 8 h/day) or (ii) 12 days (chronic stimulation daily for 8 h/day) using a portable stimulator (ANS model 3510) to different groups of rats	Frequency: 130 Hz Amplitude: 200 µA Pulse Width: 90 µs	N.A.	Both treatments increase serotonin (5-HT) release, although fluoxetine resulted in a higher sustained concentration, even upon chronic treatment. Chronic DBS resulted in lowered 5HT release by Day 12. DBS reduced raphe SERT expression. DBS induced changes in 5-HT1B receptor expression, whereas fluoxetine induced changes in 5-HT1A receptors expression in the prefrontal cortex. Research highlighted different effects of both treatments on the serotonergic system.

Table 3. *Cont.*

Authors	Target	Animal	Animal Models & DBS Design	Stimulation Parameters	Behavioral Tests	Outcomes
Reznikov et al. (2017) [108]	IL	Sprague-Dawley rats, male.	Posttraumatic stress disorder animal model. 3-day fear conditioning. DBS from 1 week after extinction recall to the end of experiment, 8 h/day, or 2 h before and 4 h after behavioral tests.	Frequency: 130 Hz Amplitude: 100 μA Pulse Width: 90 μs	Extinction recall test	Higher freezing scores in DBS-weak extinction than DBS-strong extinction.
					Open field test	No significant difference between groups.
					Novelty suppressed feeding test	Reduced latency to feeding in DBS-weak extinction, but not strong extinction.
					Elevated plus maze	No significant difference observed between groups.
Bruchim-Samuel et al. (2016) [96]	vmPFC VTA	Flinders Sensitive Line rats, male. Sprague-Dawley rats, male. (Control)	Flinders Sensitive Line model. DBS for 15 min/day, for 10 days.	Bilateral, Monopolar vmPFC Stimulation Frequency: 20 Hz Amplitude: 400 μA Pulse Width: 200 μs VTA Stimulation (control) Frequency: 10 Hz Amplitude: 300 μA Pulse Width: 200 μs	Sweetened condensed milk intake test	No significant difference between vmPFC groups. Significant difference between VTA groups for Flinders Sensitive Line rats.
					Novelty Exploration Test	No significant difference between vmPFC groups. Significant difference between VTA groups for Flinders sensitive line rats.
					Forced swim test	Decreased immobility for vmPFC-stimulated rats after DBS for 10 days, half relapsed at day 28. VTA-stimulated Sprague-Dawley rats had persistently reduced immobility until the end of the experiment.
Jiménez-Sánchez et al. (2016) [33]	IL	Wistar rats, male.	Olfactory bulbectomized model animal model. DBS 1 h daily stimulation, beginning 2 days after electrode implantation before behavioral testing.	Bipolar Biphasic Frequency: 130 Hz Amplitude: 200 μA Pulse Width: 90 μs	Social interaction test	Increased duration of active contact.

Table 3. Cont.

Authors	Target	Animal	Animal Models & DBS Design	Stimulation Parameters	Behavioral Tests	Outcomes
Jiménez-Sánchez et al. (2016) [81]	IL PrL	Wistar rats, male.	Naïve animal model. DBS for 1 h daily before behavioral testing.	Bipolar Biphasic Frequency: 130 Hz Amplitude: 200 μA Pulse Width: 90 μs	Sucrose preference test	Increased percentage of sucrose consumption in total liquid consumption.
					Forced swim test	Reduced immobility and increased climbing but not swimming.
					Hyperemotionality test	Reduced total behavioral scores when compared to olfactory bulbectomized sham rats.
					Forced swim test	Reduced immobility and increased climbing in IL-DBS. No significant behavioral changes in PrL-DBS.
					Open field test	Insignificant locomotor changes in IL-DBS.
					Novelty suppressed feeding test	Decreased latency to feed in IL-DBS.
Rummel et al. (2016) [113]	vmPFC	Flinders Sensitive Line rats, male. Congenitally learned helplessness rats, Male.	Experiment 1: Chronic intermittent DBS 1 week after surgery in Flinders sensitive line rats, 30 min each morning and extra 30-min stimulation on afternoons before the day of behavioral test. Experiment 2: Chronic continuous DBS 1 week after surgery for 16 days. Experiment 3: Chronic intermittent DBS in congenitally learned helpless rats, procedures followed that in experiment 1.	Chronic intermittent DBS Frequency: 130 Hz Amplitude: 300 μA Pulse Width: 100 μs Chronic continuous DBS Frequency: 130 Hz Amplitude: 150 μA Pulse Width: 100 μs	Sucrose consumption test	Chronic intermittent DBS increased sucrose intake in Flinders sensitive line rats but not in congenitally learned helplessness rats. Chronic continuous DBS did not affect sucrose intake in Flinders sensitive line rats and congenitally learned helplessness rats.

Table 3. Cont.

Authors	Target	Animal	Animal Models & DBS Design	Stimulation Parameters	Behavioral Tests	Outcomes
					Forced swim test	Chronic intermittent DBS and chronic continuous DBS increased latency to immobility in Flinders sensitive line rats but not congenitally learned helplessness rats.
					Learned helplessness paradigm	Chronic intermittent DBS and chronic continuous DBS decreased helplessness in Flinders sensitive line rats but not cLH rats.
					Sucrose intake test	No significant difference observed.
					Novelty exploration test	No significant difference observed.
Bambico et al. (2015) [98]	vmPFC	Fisher rats, Male.	CUS animal model CUS for ~4 weeks until anhedonia inferred by SPT scores, then performed implantation DBS for 3 weeks after implantation, 8 h per day, 7 days per week	Frequency: 130 Hz Amplitude: 100 µA Pulse Width: 90 µs	Novelty-suppressed feeding test	Reduced latency to feeding in CUS-DBS animals compared to CUS-sham animals.

Table 3. Cont.

Authors	Target	Animal	Animal Models & DBS Design	Stimulation Parameters	Behavioral Tests	Outcomes
					Open field test	No significant difference observed.
					Elevated plus maze test	More time in open arms in CUS-DBS animals compared to CUS-sham animals.
					Forced swim test	Reduced immobility time in CUS-DBS animals compared to CUS-sham animals.
Edemann-Callesen et al. (2015) [94]	vmPFC; Medial forebrain bundle.	Flinders sensitive line rats, male. Sprague-Dawley rats, male.	Naïve animal model. DBS was applied in an Intra-cranial self-stimulation protocol.	Bilateral. Monopolar Frequency: 20–200 Hz Amplitude: 170–560 µA Pulse Width: 100 µs	Intra-cranial self-stimulation	For Flinders Sensitive Line rats, vmPFC-DBS did not affect the reward-seeking behavior compared to medial forebrain bundle DBS.
Etiévant et al. (2015) [103]	IL	Sprague-Dawley rats, male.	Naïve animal model. DBS for 4 h after forced swim pre-test and 2 h before forced swim test.	Bipolar Unilateral Frequency: 130 Hz Amplitude: 150 µA Pulse Width: 60 µs	Forced swim test	Reduced immobility duration in IL-DBS compared to control.
Insel et al. (2015) [111]	IL	Sprague-Dawley rats, male.	Naïve animal model. DBS for 8 h per day, for 10 days.	Monopolar Bilateral Frequency: 130 Hz Amplitude: 100 µA Pulse Width: 90 µs	Spontaneous behavior recording	Coherence between ventral hippocampus and IL was reduced after 10-day DBS compared to sham in 2–4 Hz brain activity range, but was not reduced after only 1 day of treatment. Coherence was not affected by fluoxetine, indicating that IL-DBS observations were independent of the serotonergic pathways.

Table 3. Cont.

Authors	Target	Animal	Animal Models & DBS Design	Stimulation Parameters	Behavioral Tests	Outcomes
Lim et al. (2015) [102]	vmPFC	Sprague-Dawley rats, male.	Experiment 1 Naïve animal model. Experiment 2 CUS animal model. CUS for 3 weeks, each stressor lasted for 10-14 h DBS for 15 min before home-cage emergence test, before and during open field test.	Bipolar Biphasic Experiment 1 Frequency:10/100 Hz Amplitude: 100 µA Pulse Width: 100 µs Experiment 2 Frequency: 100 Hz Amplitude: 100µA Pulse Width: 100µs	Home-cage emergence test	HFS reduced escape latency time in Naïve and CUS animal model.
					Open-field test	Insignificant effect in Naïve animals for both HFS and LFS. Increased time spent in the central zone for HFS-CUS.
					Food-intake test	HFS increased food intake in naïve animals. No significance difference observed in CUS animals.
					Sucrose-intake test	Insignificant in Naïve animals for both HFS and LFS. Increased sucrose intake in HFS-CUS.
					Forced swim test	Insignificant in Naïve for both HFS and LFS. Reduced immobility duration in HFS-CUS.
Lim et al. (2015) [108]	PrL	Sprague-Dawley rats, male.	Naïve animal model. DBS for 15 min before and during sucrose intake test (same for forced swim test) and before sacrifice for 1 h.	Bipolar Biphasic Frequency: 100 Hz Amplitude: 100 µA Pulse Width: 100 µs	Sucrose intake test	Increased sucrose consumption.
					Forced swim test	Reduced immobility.
Liu et al. (2015) [99]	vmPFC	Sprague-Dawley rats, male. 4 months old and 12 months old.	Acute DBS Naïve animal model. DBS for 30 min before the behavioral tests. Chronic DBS Naïve animal model. DBS for 1 h daily including days of behavioral tests.	Bipolar Biphasic Acute DBS Frequency: 10/100 Hz Amplitude: 50/100/200/400 µA Pulse Width: 100 µs Chronic DBS Frequency: 100 Hz Amplitude: 100 µA Pulse Width: 100 µs	Novel object recognition test	Acute HFS at 200 µA produced higher novel object exploration than familiar object in short-term memory test. Chronic HFS increased novel object exploration in short- and long-term memory than familiar object, as well as the durations.

Table 3. *Cont.*

Authors	Target	Animal	Animal Models & DBS Design	Stimulation Parameters	Behavioral Tests	Outcomes
					Morris water maze	Shorter latency to reach platform on day 1 and 2 in chronic HFS compared to sham. More time spent in the target quadrant and less in the opposite quadrant in chronic HFS compared to sham.
Hamani et al. (2014) [100]	vmPFC	Sprague-Dawley rats, male.	Naïve animal model. DBS for 4 h after FST on day 1, 2 h before swimming on day 2 DBS 1 week after forced swim test, 4 h on day 1, 2 h on day 2, then assessed in open field test	Monopolar Frequency: 130 Hz Amplitude: 100 µA Pulse Width: 90 µs	Forced swim test	Reduced immobility and increased climbing frequency between groups.
					Open field test	No significant difference in locomotion observed.
Laver et al. (2014) [112]	vmPFC	Sprague-Dawley rats, male.	Naïve animal model. Serotonin reuptake inhibitors/vehicle were injected i.p. 1 h and 5 h after forced swim test on day 1 and 1 h before forced swim test on day 2. DBS for 4 h on day 1 of forced swim pre-test and 2 h before forced swim test on day 2.	Monopolar Bilateral Frequency: 130 Hz Amplitude: 100 µA Pulse Width: 90 µs	Forced swim test	DBS-saline, DBS-buspirone, DBS-Risperidone, DBS-pindolol-treated animals had higher observed swimming and lower observed immobility frequencies.
					Open field test	No significant difference observed
Perez-Caballero et al. (2013) [45]	IL	Wistar rats, male.	CUS animal model. Electrode implantation after week 4 of CUS, then CUS resumed. DBS for 4 h after forced swim pre-test and 2 h before forced swim test. Some animals received pre-treatment with indomethacin or ibuprofen.	Bipolar Monophasic Frequency: 130 Hz Amplitude: 100 µA Pulse Width: 90 µs	Forced swim test	Reduced immobility and increased swimming in DBS-off-IL and DBS-on-IL compared to sham- and naive-animals. Increased immobility and reduced swimming in DBS-off-IL animals treated with NSAIDs.

Table 3. *Cont.*

Authors	Target	Animal	Animal Models & DBS Design	Stimulation Parameters	Behavioral Tests	Outcomes
Rea et al. (2014) [95]	vmPFC	Flinders sensitive line rats, male. Flinders resistant line rats, male. (Control)	DBS for 30 min each morning for 2 weeks. Extra DBS for 30 min in the afternoon before the day of behavioral tests and during behavioral tests.	Monopolar Frequency: 130 Hz Amplitude: 300 µA Pulse Width: 100 µs	Open field test	No significant difference.
					Forced swim test	DBS reduced immobility in both groups of rats.
					Sucrose consumption test	DBS increased sucrose consumption in both groups of rats.
Veerakumar et al. (2014) [104]	vmPFC	C57BL/6 mice, male.	Chronic social defeat stress animal model. DBS for 5 h/day, for 7 days.	Bipolar Unilateral Frequency: 160 Hz Amplitude: 150 µA Pulse Width: 60 µs	Social interaction test	Before DBS, defeat-susceptible mice showed lower interaction times. Defeated animals with DBS spent longer in the interaction zone than sham and similar to non-stressed animals. DBS increased the total distance traveled.
Hamani et al. (2012) [92]	vmPFC	Wistar rats, male.	CUS animal model. DBS for 8 h/day, for 2 weeks	Monopolar Frequency: 130 Hz Amplitude: 200 µA Pulse Width: 90 µs	Sucrose preference test	Higher preference observed in CUS-treated DBS animals when compared to CUS-sham animals. Higher sucrose consumption in CUS-treated DBS than CUS-sham alone.
Hamani et al. (2010) [93]	vmPFC, IL, PrL	Sprague-Dawley rats, male	Naïve animal model DBS for 4 h after FST on day 1, 2 h before swimming on day 2	Frequency: 20 Hz/130 Hz Amplitude: 100/200/300/400 µA Pulse Width: 90 µs	Forced swim test	Parameters of 130 Hz, 90 µs, 200 µA reduced immobility the most in vmPFC-DBS, also at 100 µA and 300 µA. PrL stimulation at 130 Hz, 90 µs, 200 µA reduced immobility, but IL stimulation was insignificant.

Table 3. Cont.

Authors	Target	Animal	Animal Models & DBS Design	Stimulation Parameters	Behavioral Tests	Outcomes
Hamani et al. (2010) [91]	vmPFC	Sprague-Dawley rats, male	Naïve animal model, with serotonergic depletion, or norepinephrine lesion. DBS for Forced Swim Test Day 1: 4 h after forced swim test Day 2: 2 h before forced swim test DBS for open field test, novelty suppressed feeding test, and learned helplessness. Pre-test Day 1: 4 h Pre-test Day 2: 2 h	Monopolar Frequency: 130 Hz Amplitude: 100 µA Pulse Width: 90 µs	Forced swim test	DBS reduced immobility and increased swimming counts in naïve animals. DBS in animals with ibotenic acid injection had lower immobility and higher swimming counts than control. Rats with DBS without serotonergic depletion exhibited lower immobility than DBS animals with serotonergic depletion. Rats with DBS without norepinephrine lesion had lower immobility than control, similar reduction in immobility was shown in animals with DBS and norepinephrine lesion.
					Open field test	No significant difference.
					Novelty suppressed feeding test	DBS reduced latency to feed compared to control.
					Learned helplessness paradigm	Insignificant difference in escape latency between DBS and control.

Table 3. *Cont.*

Authors	Target	Animal	Animal Models & DBS Design	Stimulation Parameters	Behavioral Tests	Outcomes
			Animals predisposed to helplessness. DBS for 2 h before baseline assessment, 2 h before footshock at 2 days after baseline test, and DBS for 2 h before sucrose consumption test on the next day	Monopolar Frequency: 130 Hz Amplitude: 100 µA Pulse Width: 90 µs	Sucrose consumption test	DBS reduced the sucrose drinking time in animals after footshock, but this was insignificant.

Abbreviations: Cg, cingulate cortex; CUS, chronic unpredictable stress; EPM, elevated plus maze; FST, forced swim test; HFS, high-frequency stimulation; IL, infralimbic cortex; LFS, low-frequency stimulation; MWM, Morris water maze test; NORT, novel object recognition test; NSFT, novelty-suppressed feeding test; OBX, olfactory bulbectomy; OFT, open field test; PrL, prelimbic cortex; SD, Sprague-Dawley; SPI, sucrose preference index; vmPFC, ventromedial prefrontal cortex.

Preclinical studies have progressed from studying the behavioral effects of DBS to understanding the accompanying cellular and molecular changes, be they local or distal nodes in the neurocircuitry. However, issues concerning the rodent homologs of SCC and the effect of stimulation in the subdivisions of vmPFC have yet to be resolved and are discussed in the later part of the review.

6. Potential Mechanisms of Stimulation-Induced Antidepressant-Like Activities

Several preclinical studies reported that DBS modulates neuronal activities in different brain regions, leading to antidepressant-like behaviors (Figure 1A). The network-wide cellular and molecular changes caused by vmPFC-DBS can be classified into neuroplasticity-dependent and -independent changes (Figure 1B). Neuroplasticity-dependent effects included neurogenesis, increased synaptic plasticity, enhanced neurotrophin signaling, and potential activation of glial cell-mediated changes, whereas neuroplasticity-independent effects included changes in serotonergic (5-HT) and glutamatergic neurotransmission patterns, either locally or in distal structures. Other changes outside the scope of this review might also be relevant.

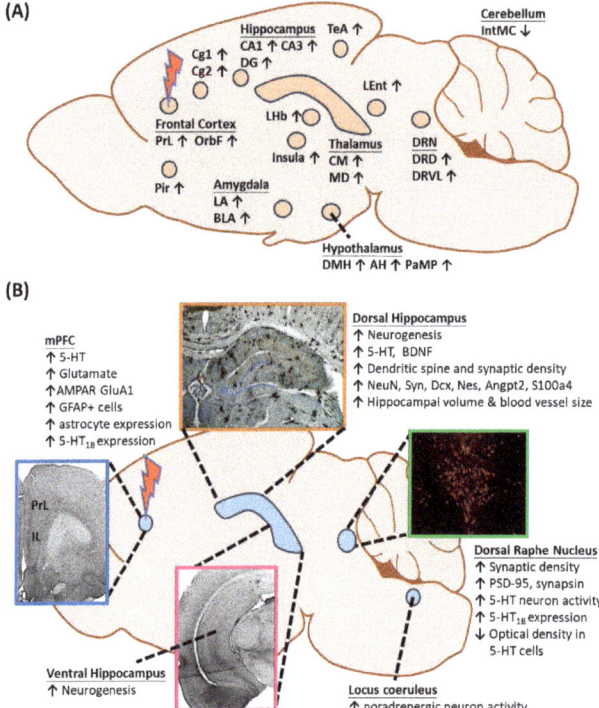

Figure 1. (**A**) Changes in local and distal neuronal activity after electrical stimulation of the ventromedial prefrontal cortex. (**B**) Neuroplasticity-dependent and -independent changes in different structures following vmPFC-DBS. Abbreviations: AH, anterior hypothalamus; AMPAR, α-amino-3-hydroxy-5-methyl-4-isoxazolepropionic acid receptor; BDNF, brain-derived neurotrophic factor; BLA, basolateral amygdaloid nucleus; Cg1,2, cingulate gyrus area 1, 2; CM, centromedial thalamic nucleus; DG, dentate gyrus; DMH, dorsomedial hypothalamus; DRD, dorsal raphe nucleus, dorsal part; DRVL, dorsal raphe nucleus, ventrolateral part; IntMC, interposed cerebellar nucleus, magnocellular part; LA, lateral amygdaloid nucleus; LEnt, lateral entorhinal cortex; LHb, lateral habenula; MD, mediodorsal thalamic nucleus; mPFC, medial prefrontal cortex; OrbF, orbitofrontal cortex; PaMP, paraventricular hypothalamic nucleus, medial parvicellular; Pir, piriform cortex; PrL, prelimbic cortex; TeA, temporal association area; and 5-HT, serotonin.

Neuroplasticity-Dependent Effects of Electrical Stimulation

(i) Neurogenesis is a Long-Term Cellular Change Brought About by Electrical Stimulation

Post-mortem studies, pharmacological analyses, and electroconvulsive therapy reports have led to the neurogenic hypothesis of the pathogenesis of depression, whereby atrophy and apoptosis of hippocampal neurons correlated with depression and neurogenesis induce antidepressant-like effects [120,121]. As CA1 and subiculum in the hippocampus project substantially to the IL and the latter feeds back to the hippocampus via the relay nucleus reuniens in the thalamus [102,122], vmPFC-DBS induces a corollary of hippocampal neuromodulation that may mediate the antidepressant-like outcome. Etiévant et al. found that there was increased neurogenesis in the dentate gyrus of the dorsal and ventral hippocampus in rodents after 1-h IL-DBS, as detected by positive BrdU cells, and this was accompanied by reduced immobility in FST [103]. Similarly, Liu et al. reported proliferation of neuronal progenitors after chronic vmPFC-DBS, as demonstrated by increased positive BrdU and Dcx cell counts, as well as upregulated expressions of genes related to neurogenesis (NeuN, Syn, Dcx, Nes) and neuronal differentiation and protective functions (Angpt2, S100a4). These results were correlated with enhanced memory function, which may serve as another indication of vmPFC-DBS [99]. Bambico et al. confirmed that new cells with mature neuronal phenotype were found in the hippocampus after vmPFC-DBS, as detected by BrdU and NeuN co-expression. They also reported that temozolomide-induced reduction of these cells led to a longer latency to feed in a novelty-suppressed feeding test, but did not significantly change immobility in FST. This prompted the authors to further examine the anxiolytic-like and anti-anhedonic-like effects of vmPFC-DBS. In contrast, Winter et al. showed that 1 h of vmPFC-DBS with established DBS parameters in rodents did not increase the percentage of BrdU and Dcx double-stained cells in the dentate gyrus compared to the control [123]. Although research on the interaction between neurogenesis and substrates such as serotonin is ongoing, BDNF may be required to exert this antidepressant-like effect [98]. Neurogenesis is a widely investigated mechanism of DBS and these results indicate positive effects in the hippocampal region.

(ii) Synaptic Plasticity is Altered More Rapidly by Electrical Stimulation than by Neurogenesis

Disruption in synaptic functions and signaling are implicated in the pathophysiology of MDD, considering their importance in neurotransmission and ultimately, in cell survival [20]. Chronic stress, a risk factor of MDD, was shown to cause retraction of dendrites in the medial prefrontal cortex [124] and CA3 of the hippocampus [125] in rodents. In the latter, the long-term potentiation (LTP) of synapses was compromised, affecting long-term memory formation [126]. Regarding the changes in synaptic plasticity caused by vmPFC-DBS, Liu et al. reported denser secondary dendritic spines in the dentate gyrus, as demonstrated by upregulated Syn expression correlated with Nes and Dcx. The authors also reported a slight (1.2 fold) increase in hippocampal BDNF gene expression, a regulator of synaptic plasticity [99]. More recently, Bezchlibnyk et al. found that 1 h of IL-DBS resulted in longer dendritic length and branch points localized in the basal and apical regions of hippocampal CA1 neurons, respectively. These results indicated that the acute stimulation stressed the indispensable connections between the hippocampus and vmPFC, which may have implications in MDD and its treatment [127].

Chakravarty et al. found that 5 days of 6-h vmPFC-DBS daily in 9-week-old C57Bl/6 mice resulted in a larger hippocampal volume and increased hippocampal synaptic density, as indicated by upregulated synaptophysin expression, a presynaptic marker [128]. Similarly, Veerakumar et al. found that chronic vmPFC-DBS in transgenic mice increased dendrite length and complexity of the 5-HT DRN neurons and upregulated the expression of postsynaptic markers synaptophysin and PSD-95 [104]. Moreover, Etiévant et al. reported synaptogenesis in the DRN, as indicated by higher expressions of PSD-95 and synapsin. This may explain the prolonged DRN neuronal activation during and after vmPFC-DBS, leading to an antidepressant-like effect [103]. According to earlier reviews, dendritic spines can respond swiftly and provide surfaces for synapse formation [126,129]. Given the more dynamic properties of synapses compared to neurogenesis, synaptic plasticity may serve as an early indicator of vmPFC-DBS efficacy. More preclinical studies characterizing the dynamics of synaptic plasticity under vmPFC-DBS are anticipated.

(iii) Neurotrophin Signaling Underlies the Antidepressant-Like Effect of Electrical Stimulation

The neurotrophin BDNF is important in synaptic regulation, neuronal survival, and differentiation of new neuron terminals in the adult brain [130–132]. Preclinical studies reported that depressive-like rats subjected to chronic unpredictable stress [92,98] or olfactory bulbectomy [33] had lower BDNF levels, whereas DBS increased BDNF levels, thus preventing the development of depressive-like behaviors. Extracellularly, pro-BDNF is cleaved by tissue plasminogen activator/plasmin to form mature BDNF. The high-affinity tropomyosin-related kinase B (TrkB) receptor is activated by BDNF [133], leading to downstream phosphorylation of kinases, including protein kinase B (Akt) and extracellular signal-regulated kinases (ERK), which are important mediators of anti-apoptosis and proliferation, respectively [134]. Moreover, BDNF-TrkB triggers Serine 133 phosphorylation of transcription factor cAMP response element binding (CREB), leading to the formation of the dimer. The phosphorylated CREB dimer forms a larger transcriptional complex and alters multiple gene expressions including BDNF itself [135]. Encouragingly, Jiménez-Sánchez et al. showed that IL-DBS administered to olfactory bulbectomized rats activated these signaling pathways, as demonstrated by lowered Akt/pAkt, ERK/pERK, and CREB/pCREB ratios during 1 h of stimulation that increased again after stopping the stimulation, which was similar to the expression pattern of BDNF [33]. Further molecular studies are needed to characterize the action of vmPFC-DBS toward different targets in this signaling cascade.

(iv) Potential Involvement of Glial Cells in Mediating the Outcome of Electrical Stimulation

Glial cells may be involved in the pathogenesis of depression, as revealed by post-mortem studies of MDD patients, which found lower densities in the prefrontal cortex and amygdala, but increased levels in the hippocampal hilus [136–138]. The latter may be activated as a result of neuronal injury and decreasing neuronal populations [139,140]. Glial cells metabolically support neurons and regulate glutamate synthesis and thus, regulate synaptic plasticity. They may be modulated by DBS to potentiate the therapeutic effects [136]. This mechanism was supported in a study by Etiévant et al., which found that glial lesion by L-alpha-aminoadipic acid injection diminished antidepressant-like behaviors, hippocampal neurogenesis, and LTP induced by IL-DBS [103]. These findings led to the hypothesis that the neuronal-glial relationship is a determinant of the antidepressant-like efficacy of DBS, but this requires further study. Perez-Caballero et al. also studied the effects of electrode implantation and analgesic supplements [115]. They found that implantation with non-NSAID analgesic treatments, like tramadol and morphine, did not ameliorate the anti-depressant effects of the electrode implantation. This observation was accompanied by an increase in glial marker GFAP-positive cells. This finding suggests that the supplementation of non-NSAIDs postoperatively could improve the comfort of patients.

Neuroplasticity-Independent Effects of Electrical Stimulation

Besides modulating neuroplasticity-dependent mechanisms, DBS may manipulate some neuroplasticity-independent pathways to induce antidepressant-like effects. In a chronic mild stress model, depressive-like behaviors developed without significant deterioration of hippocampal neurogenesis or neuronal survival [141]. There are two likely inter-related neurotransmission systems that potentiate DBS efficacy, namely serotonergic and glutamatergic systems.

(i) An Alternative Action of the Serotonergic System by Electrical Stimulation

Results from preclinical studies have established an important role of the vmPFC-DRN axis and downstream 5-HT neurotransmission in the treatment of depression. Hamani et al. first reported that 5-HT neurotransmission was augmented by DBS, as shown by a four-fold increase in hippocampal

5-HT after 1 h of vmPFC-DBS [91]. The authors also suggested a relationship between the integral 5-HT system and DBS efficacy, as 5-HT depletion induced by DRN lesions with 5,7-dihydroxytryptamine injection diminished the antidepressant-like effects of vmPFC-DBS [91,92]. Similarly, a study by Perez-Caballero et al. showed that the administration of para-chlorophenylalanine ester impeded 5-HT biosynthesis and diminished the antidepressant-like behaviors in early DBS among IL sham-treated animals [59]. Interestingly, Volle et al. showed that DBS and fluoxetine could rescue the 5-HT system via different mechanisms [119]. Both treatments increased the amount of 5-HT at the end of the chronic treatments, but chronic fluoxetine treatment was associated with decreased expression of $5-HT_{1A}$ in the prefrontal cortex and the hippocampus, whereas chronic DBS increased $5-HT_{1B}$ expression in the prefrontal cortex, globus pallidus, substantia nigra, and raphe nuclei.

A study by Veerakumar et al. in a transgenic mouse model of chronic social defeat stress revealed normalization of 5-HT neuron excitability in DRN after vmPFC-DBS [104]. Moreover, Jiménez-Sánchez et al. found increased prefrontal 5-HT efflux after 1 h of IL-DBS in olfactory bulbectomized rats [33] and in naive rats [81]. Etiévant et al. also found spontaneous DRN 5-HT neuron activity increased with IL-DBS [103]. Strikingly, an electrophysiological study performed by Srejic et al. showed that IL-DBS decreased the firing rate of DRN neurons, including serotonergic subtypes via the activation of GABAergic interneurons and possibly by the inhibition of excitatory glutamatergic neurons that modulate the firing of 5-HT [142]. Hence, the positive response to DBS could be enhanced by more selective targeting of the neuronal population by pharmacological adjuncts or coupling with optogenetic techniques. A study by Bregman et al. in 2018 using a serotonin transporter knockout mouse model found that DBS increased hippocampal 5-HT concentration, despite mice responding poorly to fluoxetine, a conventional selective serotonin reuptake inhibitor that acts on serotonin transporter [97]. These findings revealed a novel antidepressant-like activity of DBS involving the 5-HT system primarily in the DRN [79].

(ii) Glutamatergic Neurotransmission is a Promising Target of Electrical Stimulation

Jiménez-Sánchez et al. showed that there was enhanced prefrontal glutamatergic efflux together with changes in the local 5-HT profile [33,81]. The administration of AMPAR agonist and antagonist and subsequent FST showed that the increased glutamate led to antidepressant-like behaviors in animals [81]. The authors also found increased synthesis of the GluA1 subunit of AMPAR and postulated that their postsynaptic membrane insertion may explain the antidepressant-like outcome after 1 h of IL-DBS [33]. The activated glutamate output from the medial prefrontal cortex and frontal cortex enhanced 5-HT neuronal firing in the DRN [143], resulting in the antidepressant-like effect. However, Etiévant et al. argued that their activation was attributed to increased synaptogenesis in the DRN as previously described [103]. Nevertheless, Lim et al. hypothesized that a glutamatergic projection from the vmPFC to the medial subthalamic nucleus [144] may account for the antidepressant-like effects of vmPFC-DBS, as seen by increased c-Fos-immunoreactive cells in the medial subthalamic nucleus, increased sucrose consumption, and reduced immobility duration in FST [108]. With the emergence of glutamate-targeting pharmacotherapy [81], the ability to modulate glutamatergic transmission of DBS would add to the therapeutic novelty.

7. Concerns and Limitations of the Electrical Stimulation Studies

The small sample sizes in several clinical studies might compromise the credibility of the DBS efficacy, even in studies with similar recruited DBS subjects or consistent outcomes [18,56]. Most of the clinical studies were open-label, which means the responses could be prone to the placebo effect, despite the early response characterized by Perez-Caballero [59]. Efficacy of DBS treatment could be overestimated, unless countered by long stimulation, randomization, and blinding [18,145], such as double-blinded and sham-controlled studies [55]. A major criterion in preclinical studies is that they should mimic clinical studies. As it is unfeasible to stimulate animals for 24 h a day as in clinical designs [128], the scheduling of the stimulations and behavioral assessments will thus be relevant to the validity of the outcomes. Stimulation during behavioral tests will be most similar to clinical studies, but this may interfere with the physiological functions of the animals [79]. Besides, DBS is normally carried out in animals for relatively short periods and the effects might not correlate well with chronic stimulation [33]. Some preclinical studies were conducted in naive animal models and would not be compatible with clinical trials as TRD patients will be recruited exclusively in clinical settings [33,93]. Moreover, carry-over effects and lesion effects may interfere with the results in both settings. Carry-over effects refer to behavioral or neurochemical changes after DBS ceases. This needs to be counteracted by a washout period to allow the subjects to resume their baseline physiological states before the next stimulation [79]. Lesion effects occur where responses are observed after electrode implantation [19,60,72]. This needs to be differentiated from true responses observed in preclinical studies by sham-treatment [67], otherwise, the therapeutic effect will be over-estimated. Generally speaking, care must be taken in the design of experiments and data analysis of preclinical studies to increase their translational value to clinical studies.

8. Prospective Approaches to Enhance Deep Brain Stimulation Safety and Efficacy

Clinical response to SCC-DBS and various predictors can facilitate precise patient selection and customize the stimulation targets, thereby yielding maximal therapeutic outcomes with minimal adverse effects. For example, a lower baseline frontal theta cordance and incremental increase in the early stage of DBS indicates a clinical response [63]. Efforts have been made toward a more standardized approach to localize SCG in DBS responders [70]. Recently, real-time recording of the local field potential at the site of electrode implantation coupled with electroencephalogram have revealed network-wide clinical changes in DBS, which may improve the surgical precision [146]. Tractography-guided localization of electrodes, being more customized and precise, can improve the response rate [49]. A rechargeable DBS system should also be considered for long-term stimulation to reduce the need for surgery to replace batteries [17]. Lastly, given the high cost and invasiveness of DBS, more stringent regulation and evidence from randomized controlled studies are necessary to justify the benefits in TRD patients [147,148].

9. Conclusions

Major depressive disorder is a debilitating psychiatric condition, which is affected by treatment resistance. Although safety concerns were raised on the risks of ablative treatment, it paved the way for deep brain stimulation as an adjustable therapy against depression. This review summarized the efficacies of deep brain stimulation in the subcallosal cingulate, one of the most extensively studied targets of stimulation, and in the ventromedial prefrontal cortex, which is the rodent homolog. Research on DBS initially focused on symptomatic relief. As the decades have progressed, studies have started to branch out and utilize modern technology to improve targeting of brain regions and to investigate a broader list of symptoms in patients. This has allowed us to better understand the impact of DBS on underreported parameters, such as heart rate, skin conductance, and brain waveforms. Additionally, preclinical research has expanded our understanding of the molecular factors modulated by stimulation. Besides the local effects, DBS has been shown to modulate distal structures, which can involve numerous projections to and from the stimulated targets, and can contribute to the antidepressant effects. This review also described some of the neuroplasticity-dependent and -independent changes brought about by DBS. Progress in different areas of research has helped lay the groundwork for the next wave of DBS research investigating more targeted and more effective applications of DBS for treating MDD. Last but not least, with further customization, more precise approaches, and more stringent regulation, it is anticipated that deep brain stimulation has great promise to treat severe, refractory depressive disorders in the near future.

Author Contributions: Methodology, Investigation, Formal Analysis, Data Curation, Visualization, & Writing-Original Draft Preparation, Review & Editing: S.K., F.Y.N. and L.W.L.; Conceptualization, Supervision, Project Administration, Resources, & Funding Acquisition: L.W.L.; Validation: S.K., L.A., W.L.L. & L.W.L.;

Manuscript Intellectual Inputs: W.L.L., L.A., N.A.K., M.-L.F., Y.-S.C. and Y.T. All authors have read and agreed to the published version of the manuscript.

Funding: This scientific work was funded by grants from the Hong Kong Research Grants Council (27104616; 17119420) and the University of Hong Kong Seed Funding for Basic Research awarded to L.W.L.

Conflicts of Interest: The authors declare no conflict of interest.

References

1. Collaborators. GBD 2017 Disease and Injury Incidence and Prevalence. Global, regional, and national incidence, prevalence, and years lived with disability for 354 diseases and injuries for 195 countries and territories, 1990–2017: A systematic analysis for the Global Burden of Disease Study 2017. *Lancet* **2018**, *392*, 1789–1858.
2. Ferrari, A.J.; Charlson, F.J.; Norman, R.E.; Patten, S.B.; Freedman, G.; Murray, C.J.; Vos, T.; Whiteford, H.A. Burden of depressive disorders by country, sex, age, and year: Findings from the global burden of disease study 2010. *PloS Med.* **2013**, *10*, e1001547. [CrossRef] [PubMed]
3. Greenberg, P.E.; Fournier, A.-A.; Sisitsky, T.; Pike, C.T.; Kessler, R.C. The economic burden of adults with major depressive disorder in the United States (2005 and 2010). *J. Clin. Psychiatry* **2015**, *76*, 155–162. [CrossRef] [PubMed]
4. American Psychiatric Association. *Diagnostic and Statistical Manual of Mental Disorders*, 5th ed.; American Psychiatric Association Publishing: Washington, DC, USA, 2013.
5. Kendler, K.S.; Walters, E.E.; Neale, M.C.; Kessler, R.C.; Heath, A.C.; Eaves, L.J. The Structure of the Genetic and Environmental Risk Factors for Six Major Psychiatric Disorders in Women: Phobia, Generalized Anxiety Disorder, Panic Disorder, Bulimia, Major Depression, and Alcoholism. *Arch. Gen. Psychiatry* **1995**, *52*, 374–383. [CrossRef] [PubMed]
6. Kendler, K.S.; Gardner, C.O.; Lichtenstein, P. A developmental twin study of symptoms of anxiety and depression: Evidence for genetic innovation and attenuation. *Psychol. Med.* **2008**, *38*, 1567–1575. [CrossRef]
7. Rudolph, M.; Rosanowski, F.; Eysholdt, U.; Kummer, P. Anxiety and depression in mothers of speech impaired children. *Int. J. Pediatric Otorhinolaryngol.* **2003**, *67*, 1337–1341. [CrossRef]
8. Montero-Pedrazuela, A.; Venero, C.; Lavado-Autric, R.; Fernández-Lamo, I.; García-Verdugo, J.M.; Bernal, J.; Guadaño-Ferraz, A. Modulation of adult hippocampal neurogenesis by thyroid hormones: Implications in depressive-like behavior. *Mol. Psychiatry* **2006**, *11*, 361–371. [CrossRef]
9. Monteagudo, P.T.; Falcão, A.A.; Verreschi, I.T.N.; Zanella, M.-T. The imbalance of sex-hormones related to depressive symptoms in obese men. *Aging Male* **2016**, *19*, 20–26. [CrossRef]
10. Rohr, U.D. The impact of testosterone imbalance on depression and women's health. *Maturitas* **2002**, *41*, 25–46. [CrossRef]
11. Malhi, G.S.; Bridges, P.K.; Malizia, A.L. Neurosurgery for mental disorders (NMD) A clinical worldwide perspective: Past, present and future. *Int. J. Psychiatry Clin. Pract.* **1997**, *1*, 119–129. [CrossRef]
12. López-Muñoz, F.; Alamo, C. Monoaminergic Neurotransmission: The History of the Discovery of Antidepressants from 1950s Until Today. *Curr. Pharm. Des.* **2009**, *15*, 1563–1586. [CrossRef]
13. Baghai, T.C.; Blier, P.; Baldwin, D.S.; Bauer, M.; Goodwin, G.M.; Fountoulakis, K.N.; Kasper, S.; Leonard, B.E.; Malt, U.F.; Stein, D.; et al. General and comparative efficacy and effectiveness of antidepressants in the acute treatment of depressive disorders: A report by the WPA section of pharmacopsychiatry. *Eur. Arch. Psychiatry Clin. Neurosci.* **2011**, *261*, 207–245. [CrossRef]
14. McInerney, S.J.; McNeely, H.E.; Geraci, J.; Giacobbe, P.; Rizvi, S.J.; Ceniti, A.K.; Cyriac, A.; Mayberg, H.S.; Lozano, A.M.; Kennedy, S.H. Neurocognitive Predictors of Response in Treatment Resistant Depression to Subcallosal Cingulate Gyrus Deep Brain Stimulation. *Front. Hum. Neurosci.* **2017**, *11*, 74. [CrossRef] [PubMed]
15. Holtzheimer, P.E.; Husain, M.M.; Lisanby, S.H.; Taylor, S.F.; Whitworth, L.A.; McClintock, S.; Slavin, K.V.; Berman, J.; McKhann, G.M.; Patil, P.G.; et al. Subcallosal cingulate deep brain stimulation for treatment-resistant depression: A multisite, randomised, sham-controlled trial. *Lancet Psychiatry* **2017**, *4*, 839–849. [CrossRef]

16. Temel, Y.; Hescham, S.A.; Jahanshahi, A.; Janssen, M.L.; Tan, S.K.; van Overbeeke, J.J.; Ackermans, L.; Oosterloo, M.; Duits, A.; Leentjens, A.F.; et al. Neuromodulation in psychiatric disorders. *Int. Rev. Neurobiol.* **2012**, *107*, 283–314. [PubMed]
17. Morishita, T.; Fayad, S.M.; Higuchi, M.-a.; Nestor, K.A.; Foote, K.D. Deep Brain Stimulation for Treatment-resistant Depression: Systematic Review of Clinical Outcomes. *Neurotherapeutics* **2014**, *11*, 475–484. [CrossRef]
18. Kennedy, S.H.; Giacobbe, P.; Rizvi, S.J.; Placenza, F.M.; Nishikawa, Y.; Mayberg, H.S.; Lozano, A.M. Deep Brain Stimulation for Treatment-Resistant Depression: Follow-Up After 3 to 6 Years. *Am. J. Psychiatry* **2011**, *168*, 502–510. [CrossRef] [PubMed]
19. Mayberg, H.S.; Lozano, A.M.; Voon, V.; McNeely, H.E.; Seminowicz, D.; Hamani, C.; Schwalb, J.M.; Kennedy, S.H. Deep Brain Stimulation for Treatment-Resistant Depression. *Neuron* **2005**, *45*, 651–660. [CrossRef]
20. Duman, R.S.; Aghajanian, G.K.; Sanacora, G.; Krystal, J.H. Synaptic plasticity and depression: New insights from stress and rapid-acting antidepressants. *Nat. Med.* **2016**, *22*, 238–249. [CrossRef]
21. Gardner, J. A history of deep brain stimulation: Technological innovation and the role of clinical assessment tools. *Soc. Stud. Sci.* **2013**, *43*, 707–728. [CrossRef]
22. Benabid, A.L.; Pollak, P.; Louveau, A.; Henry, S.; de Rougemont, J. Combined (thalamotomy and stimulation) stereotactic surgery of the VIM thalamic nucleus for bilateral Parkinson disease. *Appl. Neurophysiol.* **1987**, *50*, 344–346. [CrossRef] [PubMed]
23. Faria, M.A. Violence, mental illness, and the brain—A brief history of psychosurgery: Part 2—From the limbic system and cingulotomy to deep brain stimulation. *Surg. Neurol. Int.* **2013**, *4*, 75. [CrossRef] [PubMed]
24. Krüger, S.; Seminowicz, D.; Goldapple, K.; Kennedy, S.H.; Mayberg, H.S. State and trait influences on mood regulation in bipolar disorder: Blood flow differences with an acute mood challenge. *Biol. Psychiatry* **2003**, *54*, 1274–1283. [CrossRef]
25. Zald, D.H.; Mattson, D.L.; Pardo, J.V. Brain activity in ventromedial prefrontal cortex correlates with individual differences in negative affect. *Proc. Natl. Acad. Sci. USA* **2002**, *99*, 2450–2454. [CrossRef]
26. Jimenez, F.; Velasco, F.; Salin-Pascual, R.; Hernandez, J.A.; Velasco, M.; Criales, J.L.; Nicolini, H. A patient with a resistant major depression disorder treated with deep brain stimulation in the inferior thalamic peduncle. *Neurosurgery* **2005**, *57*, 585–593. [CrossRef]
27. Schlaepfer, T.E.; Cohen, M.X.; Frick, C.; Kosel, M.; Brodesser, D.; Axmacher, N.; Joe, A.Y.; Kreft, M.; Lenartz, D.; Sturm, V. Deep brain stimulation to reward circuitry alleviates anhedonia in refractory major depression. *Neuropsychopharmacology* **2008**, *33*, 368–377. [CrossRef]
28. Schlaepfer, T.E.; Bewernick, B.H.; Kayser, S.; Madler, B.; Coenen, V.A. Rapid effects of deep brain stimulation for treatment-resistant major depression. *Biol. Psychiatry* **2013**, *73*, 1204–1212. [CrossRef]
29. Kringelbach, M.L.; Aziz, T.Z. Deep brain stimulation: Avoiding the errors of psychosurgery. *JAMA* **2009**, *301*, 1705–1707. [CrossRef]
30. Holtzheimer, P.E.; Mayberg, H.S. Neuromodulation for treatment-resistant depression. *F1000 Med. Rep.* **2012**, *4*, 22. [CrossRef]
31. Philip, M.L.; Richard, H.T.; Jeffrey, V.R.; Paul, B.F. Brain Neuromodulation Techniques: A Review. *Neuroscientist* **2016**, *22*, 406–421.
32. Blomstedt, P.; Hariz, M.I. Deep brain stimulation for movement disorders before DBS for movement disorders. *Parkinsonism Relat. Disord.* **2010**, *16*, 429–433. [CrossRef] [PubMed]
33. Jiménez-Sánchez, L.; Linge, R.; Campa, L.; Valdizán, E.M.; Pazos, Á.; Díaz, Á.; Adell, A. Behavioral, neurochemical and molecular changes after acute deep brain stimulation of the infralimbic prefrontal cortex. *Neuropharmacology* **2016**, *108*, 91–102. [CrossRef] [PubMed]
34. Greenberg, B.D.; Gabriels, L.A.; Malone, D.A.; Friehs, G.M.; Okun, M.S.; Shapira, N.A.; Foote, K.D.; Cosyns, P.R.; Kubu, C.S.; Malloy, P.F.; et al. Deep brain stimulation of the ventral internal capsule/ventral striatum for obsessive-compulsive disorder: Worldwide experience. *Mol. Psychiatry* **2010**, *15*, 64–79.
35. Kriston, L.; von Wolff, A. Not as golden as standards should be: Interpretation of the Hamilton Rating Scale for Depression. *J. Affect. Disord.* **2011**, *128*, 175–177. [CrossRef]
36. Hamani, C.; Mayberg, H.; Stone, S.; Laxton, A.; Haber, S.; Lozano, A.M. The subcallosal cingulate gyrus in the context of major depression. *Biol. Psychiatry* **2011**, *69*, 301–308. [CrossRef]

37. Andrade, P.; Noblesse, L.H.M.; Temel, Y.; Ackermans, L.; Lim, L.W.; Steinbusch, H.W.M.; Visser-Vandewalle, V. Neurostimulatory and ablative treatment options in major depressive disorder: A systematic review. *Acta Neurochir.* **2010**, *152*, 565–577. [CrossRef]
38. Fitzgerald, P.B.; Laird, A.R.; Maller, J.; Daskalakis, Z.J. A meta-analytic study of changes in brain activation in depression. *Hum. Brain Mapp.* **2008**, *29*, 683–695. [CrossRef]
39. Mayberg, S.H.; Brannan, K.S.; Mahurin, K.R.; Jerabek, A.P.; Brickman, S.J.; Tekell, L.J.; Silva, A.J.; McGinnis, G.S.; Glass, C.T.; Martin, T.C.; et al. Cingulate function in depression: A potential predictor of treatment response. *NeuroReport* **1997**, *8*, 1057–1061. [CrossRef]
40. Sankar, T.; Chakravarty, M.M.; Jawa, N.; Li, S.X.; Giacobbe, P.; Kennedy, S.H.; Rizvi, S.J.; Mayberg, H.S.; Hamani, C.; Lozano, A.M. Neuroanatomical predictors of response to subcallosal cingulate deep brain stimulation for treatment-resistant depression. *J. Psychiatry Neurosci.* **2020**, *45*, 45–54. [CrossRef]
41. Riva-Posse, P.; Inman, C.S.; Choi, K.S.; Crowell, A.L.; Gross, R.E.; Hamann, S.; Mayberg, H.S. Autonomic arousal elicited by subcallosal cingulate stimulation is explained by white matter connectivity. *Brain Stimul.* **2019**, *12*, 743–751. [CrossRef]
42. Eitan, R.; Fontaine, D.; Benoit, M.; Giordana, C.; Darmon, N.; Israel, Z.; Linesky, E.; Arkadir, D.; Ben-Naim, S.; Iserlles, M.; et al. One year double blind study of high vs low frequency subcallosal cingulate stimulation for depression. *J. Psychiatr. Res.* **2018**, *96*, 124–134. [CrossRef]
43. Merkl, A.; Aust, S.; Schneider, G.-H.; Visser-Vandewalle, V.; Horn, A.; Kühn, A.A.; Kuhn, J.; Bajbouj, M. Deep brain stimulation of the subcallosal cingulate gyrus in patients with treatment-resistant depression: A double-blinded randomized controlled study and long-term follow-up in eight patients. *J. Affect. Disord.* **2018**, *227*, 521–529. [CrossRef]
44. Howell, B.; Choi, K.S.; Gunalan, K.; Rajendra, J.; Mayberg, H.S.; McIntyre, C.C. Quantifying the axonal pathways directly stimulated in therapeutic subcallosal cingulate deep brain stimulation. *Hum. Brain Mapp.* **2019**, *40*, 889–903. [CrossRef]
45. Waters, A.C.; Veerakumar, A.; Choi, K.S.; Howell, B.; Tiruvadi, V.; Bijanki, K.R.; Crowell, A.; Riva-Posse, P.; Mayberg, H.S. Test-retest reliability of a stimulation-locked evoked response to deep brain stimulation in subcallosal cingulate for treatment resistant depression. *Hum. Brain Mapp.* **2018**, *39*, 4844–4856. [CrossRef]
46. Smart, O.; Choi, K.S.; Riva-Posse, P.; Tiruvadi, V.; Rajendra, J.; Waters, A.C.; Crowell, A.L.; Edwards, J.; Gross, R.E.; Mayberg, H.S. Initial Unilateral Exposure to Deep Brain Stimulation in Treatment-Resistant Depression Patients Alters Spectral Power in the Subcallosal Cingulate. *Front. Comput. Neurosci.* **2018**, *12*. [CrossRef]
47. Choi, K.S.; Noecker, A.M.; Riva-Posse, P.; Rajendra, J.K.; Gross, R.E.; Mayberg, H.S.; McIntyre, C.C. Impact of brain shift on subcallosal cingulate deep brain stimulation. *Brain Stimul.* **2018**, *11*, 445–453. [CrossRef]
48. Conen, S.; Matthews, J.C.; Patel, N.K.; Anton-Rodriguez, J.; Talbot, P.S. Acute and chronic changes in brain activity with deep brain stimulation for refractory depression. *J. Psychopharmacol.* **2018**, *32*, 430–440. [CrossRef]
49. Riva-Posse, P.; Choi, K.S.; Holtzheimer, P.E.; Crowell, A.L.; Garlow, S.J.; Rajendra, J.K.; McIntyre, C.C.; Gross, R.E.; Mayberg, H.S. A connectomic approach for subcallosal cingulate deep brain stimulation surgery: Prospective targeting in treatment-resistant depression. *Mol. Psychiatry* **2017**. [CrossRef]
50. Tsolaki, E.; Espinoza, R.; Pouratian, N. Using probabilistic tractography to target the subcallosal cingulate cortex in patients with treatment resistant depression. *Psychiatry Res. Neuroimaging* **2017**, *261*, 72–74. [CrossRef]
51. Accolla, E.A.; Aust, S.; Merkl, A.; Schneider, G.-H.; Kühn, A.A.; Bajbouj, M.; Draganski, B. Deep brain stimulation of the posterior gyrus rectus region for treatment resistant depression. *J. Affect. Disord.* **2016**, *194*, 33–37. [CrossRef]
52. Richieri, R.; Borius, P.Y.; Lagrange, G.; Faget-Agius, C.; Guedj, E.; Mc Gonigal, A.; Régis, J.M.; Lançon, C.; Bartolomei, F. Unmasking Partial Seizure after Deep Brain Stimulation for Treatment-Resistant Depression: A Case Report. *Brain Stimul.* **2016**, *9*, 636–638. [CrossRef]
53. Hilimire, M.R.; Mayberg, H.S.; Holtzheimer, P.E.; Broadway, J.M.; Parks, N.A.; DeVylder, J.E.; Corballis, P.M. Effects of Subcallosal Cingulate Deep Brain Stimulation on Negative Self-Bias in Patients with Treatment-Resistant Depression. *Brain Stimul.* **2015**, *8*, 185–191. [CrossRef]

54. Martin-Blanco, A.; Serra-Blasco, M.; Perez-Egea, R.; de Diego-Adelino, J.; Carceller-Sindreu, M.; Puigdemont, D.; Molet, J.; Alvarez, E.; Perez, V.; Portella, M.J. Immediate cerebral metabolic changes induced by discontinuation of deep brain stimulation of subcallosal cingulate gyrus in treatment-resistant depression. *J. Affect. Disord.* **2015**, *173*, 159–162. [CrossRef]
55. Puigdemont, D.; Portella, M.J.; Pérez-Egea, R.; Molet, J.; Gironell, A.; de Diego-Adeliño, J.; Martín, A.; Rodríguez, R.; Àlvarez, E.; Artigas, F.; et al. A randomized double-blind crossover trial of deep brain stimulation of the subcallosal cingulate gyrus in patients with treatment-resistant depression: A pilot study of relapse prevention. *J. Psychiatry Neurosci. Jpn.* **2015**, *40*, 224–231. [CrossRef]
56. Serra-Blasco, M.; de Vita, S.; Rodriguez, M.R.; de Diego-Adelino, J.; Puigdemont, D.; Martin-Blanco, A.; Perez-Egea, R.; Molet, J.; Alvarez, E.; Perez, V.; et al. Cognitive functioning after deep brain stimulation in subcallosal cingulate gyrus for treatment-resistant depression: An exploratory study. *Psychiatry Res.* **2015**, *225*, 341–346. [CrossRef]
57. Choi, K.S.; Riva-Posse, P.; Gross, R.E.; Mayberg, H.S. Mapping the "Depression Switch" During Intraoperative Testing of Subcallosal Cingulate Deep Brain Stimulation. *JAMA Neurol.* **2015**, *72*, 1252–1260. [CrossRef]
58. Sun, Y.; Giacobbe, P.; Tang, C.W.; Barr, M.S.; Rajji, T.; Kennedy, S.H.; Fitzgerald, P.B.; Lozano, A.M.; Wong, W.; Daskalakis, Z.J. Deep Brain Stimulation Modulates Gamma Oscillations and Theta-Gamma Coupling in Treatment Resistant Depression. *Brain Stimul.* **2015**, *8*, 1033–1042. [CrossRef]
59. Perez-Caballero, L.; Pérez-Egea, R.; Romero-Grimaldi, C.; Puigdemont, D.; Molet, J.; Caso, J.R.; Mico, J.A.; Pérez, V.; Leza, J.C.; Berrocoso, E. Early responses to deep brain stimulation in depression are modulated by anti-inflammatory drugs. *Mol. Psychiatry* **2013**, *19*, 607. [CrossRef]
60. Merkl, A.; Schneider, G.-H.; Schönecker, T.; Aust, S.; Kühl, K.-P.; Kupsch, A.; Kühn, A.A.; Bajbouj, M. Antidepressant effects after short-term and chronic stimulation of the subgenual cingulate gyrus in treatment-resistant depression. *Exp. Neurol.* **2013**, *249*, 160–168. [CrossRef]
61. Ramasubbu, R.; Anderson, S.; Haffenden, A.; Chavda, S.; Kiss, Z.H. Double-blind optimization of subcallosal cingulate deep brain stimulation for treatment-resistant depression: A pilot study. *J. Psychiatry Neurosci.* **2013**, *38*, 325–332. [CrossRef] [PubMed]
62. Torres, C.V.; Ezquiaga, E.; Navas, M.; Sola, R.G. Deep brain stimulation of the subcallosal cingulate for medication-resistant type I bipolar depression: Case report. *Bipolar. Disord.* **2013**, *15*, 719–721. [CrossRef] [PubMed]
63. Broadway, J.M.; Holtzheimer, P.E.; Hilimire, M.R.; Parks, N.A.; DeVylder, J.E.; Mayberg, H.S.; Corballis, P.M. Frontal Theta Cordance Predicts 6-Month Antidepressant Response to Subcallosal Cingulate Deep Brain Stimulation for Treatment-Resistant Depression: A Pilot Study. *Neuropsychopharmacology* **2012**, *37*, 1764–1772. [CrossRef] [PubMed]
64. Hamani, C.; Giacobbe, P.; Diwan, M.; Balbino, E.S.; Tong, J.; Bridgman, A.; Lipsman, N.; Lozano, A.M.; Kennedy, S.H.; Nobrega, J.N. Monoamine oxidase inhibitors potentiate the effects of deep brain stimulation. *Am. J. Psychiatry* **2012**, *169*, 1320–1321. [CrossRef] [PubMed]
65. Holtzheimer, P.E.; Kelley, M.E.; Gross, R.E.; Filkowski, M.M.; Garlow, S.J.; Barrocas, A.; Wint, D.; Craighead, M.C.; Kozarsky, J.; Chismar, R.; et al. Subcallosal Cingulate Deep Brain Stimulation for Treatment-Resistant Unipolar and Bipolar Depression. *Arch. Gen. Psychiatry* **2012**, *69*, 150–158. [CrossRef] [PubMed]
66. Lozano, A.M.; Giacobbe, P.; Hamani, C.; Rizvi, S.J.; Kennedy, S.H.; Kolivakis, T.T.; Debonnel, G.; Sadikot, A.F.; Lam, R.W.; Howard, A.K.; et al. A multicenter pilot study of subcallosal cingulate area deep brain stimulation for treatment-resistant depression. *J. Neurosurg.* **2011**, *116*, 315–322. [CrossRef] [PubMed]
67. Puigdemont, D.; Pérez-Egea, R.; Portella, M.J.; Molet, J.; de Diego-Adeliño, J.; Gironell, A.; Radua, J.; Gómez-Anson, B.; Rodríguez, R.; Serra, M.; et al. Deep brain stimulation of the subcallosal cingulate gyrus: Further evidence in treatment-resistant major depression. *Int. J. Neuropsychopharmacol.* **2012**, *15*, 121–133. [CrossRef]
68. Guinjoan, S.M.; Mayberg, H.S.; Costanzo, E.Y.; Fahrer, R.D.; Tenca, E.; Antico, J.; Cerquetti, D.; Smyth, E.; Leiguarda, R.C.; Nemeroff, C.B. Asymmetrical contribution of brain structures to treatment-resistant depression as illustrated by effects of right subgenual cingulum stimulation. *J. Neuropsychiatry Clin. Neurosci.* **2010**, *22*, 265–277. [CrossRef] [PubMed]
69. Holtzheimer, P.E., 3rd; Mayberg, H.S. Deep brain stimulation for treatment-resistant depression. *Am. J. Psychiatry* **2010**, *167*, 1437–1444. [CrossRef]

70. Hamani, C.; Mayberg, H.; Snyder, B.; Giacobbe, P.; Kennedy, S.; Lozano, A.M. Deep brain stimulation of the subcallosal cingulate gyrus for depression: Anatomical location of active contacts in clinical responders and a suggested guideline for targeting. *J. Neurosurg.* **2009**, *111*, 1209. [CrossRef]
71. Puigdemont, D.; Portella, M.J.; Pérez-Egea, R.; de Diego-Adeliño, J.; Gironell, A.; Molet, J.; Duran-Sindreu, S.; Álvarez, E.; Pérez, V. Depressive Relapse After Initial Response to Subcallosal Cingulate Gyrus-Deep Brain Stimulation in a Patient with a Treatment-Resistant Depression: Electroconvulsive Therapy as a Feasible Strategy. *Biol. Psychiatry* **2009**, *66*, e11–e12. [CrossRef]
72. Lozano, A.M.; Mayberg, H.S.; Giacobbe, P.; Hamani, C.; Craddock, R.C.; Kennedy, S.H. Subcallosal Cingulate Gyrus Deep Brain Stimulation for Treatment-Resistant Depression. *Biol. Psychiatry* **2008**, *64*, 461–467. [CrossRef] [PubMed]
73. McNeely, E.H.; Mayberg, S.H.; Lozano, M.A.; Kennedy, H.S. Neuropsychological Impact of Cg25 Deep Brain Stimulation for Treatment-Resistant Depression: Preliminary Results Over 12 Months. *J. Nerv. Ment. Dis.* **2008**, *196*, 405–410. [CrossRef] [PubMed]
74. Neimat, J.S.; Hamani, C.; Giacobbe, P.; Merskey, H.; Kennedy, S.H.; Mayberg, H.S.; Lozano, A.M. Neural stimulation successfully treats depression in patients with prior ablative cingulotomy. *Am. J. Psychiatry* **2008**, *165*, 687. [CrossRef] [PubMed]
75. Bari, A.A.; Mikell, C.B.; Abosch, A.; Ben-Haim, S.; Buchanan, R.J.; Burton, A.W.; Carcieri, S.; Cosgrove, G.R.; D'Haese, P.-F.; Daskalakis, Z.J.; et al. Charting the road forward in psychiatric neurosurgery: Proceedings of the 2016 American Society for Stereotactic and Functional Neurosurgery workshop on neuromodulation for psychiatric disorders. *J. Neurol. Neurosurg. Psychiatry* **2018**, *89*, 886–896. [CrossRef]
76. Moreines, J.L.; McClintock, S.M.; Kelley, M.E.; Holtzheimer, P.E.; Mayberg, H.S. Neuropsychological function before and after subcallosal cingulate deep brain stimulation in patients with treatment-resistant depression. *Depress. Anxiety* **2014**, *31*, 690–698. [CrossRef]
77. Nyandege, A.N.; Slattum, P.W.; Harpe, S.E. Risk of Fracture and the Concomitant Use of Bisphosphonates With Osteoporosis-Inducing Medications. *Ann. Pharmacother.* **2015**, *49*, 437–447. [CrossRef]
78. Cox, G.R.; Callahan, P.; Churchill, R.; Hunot, V.; Merry, S.N.; Parker, A.G.; Hetrick, S.E. Psychological therapies versus antidepressant medication, alone and in combination for depression in children and adolescents. *Cochrane Database Syst. Rev.* **2014**, *11*, CD008324. [CrossRef]
79. Hamani, C.; Nobrega, J.N. Preclinical Studies Modeling Deep Brain Stimulation for Depression. *Biol. Psychiatry* **2012**, *72*, 916–923. [CrossRef]
80. Vertes, R.P. Interactions among the medial prefrontal cortex, hippocampus and midline thalamus in emotional and cognitive processing in the rat. *Neuroscience* **2006**, *142*, 1–20. [CrossRef]
81. Jiménez-Sánchez, L.; Castañé, A.; Pérez-Caballero, L.; Grifoll-Escoda, M.; López-Gil, X.; Campa, L.; Galofré, M.; Berrocoso, E.; Adell, A. Activation of AMPA Receptors Mediates the Antidepressant Action of Deep Brain Stimulation of the Infralimbic Prefrontal Cortex. *Cereb. Cortex* **2016**, *26*, 2778–2789. [CrossRef]
82. Ferry, A.T.; Öngür, D.; An, X.; Price, J.L. Prefrontal cortical projections to the striatum in macaque monkeys: Evidence for an organization related to prefrontal networks. *J. Comp. Neurol.* **2000**, *425*, 447–470. [CrossRef]
83. McFarland, N.R.; Haber, S.N. Thalamic Relay Nuclei of the Basal Ganglia Form Both Reciprocal and Nonreciprocal Cortical Connections, Linking Multiple Frontal Cortical Areas. *J. Neurosci.* **2002**, *22*, 8117–8132. [CrossRef]
84. Parthoens, J.; Verhaeghe, J.; Stroobants, S.; Staelens, S. Deep Brain Stimulation of the Prelimbic Medial Prefrontal Cortex: Quantification of the Effect on Glucose Metabolism in the Rat Brain Using [18 F] FDG MicroPET. *Mol. Imaging Biol.* **2014**, *16*, 838–845. [CrossRef]
85. Hajós, M.; Richards, C.D.; Székely, A.D.; Sharp, T. An electrophysiological and neuroanatomical study of the medial prefrontal cortical projection to the midbrain raphe nuclei in the rat. *Neuroscience* **1998**, *87*, 95–108. [CrossRef]
86. Wood, M.; Adil, O.; Wallace, T.; Fourman, S.; Wilson, S.P.; Herman, J.P.; Myers, B. Infralimbic prefrontal cortex structural and functional connectivity with the limbic forebrain: A combined viral genetic and optogenetic analysis. *Brain Struct. Funct.* **2019**, *224*, 73–97. [CrossRef] [PubMed]
87. Sesack, S.R.; Deutch, A.Y.; Roth, R.H.; Bunney, B.S. Topographical organization of the efferent projections of the medial prefrontal cortex in the rat: An anterograde tract-tracing study with Phaseolus vulgaris leucoagglutinin. *J. Comp. Neurol.* **1989**, *290*, 213–242. [CrossRef] [PubMed]

88. Chandler, L.J.; Gass, J.T. The plasticity of extinction: Contribution of the prefrontal cortex in treating addiction though inhibitory learning. *Front. Psychiatry* **2013**, *4*. [CrossRef]
89. Uylings, H.B.; van Eden, C.G. Qualitative and quantitative comparison of the prefrontal cortex in rat and in primates, including humans. *Prog. Brain Res.* **1990**, *85*, 31–62. [PubMed]
90. Lim, L.W.; Tan, S.K.; Groenewegen, H.J.; Temel, Y. Electrical brain stimulation in depression: Which target(s)? *Biol. Psychiatry* **2011**, *69*, e5–e6, author reply e7–e8. [CrossRef] [PubMed]
91. Hamani, C.; Diwan, M.; Macedo, C.E.; Brandao, M.L.; Shumake, J.; Gonzalez-Lima, F.; Raymond, R.; Lozano, A.M.; Fletcher, P.J.; Nobrega, J.N. Antidepressant-like effects of medial prefrontal cortex deep brain stimulation in rats. *Biol. Psychiatry* **2010**, *67*, 117–124. [CrossRef]
92. Hamani, C.; Machado, D.C.; Hipólide, D.C.; Dubiela, F.P.; Suchecki, D.; Macedo, C.E.; Tescarollo, F.; Martins, U.; Covolan, L.; Nobrega, J.N. Deep Brain Stimulation Reverses Anhedonic-Like Behavior in a Chronic Model of Depression: Role of Serotonin and Brain Derived Neurotrophic Factor. *Biol. Psychiatry* **2012**, *71*, 30–35. [CrossRef] [PubMed]
93. Hamani, C.; Diwan, M.; Isabella, S.; Lozano, A.M.; Nobrega, J.N. Effects of different stimulation parameters on the antidepressant-like response of medial prefrontal cortex deep brain stimulation in rats. *J. Psychiatr. Res.* **2010**, *44*, 683–687. [CrossRef] [PubMed]
94. Edemann-Callesen, H.; Voget, M.; Empl, L.; Vogel, M.; Wieske, F.; Rummel, J.; Heinz, A.; Mathé, A.A.; Hadar, R.; Winter, C. Medial Forebrain Bundle Deep Brain Stimulation has Symptom-specific Anti-depressant Effects in Rats and as Opposed to Ventromedial Prefrontal Cortex Stimulation Interacts With the Reward System. *Brain Stimul.* **2015**, *8*, 714–723. [CrossRef] [PubMed]
95. Rea, E.; Rummel, J.; Schmidt, T.T.; Hadar, R.; Heinz, A.; Mathé, A.A.; Winter, C. Anti-Anhedonic Effect of Deep Brain Stimulation of the Prefrontal Cortex and the Dopaminergic Reward System in a Genetic Rat Model of Depression: An Intracranial Self-Stimulation Paradigm Study. *Brain Stimul.* **2014**, *7*, 21–28. [CrossRef] [PubMed]
96. Bruchim-Samuel, M.; Lax, E.; Gazit, T.; Friedman, A.; Ahdoot, H.; Bairachnaya, M.; Pinhasov, A.; Yadid, G. Electrical stimulation of the vmPFC serves as a remote control to affect VTA activity and improve depressive-like behavior. *Exp. Neurol.* **2016**, *283*, 255–263. [CrossRef] [PubMed]
97. Bregman, T.; Nona, C.; Volle, J.; Diwan, M.; Raymond, R.; Fletcher, P.J.; Nobrega, J.N.; Hamani, C. Deep brain stimulation induces antidepressant-like effects in serotonin transporter knockout mice. *Brain Stimul.* **2018**, *11*, 423–425. [CrossRef]
98. Bambico, F.R.; Bregman, T.; Diwan, M.; Li, J.; Darvish-Ghane, S.; Li, Z.; Laver, B.; Amorim, B.O.; Covolan, L.; Nobrega, J.N.; et al. Neuroplasticity-dependent and -independent mechanisms of chronic deep brain stimulation in stressed rats. *Transl. Psychiatry* **2015**, *5*, e674. [CrossRef]
99. Liu, A.; Jain, N.; Vyas, A.; Lim, L.W. Ventromedial prefrontal cortex stimulation enhances memory and hippocampal neurogenesis in the middle-aged rats. *eLife* **2015**, *4*, e04803. [CrossRef]
100. Hamani, C.; Amorim, B.O.; Wheeler, A.L.; Diwan, M.; Driesslein, K.; Covolan, L.; Butson, C.R.; Nobrega, J.N. Deep brain stimulation in rats: Different targets induce similar antidepressant-like effects but influence different circuits. *Neurobiol. Dis.* **2014**, *71*, 205–214. [CrossRef]
101. Bregman, T.; Reznikov, R.; Diwan, M.; Raymond, R.; Butson, C.R.; Nobrega, J.N.; Hamani, C. Antidepressant-like Effects of Medial Forebrain Bundle Deep Brain Stimulation in Rats are not Associated With Accumbens Dopamine Release. *Brain Stimul.* **2015**, *8*, 708–713. [CrossRef]
102. Lim, L.W.; Prickaerts, J.; Huguet, G.; Kadar, E.; Hartung, H.; Sharp, T.; Temel, Y. Electrical stimulation alleviates depressive-like behaviors of rats: Investigation of brain targets and potential mechanisms. *Transl. Psychiatry* **2015**, *5*, e535. [CrossRef] [PubMed]
103. Etiévant, A.; Oosterhof, C.; Bétry, C.; Abrial, E.; Novo-Perez, M.; Rovera, R.; Scarna, H.; Devader, C.; Mazella, J.; Wegener, G.; et al. Astroglial Control of the Antidepressant-Like Effects of Prefrontal Cortex Deep Brain Stimulation. *EBioMedicine* **2015**, *2*, 898–908. [CrossRef] [PubMed]
104. Veerakumar, A.; Challis, C.; Gupta, P.; Da, J.; Upadhyay, A.; Beck, S.G.; Berton, O. Antidepressant-like effects of cortical deep brain stimulation coincide with pro-neuroplastic adaptations of serotonin systems. *Biol. Psychiatry* **2014**, *76*, 203–212. [CrossRef] [PubMed]
105. Bhaskar, Y.; Lim, L.W.; Mitra, R. Enriched Environment Facilitates Anxiolytic Efficacy Driven by Deep-Brain Stimulation of Medial Prefrontal Cortex. *Front. Behav. Neurosci.* **2018**, *12*, 204. [CrossRef] [PubMed]

106. Creed, M.C.; Hamani, C.; Nobrega, J.N. Effects of repeated deep brain stimulation on depressive- and anxiety-like behavior in rats: Comparing entopeduncular and subthalamic nuclei. *Brain Stimul.* **2013**, *6*, 506–514. [CrossRef]
107. Meng, H.; Wang, Y.; Huang, M.; Lin, W.; Wang, S.; Zhang, B. Chronic deep brain stimulation of the lateral habenula nucleus in a rat model of depression. *Brain Res.* **2011**, *1422*, 32–38. [CrossRef]
108. Lim, L.W.; Janssen, M.L.F.; Kocabicak, E.; Temel, Y. The antidepressant effects of ventromedial prefrontal cortex stimulation is associated with neural activation in the medial part of the subthalamic nucleus. *Behav. Brain Res.* **2015**, *279*, 17–21. [CrossRef]
109. Reznikov, R.; Bambico, F.R.; Diwan, M.; Raymond, R.J.; Nashed, M.G.; Nobrega, J.N.; Hamani, C. Prefrontal Cortex Deep Brain Stimulation Improves Fear and Anxiety-Like Behavior and Reduces Basolateral Amygdala Activity in a Preclinical Model of Posttraumatic Stress Disorder. *Neuropsychopharmacology* **2017**, *43*, 1099–1106. [CrossRef]
110. Torres-Sanchez, S.; Perez-Caballero, L.; Mico, J.A.; Celada, P.; Berrocoso, E. Effect of Deep Brain Stimulation of the ventromedial prefrontal cortex on the noradrenergic system in rats. *Brain Stimul.* **2018**, *11*, 222–230. [CrossRef]
111. Insel, N.; Pilkiw, M.; Nobrega, J.N.; Hutchison, W.D.; Takehara-Nishiuchi, K.; Hamani, C. Chronic deep brain stimulation of the rat ventral medial prefrontal cortex disrupts hippocampal–prefrontal coherence. *Exp. Neurol.* **2015**, *269*, 1–7. [CrossRef]
112. Laver, B.; Diwan, M.; Nobrega, J.N.; Hamani, C. Augmentative therapies do not potentiate the antidepressant-like effects of deep brain stimulation in rats. *J. Affect. Disord.* **2014**, *161*, 87–90. [CrossRef]
113. Rummel, J.; Voget, M.; Hadar, R.; Ewing, S.; Sohr, R.; Klein, J.; Sartorius, A.; Heinz, A.; Mathé, A.A.; Vollmayr, B.; et al. Testing different paradigms to optimize antidepressant deep brain stimulation in different rat models of depression. *J. Psychiatr. Res.* **2016**, *81*, 36–45. [CrossRef] [PubMed]
114. Lehto, L.J.; Filip, P.; Laakso, H.; Sierra, A.; Slopsema, J.P.; Johnson, M.D.; Eberly, L.E.; Low, W.C.; Grohn, O.; Tanila, H.; et al. Tuning Neuromodulation Effects by Orientation Selective Deep Brain Stimulation in the Rat Medial Frontal Cortex. *Front. Neurosci.* **2018**, *12*, 899. [CrossRef] [PubMed]
115. Perez-Caballero, L.; Soto-Montenegro, M.L.; Hidalgo-Figueroa, M.; Mico, J.A.; Desco, M.; Berrocoso, E. Deep brain stimulation electrode insertion and depression: Patterns of activity and modulation by analgesics. *Brain Stimul.* **2018**, *11*, 1348–1355. [CrossRef] [PubMed]
116. Jia, L.; Sun, Z.; Shi, D.; Wang, M.; Jia, J.; He, Y.; Xue, F.; Ren, Y.; Yang, J.; Ma, X. Effects of different patterns of electric stimulation of the ventromedial prefrontal cortex on hippocampal–prefrontal coherence in a rat model of depression. *Behav. Brain Res.* **2019**, *356*, 179–188. [CrossRef]
117. Papp, M.; Gruca, P.; Lason, M.; Niemczyk, M.; Willner, P. The role of prefrontal cortex dopamine D2 and D3 receptors in the mechanism of action of venlafaxine and deep brain stimulation in animal models of treatment-responsive and treatment-resistant depression. *J. Psychopharmacol.* **2019**, *33*, 748–756. [CrossRef]
118. Papp, M.; Gruca, P.; Lason, M.; Tota-Glowczyk, K.; Niemczyk, M.; Litwa, E.; Willner, P. Rapid antidepressant effects of deep brain stimulation of the pre-frontal cortex in an animal model of treatment-resistant depression. *J. Psychopharmacol* **2018**, *32*, 1133–1140. [CrossRef]
119. Volle, J.; Bregman, T.; Scott, B.; Diwan, M.; Raymond, R.; Fletcher, P.J.; Nobrega, J.N.; Hamani, C. Deep brain stimulation and fluoxetine exert different long-term changes in the serotonergic system. *Neuropharmacology* **2018**, *135*, 63–72. [CrossRef]
120. Santarelli, L.; Saxe, M.; Gross, C.; Surget, A.; Battaglia, F.; Dulawa, S.; Weisstaub, N.; Lee, J.; Duman, R.; Arancio, O.; et al. Requirement of Hippocampal Neurogenesis for the Behavioral Effects of Antidepressants. *Science* **2003**, *301*, 805. [CrossRef]
121. Pittenger, C.; Duman, R.S. Stress, depression, and neuroplasticity: A convergence of mechanisms. *Neuropsychopharmacology* **2008**, *33*, 88–109. [CrossRef]
122. Vertes, R.P.; Hoover, W.B.; Szigeti-Buck, K.; Leranth, C. Nucleus reuniens of the midline thalamus: Link between the medial prefrontal cortex and the hippocampus. *Brain Res. Bull.* **2007**, *71*, 601–609. [CrossRef]
123. Winter, C.; Bregman, T.; Voget, M.; Raymond, R.; Hadar, R.; Nobrega, J.N.; Hamani, C. Acute high frequency stimulation of the prefrontal cortex or nucleus accumbens does not increase hippocampal neurogenesis in rats. *J. Psychiatr. Res.* **2015**, *68*, 27–29. [CrossRef] [PubMed]

124. Cook, S.C.; Wellman, C.L. Chronic stress alters dendritic morphology in rat medial prefrontal cortex. *J. Neurobiol.* **2004**, *60*, 236–248. [CrossRef] [PubMed]
125. Magariños, A.M.; McEwen, B.S.; Flügge, G.; Fuchs, E. Chronic psychosocial stress causes apical dendritic atrophy of hippocampal CA3 pyramidal neurons in subordinate tree shrews. *J. Neurosci. Off. J. Soc. Neurosci.* **1996**, *16*, 3534. [CrossRef]
126. Shepherd, G.M. The dendritic spine: A multifunctional integrative unit. *J. Neurophysiol.* **1996**, *75*, 2197–2210. [CrossRef] [PubMed]
127. Bezchlibnyk, Y.B.; Stone, S.S.D.; Hamani, C.; Lozano, A.M. High frequency stimulation of the infralimbic cortex induces morphological changes in rat hippocampal neurons. *Brain Stimul.* **2017**, *10*, 315–323. [CrossRef] [PubMed]
128. Chakravarty, M.M.; Hamani, C.; Martinez-Canabal, A.; Ellegood, J.; Laliberté, C.; Nobrega, J.N.; Sankar, T.; Lozano, A.M.; Frankland, P.W.; Lerch, J.P. Deep brain stimulation of the ventromedial prefrontal cortex causes reorganization of neuronal processes and vasculature. *NeuroImage* **2016**, *125*, 422–427. [CrossRef] [PubMed]
129. Hering, H.; Sheng, M. Dendritic spines: Structure, dynamics and regulation. *Nat. Rev. Neurosci.* **2001**, *2*, 880. [CrossRef]
130. Kuem-Ju, L.; Sung-Jin, K.; Suk-Won, K.; Song-Hyen, C.; You-Chan, S.; Sang-Ha, P.; Bo-Hyun, M.; Eujin, C.; Min-Soo, L.; Sang-Hyun, C.; et al. Chronic mild stress decreases survival, but not proliferation, of new-born cells in adult rat hippocampus. *Exp. Amp; Mol. Med.* **2006**, *38*, 44.
131. Gulyaeva, N.V. Molecular Mechanisms of Neuroplasticity: An Expanding Universe. *Biochem. Mosc.* **2017**, *82*, 237–242. [CrossRef]
132. Chan, J.P.; Cordeira, J.; Calderon, G.A.; Iyer, L.K.; Rios, M. Depletion of central BDNF in mice impedes terminal differentiation of new granule neurons in the adult hippocampus. *Mol. Cell. Neurosci.* **2008**, *39*, 372–383. [CrossRef] [PubMed]
133. Reichardt, L.F. Neurotrophin-Regulated Signalling Pathways. *Philos. Trans. Biol. Sci.* **2006**, *361*, 1545–1564. [CrossRef]
134. Duman, R.S.; Voleti, B. Signaling pathways underlying the pathophysiology and treatment of depression: Novel mechanisms for rapid-acting agents. *Trends Neurosci.* **2012**, *35*, 47–56. [CrossRef] [PubMed]
135. Carlezon, W.A.; Duman, R.S.; Nestler, E.J. The many faces of CREB. *Trends Neurosci.* **2005**, *28*, 436–445. [CrossRef]
136. Öngür, D.; Drevets, W.C.; Price, J.L. Glial reduction in the subgenual prefrontal cortex in mood disorders. *Proc. Natl. Acad. Sci. USA* **1998**, *95*, 13290–13295. [CrossRef]
137. Bowley, M.P.; Drevets, W.C.; Öngür, D.; Price, J.L. Low glial numbers in the amygdala in major depressive disorder. *Biol. Psychiatry* **2002**, *52*, 404–412. [CrossRef]
138. Vostrikov, V.M.; Uranova, N.A.; Orlovskaya, D.D. Deficit of perineuronal oligodendrocytes in the prefrontal cortex in schizophrenia and mood disorders. *Schizophr. Res.* **2007**, *94*, 273–280. [CrossRef]
139. Stockmeier, C.A.; Mahajan, G.J.; Konick, L.C.; Overholser, J.C.; Jurjus, G.J.; Meltzer, H.Y.; Uylings, H.B.; Friedman, L.; Rajkowska, G. Cellular changes in the postmortem hippocampus in major depression. *Biol. Psychiatry* **2004**, *56*, 640–650. [CrossRef]
140. Rajkowska, G.; Miguel-Hidalgo, J.J.; Dubey, P.; Stockmeier, C.A.; Krishnan, K.R. Prominent reduction in pyramidal neurons density in the orbitofrontal cortex of elderly depressed patients. *Biol. Psychiatry* **2005**, *58*, 297–306. [CrossRef]
141. Airan, R.D.; Meltzer, L.A.; Roy, M.; Gong, Y.; Chen, H.; Deisseroth, K. High-Speed Imaging Reveals Neurophysiological Links to Behavior in an Animal Model of Depression. *Science* **2007**, *317*, 819. [CrossRef]
142. Srejic, L.R.; Hamani, C.; Hutchison, W.D. High-frequency stimulation of the medial prefrontal cortex decreases cellular firing in the dorsal raphe. *Eur. J. Neurosci.* **2015**, *41*, 1219–1226. [CrossRef] [PubMed]
143. Celada, P.; Puig, M.; Casanovas, J.; Guillazo, G.; Artigas, F. Control of Dorsal Raphe Serotonergic Neurons by the Medial Prefrontal Cortex: Involvement of Serotonin-1A, GABA sub(A), and Glutamate Receptors. *J. Neurosci.* **2001**, *21*, 9917–9929. [CrossRef]
144. Nambu, A.; Tokuno, H.; Takada, M. Functional significance of the cortico–subthalamo–pallidal 'hyperdirect' pathway. *Neurosci. Res.* **2002**, *43*, 111–117. [CrossRef]

145. Anderson, R.J.; Frye, M.A.; Abulseoud, O.A.; Lee, K.H.; McGillivray, J.A.; Berk, M.; Tye, S.J. Deep brain stimulation for treatment-resistant depression: Efficacy, safety and mechanisms of action. *Neurosci. Biobehav. Rev.* **2012**, *36*, 1920–1933. [CrossRef]
146. Deeb, W.; Giordano, J.J.; Rossi, P.J.; Mogilner, A.Y.; Gunduz, A.; Judy, J.W.; Klassen, B.T.; Butson, C.R.; Van Horne, C.; Deny, D.; et al. Proceedings of the Fourth Annual Deep Brain Stimulation Think Tank: A Review of Emerging Issues and Technologies. *Front. Integr. Neurosci.* **2016**, *10*, 38. [CrossRef]
147. Schermer, M. Ethical Issues in Deep Brain Stimulation. *Front. Integr. Neurosci.* **2011**, *5*. [CrossRef]
148. Bell, E.; Mathieu, G.; Racine, E. Preparing the ethical future of deep brain stimulation. *Surg. Neurol.* **2009**, *72*, 577. [CrossRef]

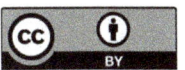

© 2020 by the authors. Licensee MDPI, Basel, Switzerland. This article is an open access article distributed under the terms and conditions of the Creative Commons Attribution (CC BY) license (http://creativecommons.org/licenses/by/4.0/).

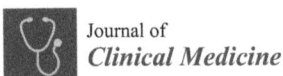

Review

Effectiveness, Timing and Procedural Aspects of Cognitive Behavioral Therapy after Deep Brain Stimulation for Therapy-Resistant Obsessive Compulsive Disorder: A Systematic Review

Meltem Görmezoğlu [1,2], Tim Bouwens van der Vlis [2], Koen Schruers [3,4], Linda Ackermans [2,4], Mircea Polosan [5] and Albert F.G. Leentjens [3,4,*]

1. Department of Psychiatry, Ondokuz Mayıs University, 55270 Samsun, Turkey; gormezoglumeltem@gmail.com
2. Department of Neurosurgery, Maastricht University Medical Centre, 6229 Maastricht, The Netherlands; tim.bouwens@mumc.nl (T.B.v.d.V.); linda.ackermans@mumc.nl (L.A.)
3. Department of Psychiatry and Neuropsychology, Maastricht University Medical Center, 6229 Maastricht, The Netherlands; koen.schruers@maastrichtuniversity.nl
4. School of Mental Health and Neuroscience, Maastricht University, 6229 Maastricht, The Netherlands
5. Grenoble Institute of Neurosciences, University of Grenoble Alpes, 38058 Grenoble, France; MPolosan@chu-grenoble.fr
* Correspondence: a.leentjens@maastrichtuniversity.nl

Received: 17 June 2020; Accepted: 22 July 2020; Published: 26 July 2020

Abstract: *Background and aim:* Deep brain stimulation (DBS) is an effective treatment for patients with severe therapy-resistant obsessive-compulsive disorder (OCD). After initiating DBS many patients still require medication and/or behavioral therapy to deal with persisting symptoms and habitual behaviors. The clinical practice of administering postoperative cognitive behavioral therapy (CBT) varies widely, and there are no clinical guidelines for this add-on therapy. The aim of this review is to assess the efficacy, timing and procedural aspects of postoperative CBT in OCD patients treated with DBS. *Method:* Systematic review of literature. *Results:* The search yielded 5 original studies, one case series and three reviews. Only two clinical trials have explicitly focused on the effectiveness of CBT added to DBS in patients with therapy-resistant OCD. These two studies both showed effectiveness of CBT. However, they had a distinctly different design, very small sample sizes and different ways of administering the therapy. Therefore, no firm conclusions can be drawn or recommendations made for administering CBT after DBS for therapy-resistant OCD. *Conclusion:* The effectiveness, timing and procedural aspects of CBT added to DBS in therapy-resistant OCD have hardly been studied. Preliminary evidence indicates that CBT has an added effect in OCD patients being treated with DBS. Since the overall treatment effect is the combined result of DBS, medication and CBT, future trials should be designed in such a way that they allow quantification of the effects of these add-on therapies in OCD patients treated with DBS. Only in this way information can be gathered that contributes to the development of an algorithm and clinical guidelines for concomitant therapies to optimize treatment effects in OCD patients being treated with DBS.

Keywords: deep brain stimulation; obsessive compulsive disorder; cognitive behavioral therapy

1. Introduction

Obsessive-compulsive disorder (OCD) is a chronic psychiatric disorder characterized by the presence of obsessions and/or compulsions. Its prevalence varies from 0.8% to 3% in the adult population [1]. The World Health Organization lists OCD as the 11th most common cause of secondary disability, accounting for 2.2% of the total years lived with disability [2]. Cognitive behavioral therapy (CBT), including exposure and response prevention (ERP), as well as pharmacotherapy with serotonergic medication, are the main forms of treatment for OCD. The effectiveness of CBT as treatment for OCD has been established in multiple studies [3,4]. However, its acceptability is limited: as much as 16% to 30% of patients offered CBT drops out during treatment [4,5]. Serotonergic medication, as well as augmentation with atypical antipsychotics, were shown to be effective, and the combination of medication and CBT is even more effective [6,7]. However, a large percentage of OCD patients show only a partial response, or are refractory to psychotherapy and pharmacotherapy. In severe therapy-resistant cases, deep brain stimulation (DBS) may be an option. Although the target and stimulation characteristics may vary across studies and clinics, DBS is generally considered safe and effective for the treatment of therapy-resistant OCD [8]. DBS received approval as treatment for OCD by the European Comission (EC) in 2009, and in the same year it was approved as a Humanitarian Device Exemption by the U.S. Food and Drug Administration (FDA).

After DBS, patients often still need medication, and CBT is often offered because it is considered useful in the treatment of remaining obsessive and compulsive symptoms, in dealing with behavior that has become habitual and persists even when the urge has subsided, and in helping to adjust to the new situation and new expectancies. In addition, CBT provides the patient with new coping styles and problem solving skills that may be important to prevent relapse and contribute to the long-term efficacy of DBS. Whereas guidelines for CBT in OCD have suggested offering CBT after DBS, clinical practice varies widely across institutions and often depends on local possibilities and traditions [9,10]. A more uniform and evidence-based approach may be beneficial for patients.

Up until now, the added effect of CBT to DBS for OCD has not been reviewed. The aim of this systematic review is to assess the literature on efficacy, timing and procedural aspects of postoperative CBT in patients being treated with DBS for therapy-resistant OCD, and to formulate clinical recommendations for future research and for offering CBT after DBS.

2. Methods

A systematic review of studies catalogued in PubMed was performed following the Preferred Reporting Items for Systematic Reviews and Meta-Analyses (PRISMA) guidelines (www.prisma-statement.org). The search was done over the full time span up until 17 April 2020. Only papers in English were included. We used the following broad Booleian search strategy: "(deep brain stimulation) AND (obsessive compulsive disorder) AND ((exposure and response prevention) OR (behavioral therapy) OR (cognitive behavioral therapy))". Given the limited yield of a narrower, exploratory search, all papers that addressed any form of postoperative CBT in patients receiving DBS for therapy-resistant OCD were included. This not only comprised clinical trials, cohort studies, case series and case studies, but also systematic and narrative reviews on DBS for OCD and position papers if they also commented on CBT after DBS. Reference lists of the included studies were checked for additional papers. The Evidence Project risk of bias tool was used to assess the quality of the included studies (not being reviews) [11]. Two authors rated the quality (MG and AL) and discrepancies were resolved by consensus. Due to the very limited yield of our search, no minimum quality score was applied for inclusion. The effectiveness of CBT added to DBS was quantified by looking at the changes in scores on the Yale–Brown Obsessive Compulsive Scale (Y-BOCS) before and after CBT. Although the initial intention was to perform a meta-analysis, this was not possible because of the limited number of included studies that, in addition, used different indication criteria and different forms and ways of delivery of CBT. Timing and procedural aspects of CBT in the studies are reported in a descriptive way.

3. Results

3.1. Literature Search

The search yielded 181 papers. One additional paper was added after checking the reference lists of included papers [12]. Based on the title and/or abstract, 154 of these were excluded because of the following reasons: animal studies ($n = 14$), not referring to OCD ($n = 61$), not referring to DBS ($n = 15$), not referring to CBT ($n = 28$), not in English ($n = 10$) and other reasons (including the absence of an abstract) ($n = 17$). The remaining 28 papers were read in full. An additional 19 of these were excluded due to the following reasons: not referring to CBT ($n = 11$), not referring to DBS ($n = 1$) and other reasons ($n = 7$). Eventually, 9 papers were included in the review: three randomized controlled trials (RCTs) [13–15], one cohort study [16], one case series [12], one qualitative study [17], one systematic review [18] and 2 narrative reviews [19,20]. These reviews were focused on the efficacy of DBS for OCD and not on the efficacy of CBT after DBS for OCD. Two of the included papers were based on the same RCT [13,14] (see Figure 1 for a PRISMA flowchart). The quality assessment of these studies are displayed in supplementary Table S1. The included systematic and narrative reviews are not discussed in the 'results' section since they did not include other relevant papers than the ones discussed below.

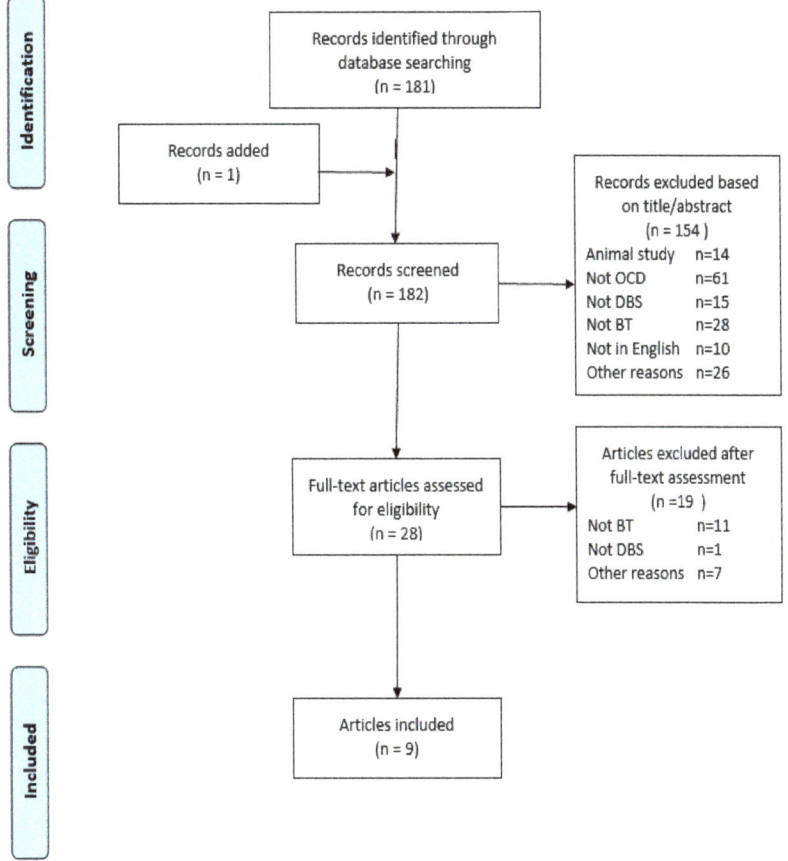

Figure 1. PRISMA flow diagramme. Abbreviations: OCD = obsessive compulsive disorder; DBS = deep brain stimulation; BT = behavioral therapy.

3.2. Description of Included Studies

The first RCT, by Denys et al. (2010) was a double-blind, sham–controlled, clinical trial of DBS of the nucleus accumbens (NA) that included 16 therapy resistant OCD patients [13]. In this study, refractoriness was defined as no or insufficient response to treatment with at least 2 different selective serotonin reuptake inhibitors (SSRIs) at maximum dosage for at least 12 weeks, treatment with clomipramine hydrochloride for at least 12 weeks with adequacy of treatment established by plasma levels, one augmentation trial with an atypical antipsychotic for 8 weeks in combination with an selective serotonin reuptake inhibitor, and at least 16 sessions of CBT [13].

Design: The study had 3 sequential treatment phases: an initial open phase, starting immediately after electrode implantation and lasting for 8 months, in which stimulation parameters were optimized and CBT was started. DBS was administered per protocol, with restricted stimulation settings at 90 μs, 130 Hz and a maximum stimulation intensity of 5.0 V. The effects of DBS were assessed with the Y-BOCS for obsessions and compulsions, with the Hamilton Anxiety Rating Scale (HAMA) for anxiety symptoms, and with the Hamilton Depression Scale (HAMD) for depression. After this open phase, a 1-month, double blind, sham-controlled phase started in which patients were randomly allocated to 2 periods of 2 weeks with the stimulators blindly turned 'on' (active stimulation) or 'off' (sham stimulation). CBT was continued throughout this phase. The double-blind phase was followed by a 12-month maintenance phase in which the stimulator was turned on for all patients and settings adjusted as required. Patients were allowed to use psychopharmacological medication during the trial.

Effectiveness: Stimulation in the initial open phase resulted in a mean decrease of 46% in Y-BOCS score from 33.7 (baseline) to 18.0 points; a mean decrease of 52% on the HAMA score from 20.9 (baseline) to 10.1 points, and a mean decrease of 46% in HAMD scores from 19.5 (baseline) to 10.5 points. Without stimulation, the improvement gained with the addition of CBT disappeared rapidly, suggesting that efficacy of CBT depends on stimulation. In this double-blind phase, the mean difference in Y-BOCS score between the active and sham condition after correction for period effects was 8.3 ($p = 0.04$). The mean difference in HAMA scores was 12.1 ($p = 0.1$) and the difference in HAMD scores was 11.3 ($p = 0.01$). It was reported that CBT was particularly effective in decreasing compulsions and avoidance behavior.

Mantione et al. (2014) performed a secondary analysis of this same RCT that was aimed at quantifying the added treatment effect of CBT after DBS, as well as to discuss the methodology of the CBT programme used (see above) [11]. The average decrease on the Y-BOCS after optimization of stimulation settings was 25%. With the addition of 24 weeks of CBT to ongoing DBS treatment, there was an additional 22% decrease of total Y-BOCS score ($p = 0.021$), without any additional effects on the HAMA or HAMD scores. The number of responders after CBT increased from 6 to 9 out of 16.

Timing: CBT was added when three conditions were fulfilled: an initial and substantial decrease (on average 6 points) in Y-BOCS score had to be obtained, there had to be no further decrease in Y-BOCS during three consecutive visits (which was usually after 8 weeks of stimulation), and it had to be observed that patients avoided resisting their compulsions or avoided anxiety-provoking exposure situations.

Procedural aspects: The CBT program consisted of 24 weekly individual face-to-face sessions of 60 min each. The protocolized treatment started with an extensive evaluation of the patient's motivation. Once motivation was established, therapy started with ERP and gradually introduced more cognitive elements at later stages [14,21].

Tyaghi et al. (2019) performed a randomized, double-blind counterbalanced comparison of DBS of the anteromedian subthalamic nucleus (STN) and ventral capsule/ventral striatal (VC/VS) stimulation in 6 patients [12]. In this study, treatment resistance was defined as no sustained benefit from treatment with at least two SSRIs for a minimum of 12 weeks at optimal doses, augmentation of SSRI treatment with an antipsychotic or extension of the SSRI dose beyond recommended limits, and at least two trials of CBT with a minimum of 10 sessions, of which one as inpatient.

Design: the study consisted of two phases: an initial randomized phase of 12 weeks with stimulation of either the STN or the VC/VS, followed by an open phase in which both targets were stimulated. Stimulation was started after a mapping session at 60 μs and 130 Hz, without restrictions for stimulation intensity and also allowing stimulation of different contact points, both monopolar and bipolar. Next, there were two additional 12-week open phases: in the first one stimulation settings were optimized using data from previous phases. In the second phase, CBT was added to optimized DBS using the combined VC/VS and STN targets.

Effectiveness: Psychopharmacological treatment was allowed and kept constant during the trial. Overall, the score on the Y-BOCS reduced by 60%, from 36.2 at baseline to 14.3 when optimal stimulation settings were administered. Adding in-patient CBT resulted in an additional decline of the Y-BOCS score by 35% to 9.3 ($p = 0.09$; total decline from baseline 74%). Although obsessions and compulsions improved significantly from baseline to optimal stimulation, there was no statistically significant added improvement after CBT. Scores on the Montgomery–Asberg Depression Rating Scale (MADRS) declined from 28 at baseline to 13 during optimal stimulation settings and further reduced to 7 after CBT (information from the authors). The authors conclude that there is no further improvement in obsessions and compulsions due to CBT after optimal stimulation settings, and that this reflects a 'floor effect' of DBS on OCD. With 'floor effect' they intend to say that no further improvement of OCD symptoms would be possible after optimization of stimulation settings.

Timing: CBT was started standard after 24 weeks

Procedural aspects: CBT, including ERP, was applied in an inpatient unit while optimal stimulation settings were maintained.

Greenberg et al. (2006) report on the long-term (>3 years) follow-up of 10 therapy-resistant OCD patients being treated with VC/VS DBS [16].

Effectiveness: The average Y-BOCS score declined by 35% from 34.6 preoperatively to 22.3 after three years of DBS. All pharmacotherapy was allowed, but kept constant up to three months after the start of DBS treatment. The information provided in the paper does not allow to calculate the added effect of behaviour therapy to DBS on OCD symptoms. Clinically, the authors describe a 'notably enhanced motivation to engage in goal directed activities' during DBS, which also included enhanced motivation for CBT, which all patients had attempted unsuccessfully before the procedure. They consider that this increased motivation may have been a key factor in the patients' clinical progress.

Timing: If patients had had behavior therapy immediately prior to DBS, this was allowed to continue after the start of DBS; if behavior therapy was newly indicated, it was allowed to start only six months after the start of DBS. No details on the number of patients that received behavioral therapy postoperatively is given, nor details about the type, frequency, duration and way of delivery of the behavioral therapy.

Procedural aspects: There is no information on procedural aspects.

Abelson et al. (2005) reported a case series of 4 therapy resistant OCD patients being treated with DBS of the anterior limb of the internal capsule, with the tip of the electrode adjacent to the nucleus accumbens [12]. After operation, a 12-week double-blind testing stage was followed by an open-ended, open stimulation phase, with efforts to optimize results by adjusting stimulation settings and by pharmacotherapy and CBT. No further details on the effectiveness, timing and procedural aspects of CBT is given.

The qualitative study by van Westen et al. (2019) reports on the results of interviews with 8 professionals involved in DBS treatment of OCD patients, as well as experiences from embedded patient observation of the author [17]. These professionals identified the process in which patients become increasingly engaged in their process of improvement as an important predictor of effect. As the patient changes, new possibilities emerge, one of which is renewed treatment with CBT, to reduce remaining symptoms and expand healthy behavioral repertoires [17].

4. Discussion

Whereas it is a common practice to offer patients with therapy-resistant OCD treated with DBS a course of CBT after their operation, its effectiveness, timing and procedural aspects, such as the preferred way of delivery of such therapy, has hardly been studied. In spite of the fact that the importance of post-operative CBT is stressed by various authors [18–20], only two trials have specifically focussed on CBT added to DBS [13–15].

4.1. Effectiveness

The two studies that assessed the effects of CBT added on to DBS both support its effectiveness. In the study by Denys et al., CBT was responsible for significant additional reduction of 22% on the Y-BOCS after optimal stimulation settings were achieved [14]. In the study by Tyagi et al., there was a trend for an additional improvement of 35% on the Y-BOCS ($p = 0.09$). Whereas this was not statistically significant, there is a clear trend towards significance for this finding and it constitutes a clinically relevant improvement. In our opinion the lack of a statistical significance may well be due to a power problem because of the very low number of included patients ($n = 6$). So contrary to the authors, who present this as a negative outcome, we consider this study in support of postoperative CBT.

In theory, the effectiveness of CBT may also depend on the preoperative cognitive state of the patient, as well as on the potential cognitive side effects of DBS. Whereas in patients with Parkinson's disease, cognitive side effects of DBS—especially of the subthalamic nucleus—have been associated with reduced processing speed and working memory [22], there is little evidence of any detrimental effect of DBS—of any target—on the cognitive performance of OCD patients [23]. Studies that do report on neuropsychological measures report no relevant change in cognitive performance after DBS [24], and in one case even an improvement in cognitive flexibility for STN DBS but not for VC/VS DBS [15]. None of the included papers report on problems administering CBT due to cognitive side effects.

There has been some discussion on whether the effects of CBT may depend on the DBS target. Mantione et al. suggest that the effect of CBT in their study may be specific to stimulation of the NA, since NA DBS has a profound effect on anxiety and depression, as opposed to, e.g., DBS of the STN, which reduces compulsions without significant effects on mood and anxiety [11]. However, in the study by Tyagi et al., the additional improvement in patients with STN and VC/VS DBS is in the same range, if not larger than in the study by Mantione et al. [15]. Based on these scarce data, we expect CBT to be effective as add-on treatment to DBS in therapy-resistant OCD patients, irrespective of the stimulation target. However, only further studies comparing the effectiveness of CBT in OCD patients with different DBS stimulation targets can reveal a potential target related effect of CBT.

4.2. Timing

The same two studies used different criteria for starting CBT. Denys et al. started CBT after partial response, defined as a substantial reduction of on average 6 points on the Y-BOCS, without further decrease during three consecutive visits [13,14]. In the study by Tyagi, CBT was started after 36 weeks in every patient, irrespective of the amount of improvement achieved by DBS [15]. In clinical practice the question of when to best start CBT is an important one. It does not seem sensible to start CBT immediately postoperatively after electrode implantation and activating the DBS system. The mental state of the patient has not changed yet, and because of that there is no reason to expect that treatments that were ineffective before DBS would now be effective. It also makes no sense to start CBT if the response to DBS is very large, since there may not be any relevant treatment goals left to work towards. The best time to start CBT is probably when there is a partial response to DBS. The altered mental state of the patient, with not only some reduction in obsessive-compulsive behavior, but usually also reduced anxiety and improved mood, provides a different starting position for CBT, and the patient may be more able and motivated to comply with therapy, as was also described by Greenberg et al., and by Van Westen et al. in their qualitative study [16,17]. The question then is when to start CBT in case of partial response? Some clinicians routinely start after a certain period (e.g., after 8 or 12 weeks). Other clinicians start CBT when it is assumed that optimal stimulation settings have been achieved. Whereas this may be preferable in a research context, in order to separate the differential contribution of DBS and CBT to the response, clinically this is debatable. On one hand, reaching optimal stimulation settings may take a long time in many patients, which would lead to an unacceptable delay for therapy and loss of momentum; on the other hand, these patients have already experienced non-effective CBT and it is important to spare them another failure because of starting CBT to soon, as this would decrease their motivation for another attempt when stimulation parameters are optimal. One option is to assess the "readiness" for CBT, as mentioned above. Another option may be to look for improvement of cognitive measures that may increase the likelihood of successful CBT. A recent intervention study showed that the effect of VC/VS DBS is explained in part by enhancement of cognitive control by the prefrontal cortex. In this study, DBS improved the patients' performance on a cognitive control task and increases theta (5–8 Hz) oscillations in both medial and lateral PFC, which predicts the clinical outcome [25]. Perhaps such indicators could be made to clinical use and help to indicate the best time to start CBT after DBS.

4.3. Procedural Aspects

In the study by Denys et al., CBT/ERP consisted of 24 weekly individual face-to-face sessions of 60 min each, administered on an outpatient basis. Tyagi et al. provided CBT/ERP for 12 weeks on an in-patient basis in a neuropsychiatry unit. In both studies, the therapy was provided by the DBS clinic. This may be feasible in a research setting, but in routine clinical practice this will be more difficult to ask from patients once the DBS settings are optimized, given the distance that many of them will have to travel to the DBS clinic. Because of this, therapy is often organized in the region where the patient lives. However, whereas many behavioral therapists from local or regional psychiatric services may have experience in treating OCD patients, few will have experience treating OCD patients with DBS. In-patient treatment is one option to let patients benefit from the expertise of therapists of the DBS clinic, but this will be costly and may not be more effective than out-patient treatment. Another way of letting patients benefit from therapists with DBS experience is to explore novel ways of administering therapy, such as by telephone, videoconferencing or online.

In addition, other indications for CBT in the peri-operative period should also be considered. CBT could be administered with different objectives and if necessary, a different procedural approach. It could for instance already be started pre-operatively with the intent to enhance motivation for change post-operatively. Such pre-operative intervention has not been studied yet. Additionally, the content of the cognitive aspects of therapy could be adapted to address some issues specific to DBS, such as specific psychoeducational purposes related to DBS and preoccupation with stimulation settings. Moreover, after substantial improvement, low frequency long term continuation therapy may be helpful in preventing relapse.

4.4. Synthesis and Recommendations

Only two studies specifically address postoperative CBT. These used different stimulation targets and stimulation protocols, as well as different approaches to administering the therapy. Both studies suffer from a number of limitations, most importantly a small sample size, and the lack of a control condition for the CBT. In addition, the focus is strongly on obsessive and compulsive symptoms, whereas a focus on quality of life and general (social) functioning may be more important to the patient [26]. The other included studies mention postoperative CBT, but do not provide any details on effectiveness, timing and procedure.

DBS is not a stand-alone treatment for therapy-resistant OCD. After their operation, many patients continue to take medication for OCD, and/or receive some form of psychotherapy to deal with remaining symptoms or problems adjusting to the new situation. The overall treatment effect is the resultant of the DBS plus adjunctive therapies, and studies into the effectiveness of DBS should also take these concurrent treatments into account.

From a clinical point of view, there is a need for an evidence based algorithm for applying concomittant therapies, both psychotherapy as well as pharmacotherapy. As far as psychotherapy is concerned, there should be clear criteria as to when to start psychotherapy and the module should be adjusted to patients being treated with DBS. In our opinion, CBT should be started after a predefined level of clinical response to DBS, which is open for dicussion. The CBT module should address issues specific to DBS patients such as a changed personal identity due to being dependent on a device for symptom control and well-being, preoccupation with stimulation settings, and having to adjust to 'real life' after a long time of therapy-resistance and severe obsessive-compulsive behaviors that rendered typical family life, social contacts or employments unfeasible [27]. In order to let patients benefit from the experience of CBT therapists working in DBS clinics, other ways of administering CBT such as by telephone, videoconferencing or online, should also be developed and evaluated.

From a research point of view, future studies into the efficacy of DBS for OCD should follow a design that also allows the evaluation of the added effect of these concurrent treatments, and helps determining the place of these concurrent treatments in a treatment algorithm of OCD patients after DBS. This implies that there should be a control condition for CBT in order to assess the placebo response of CBT treatment. It also implies that sample size should be large enough to allow evaluation of the added treatment effects of CBT. Since it is unlikely that the required sample sizes will be achieved within a reasonable amount of time in a single DBS center, multicenter studies should be initiated. It is essential that collaborating centers not only protocolize their CBT treatment, but also that they align their clinical practice with respect to DBS with respect to stimulation target, strategies to optimize stimulation parameters and follow-up assessments. This would require a closer collaboration between DBS clinics on both a national and international level.

5. Conclusions

Preliminary findings show that postoperative CBT is effective as an add-on treatment to DBS in patients with therapy-resistent OCD. Further studies are necessary to establish the place of CBT after DBS. These studies should have larger sample sizes and designs that are adequate to quantify the added effects of both CBT as well as pharmacotherapy. In order to let patients benefit optimally from the experience and expertise of behavioral therapists working in DBS clinics, novel ways of administering CBT, such as administered by telephone, videoconferencing or online, should also be studied.

Supplementary Materials: The following are available online at http://www.mdpi.com/2077-0383/9/8/2383/s1, Table S1: Quality ratings of the included studies according to the Evidence Project risk of bias tool (Kennedy 2019).

Author Contributions: Conceptualization, A.F.G.L.; methodology, A.F.G.L.; formal analysis, M.G.; writing—original draft preparation, M.G.; writing—review and editing, T.B.v.d.V., K.S., L.A., M.P.; supervision, A.F.G.L. All authors have read and agreed to the published version of the manuscript.

Funding: This research received no external funding.

Conflicts of Interest: The authors declare no conflict of interest.

References

1. Heyman, I.; Mataix-Cols, D.; Fineberg, N.A. Obsessive-compulsive disorder. *BMJ* **2006**, *333*, 424–429. [CrossRef] [PubMed]
2. Vos, S.P.; Flaxman, A.D.; Naghavi, M.; Lozano, R.; Michaud, C.; Ezzati, M.; Shibuya, K.; Salomon, J.A.; Abdalla, S.; Aboyans, V.; et al. Years lived with disability (YLD) for 1160 sequelae 289 diseases and injuries 1990–210: A systematic analysis for the Global Burden of Disease Study 2010. *Lancet* **2012**, *380*, 2163–2196. [CrossRef]
3. Law, C.; Boisseau, C.L. Exposure and Response Prevention in the Treatment of Obsessive-Compulsive Disorder: Current Perspectives. *Psychol. Res. Behav. Manag.* **2019**, *12*, 1167–1174. [CrossRef] [PubMed]

4. Olatunji, B.O.; Davis, M.L.; Powers, M.B.; Smits, J.A. Cognitive-behavioral therapy for obsessive-compulsive disorder: A meta-analysis of treatment outcome and moderators. *J. Psychiatr. Res.* **2013**, *47*, 33–41. [CrossRef]
5. Leeuwerik, T.; Cavanagh, K.; Strauss, C. Patient adherence to cognitive behavioural therapy for obsessive-compulsive disorder: A systematic review and meta-analysis. *J. Anxiety Disord.* **2019**, *68*, 102135. [CrossRef]
6. Romanelli, R.J.; Wu, F.M.; Gamba, R.; Mojtabai, R.; Segal, J.B. Behavioral therapy and serotonin reuptake inhibitor pharmacotherapy in the treatment of obsessive-compulsive disorder: A systematic review and meta-analysis of head-to-head randomized controlled trials. *Depress. Anxiety* **2014**, *31*, 641–652. [CrossRef]
7. Denys, D. Pharmacotherapy of obsessive-compulsive disorder and obsessive-compulsive spectrum disorders. *Psychiatr. Clin. N. Am.* **2006**, *29*, 553–584. [CrossRef]
8. Kisely, S.; Hall, K.; Siskind, D.; Frater, J.; Olson, S.; Crompton, D. Deep brain stimulation for obsessive-compulsive disorder: A systematic review and meta-analysis. *Psychol. Med.* **2014**, *44*, 3533–3542. [CrossRef]
9. Abramowitz, J.S. *Understanding and Treating Obsessive-Compulsive Disorder: A Cognitive Behavioral Approach*; Lawrence Erlbaum Associates Publisher: Mahwah, NJ, USA, 2006.
10. Brakoulias, V.; Starcevic, V.; Albert, U.; Arumugham, S.S.; Bailey, B.E.; Belloch, A.; Borda, T.; Dell'Osso, L.; Elias, J.A.; Falkenstein, M.J.; et al. Treatments used for obsessive-compulsive disorder: An international perspective. *Hum. Psychopharmacol.* **2019**, *34*, e2686. [CrossRef]
11. Kennedy, C.E.; Fonner, V.A.; Armstrong, K.A.; Denison, J.A.; Yeh, P.T.; O'Reilly, K.R.; Sweat, M.D. The Evidence Project risk of bias tool: Assessing study rigor for both randomized and non-randomized intervention studies. *Syst. Rev.* **2019**, *8*, 3. [CrossRef]
12. Abelson, J.L.; Curtis, G.C.; Sagher, O.; Albucher, R.C.; Harrigan, M.; Taylor, S.F.; Martis, B.; Giordani, B. Deep brain stimulation for refractory obsessive-compulsive disorder. *Biol. Psychiatry* **2005**, *57*, 510–516. [CrossRef] [PubMed]
13. Denys, D.; Mantione, M.; Figee, M.; Van Den Munckhof, P.; Koerselman, F.; Westenberg, H.; Bosch, A.; Schuurman, R. Deep brain stimulation of the nucleus accumbens for treatment-refractory obsessive-compulsive disorder. *Arch. Gen. Psychiatr.* **2010**, *67*, 1061–1068. [CrossRef]
14. Mantione, M.; Nieman, D.H.; Figee, M.; Denys, D. Cognitive-behavioural therapy augments the effects of deep brain stimulation in obsessive-compulsive disorder. *Psychol. Med.* **2014**, *44*, 3515–3522. [CrossRef] [PubMed]
15. Tyagi, H.; Apergis-Schoute, A.M.; Akram, H.; Foltynie, T.; Limousin, P.; Drummond, L.M.; Fineberg, N.A.; Matthews, K.; Jahanshahi, M.; Robbins, T.W.; et al. A Randomized Trial Directly Comparing Ventral Capsule and Anteromedial Subthalamic Nucleus Stimulation in Obsessive-Compulsive Disorder: Clinical and Imaging Evidence for Dissociable Effects. *Biol. Psychiatr.* **2019**, *85*, 726–734. [CrossRef] [PubMed]
16. Greenberg, B.D.; Malone, D.A.; Friehs, G.M.; Rezai, A.R.; Kubu, C.S.; Malloy, P.F.; Salloway, S.P.; Okun, M.S.; Goodman, W.K.; Rasmussen, S.A. Three-year outcomes in deep brain stimulation for highly resistant obsessive-compulsive disorder. *Neuropsychopharmacology* **2006**, *31*, 2384–2393. [CrossRef] [PubMed]
17. Van Westen, M.; Rietveld, E.; Denys, D. Effective Deep Brain Stimulation for Obsessive-Compulsive Disorder Requires Clinical Expertise. *Front. Psychol.* **2019**, *10*, 2294. [CrossRef] [PubMed]
18. Guzick, A.; Hunt, P.J.; Bijanki, K.R.; Schneider, S.C.; Sheth, S.A.; Goodman, W.K.; Storch, E.A. Improving long term patient outcomes from deep brain stimulation for treatment-refractory obsessive-compulsive disorder. *Expert Rev. Neurother.* **2020**, *20*, 95–107. [CrossRef] [PubMed]
19. Tastevin, M.; Spatola, G.; Régis, J.; Lançon, C.; Richieri, R. Deep brain stimulation in the treatment of obsessive-compulsive disorder: Current perspectives. *Neuropsychiatr. Dis. Treat.* **2019**, *15*, 1259–1272. [CrossRef] [PubMed]
20. Bais, M.; Figee, M.; Denys, D. Neuromodulation in obsessive-compulsive disorder. *Psychiatr. Clin. N. Am.* **2014**, *37*, 393–413. [CrossRef]
21. Verbraak, M.J.P.M.; Hoogduin, C.A.L.; Methorst, G.J.; Arts, W.J.J.M.; Hansen, A.M.D.; Keijsers, G.P.J. Protocollaire behandeling van patiënten met een obsessieve-compulsieve stoornis: Exposure, responspreventie en cognitieve therapie. In *Protocollaire Behandelingen in de Ambulante Geestelijke Gezondheidszorg I*; Keijsers, G.P.J., van Minnen, A., Hoogduin, C.A.L., Eds.; Bohn Stafleu Van Loghum: Houten, The Netherlands, 2004; pp. 63–97.

22. Rughani, A.; Schwalb, J.M.; Sidiropoulos, C.; Pilitsis, J.; Ramirez-Zamora, A.; Sweet, J.A.; Mittal, S.; Espay, A.J.; Martinez, J.G.; Abosch, A.; et al. Congress of Neurological Surgeons Systematic Review and Evidence-Based Guideline on Subthalamic Nucleus and Globus Pallidus Internus Deep Brain Stimulation for the Treatment of Patients With Parkinson's Disease: Executive Summary. *Neurosurgery* **2018**, *82*, 753–756. [CrossRef]
23. Vicheva, P.; Butler, M.; Shotbolt, P. Deep Brain Stimulation for Obsessive-Compulsive Disorder: A Systematic Review of Randomised Controlled Trials. *Neurosci. Biobehav. Rev.* **2020**, *109*, 129–138. [CrossRef] [PubMed]
24. Mallet, L.; Polosan, M.; Jaafari, N.; Baup, N.; Welter, M.-L.; Fontaine, D.; Tezenas du Montcel, S.; Yelnik, J.; Chereau, I.; Arbus, C.; et al. Subthalamic nucleus stimulation in severe obsessive-compulsive disorder. *N. Engl. J. Med.* **2008**, *359*, 2121–2134. [CrossRef] [PubMed]
25. Widge, A.S.; Zorowitz, S.; Basu, I.; Paulk, A.C.; Cash, S.S.; Eskandar, E.N.; Deckerbach, T.; Miller, E.K.; Dougherty, D.D. Deep brain stimulation of the internal capsule enhances human cognitive control and prefrontal cortex function. *Nat. Commun.* **2019**, *10*, 1536. [CrossRef]
26. Ooms, P.; Mantione, M.; Figee, M.; Schuurman, P.R.; van den Munckhof, P.; Denys, D. Deep brain stimulation for obsessive-compulsive disorders: Long-term analysis of quality of life. *J. Neurol. Neurosurg. Psychiatr.* **2014**, *85*, 153–158. [CrossRef] [PubMed]
27. Horstkötter, D.; de Wert, G. Ethical considerations. In *Fundamentals and Clinics of Deep Brain Stimulation*; Temel, Y., Leentjens, A.F.G., de Bie, R.M.A., Chabardes, S., Fasasno, A., Eds.; Springer Nature: Cham, Switzerland, 2020; pp. 145–159.

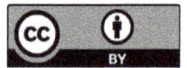

© 2020 by the authors. Licensee MDPI, Basel, Switzerland. This article is an open access article distributed under the terms and conditions of the Creative Commons Attribution (CC BY) license (http://creativecommons.org/licenses/by/4.0/).

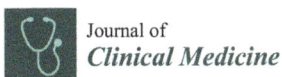

Review

The Cerebral Localization of Pain: Anatomical and Functional Considerations for Targeted Electrical Therapies

Rose M. Caston, Elliot H. Smith, Tyler S. Davis and John D. Rolston *

Department of Neurosurgery, University of Utah, Salt Lake City, UT 84106, USA; rose.caston@hsc.utah.edu (R.M.C.); e.h.smith@utah.edu (E.H.S.); tyler.davis@hsc.utah.edu (T.S.D.)
* Correspondence: john.rolston@hsc.utah.edu

Received: 13 May 2020; Accepted: 18 June 2020; Published: 22 June 2020

Abstract: Millions of people in the United States are affected by chronic pain, and the financial cost of pain treatment is weighing on the healthcare system. In some cases, current pharmacological treatments may do more harm than good, as with the United States opioid crisis. Direct electrical stimulation of the brain is one potential non-pharmacological treatment with a long history of investigation. Yet brain stimulation has been far less successful than peripheral or spinal cord stimulation, perhaps because of our limited understanding of the neural circuits involved in pain perception. In this paper, we review the history of using electrical stimulation of the brain to treat pain, as well as contemporary studies identifying the structures involved in pain networks, such as the thalamus, insula, and anterior cingulate. We propose that the thermal grill illusion, an experimental pain model, can facilitate further investigation of these structures. Pairing this model with intracranial recording will provide insight toward disentangling the neural correlates from the described anatomic areas. Finally, the possibility of altering pain perception with brain stimulation in these regions could be highly informative for the development of novel brain stimulation therapies for chronic pain.

Keywords: deep brain stimulation; closed loop; sensing; electrophysiology; neurophysiology; pain; thermal grill; imaging

1. Introduction

Pain is a unique and unorthodox sense. We reflexively respond to pain without being conscious of it, yet the conscious experience of pain can be overwhelming, debilitating, and chronic, depending on the cognitive, emotional, and allostatic context. Although the spinal reflexes mediate the rapid, unconscious avoidance of nociceptive stimuli, the experience of pain relies on the central nervous system's amplification and abstraction of nociception. In chronic pain, the healthy, adaptive relationship between experiential pain and nociception becomes disrupted. Pain-inducing contextual factors often replace pain-inducing nociception.

Two general categories of chronic hypersensitivity to pain exist. Allodynia is pain resulting from hypersensitivity to normal innocuous somatosensory (non-painful) stimuli. For example, pain resulting from brushing a hand with a feather [1]. Hyperalgesia is increased sensitivity, intensity, or duration of painful stimuli [1,2]. Both of these conditions can arise from hyperexcitability of the dorsal horn of the spinal cord (i.e., where pain fibers first synapse). However, it is thought these conditions may also be "centralized," presumably via inappropriate neuronal computations in a circuit comprised of the anterior cingulate cortex (ACC), insular cortex, and thalamus. For example, a burn can transiently cause a reduction of the pain threshold for mechanical stress, but the cognitive and affective elements of a burn can induce chronic hyperalgesia. Allodynia and hyperalgesia occur with spontaneous pain in chronic pain disorders.

Chronic and acute pain have sparked a growing interest in recent years. Chronic pain is widespread. In 2008, an estimated 100 million adults in the United States (U.S.) were affected by chronic pain. Total health care expenses attributable to pain, along with the amount associated with lower worker productivity, cost the U.S. between $560 and $635 billion per year [3]. This estimate is higher than the annual cost of heart disease ($309 billion), cancer ($243 billion), or diabetes ($188 billion) [3,4]. Pain treatment is complex and multidimensional, often involving medical providers, pain clinics, and state governments regulating narcotic drugs [5]. Narcotics, specifically opioids, are a poor treatment solution for two significant reasons—tolerance and lethality. Opioid use is associated with tolerance, as larger doses are required to achieve the same level of pain relief, yet high doses of opioids can be lethal. In 2016, 64,000 people died from drug overdoses in the U.S.—42,000 of those deaths were opioid related [6]. Opioids are not a viable long-term treatment for chronic pain. One potential solution is to design less systemic, more targeted interventions to disrupt pain signals within the brain, for example with electrical stimulation.

The use of intracranial electrical stimulation began in the mid-1900s, with the development of stereotactic frames. These devices enabled early psychologists/physiologists/psychiatrists to explore the effects before lesioning the areas of interest for a therapeutic effect [7]. Heath, a psychiatrist [8], implanted electrodes in schizophrenic patients to study the effects of intracranial stimulation. He discovered that electrical stimulation resulted in euphoria and analgesia, especially with stimulation of the septal area [9–14]. In 1954, deep brain stimulation (DBS) rat experiments alleviated pain with stimulation targeted to the septal nuclei, mammillothalamic tract, and cingulate cortex [14–16]. After these promising animal studies, stimulation of the human septum (intending to treat pain) proved less successful, with only one out of six patients with terminal cancer experiencing reduced pain [16,17].

The motivation to treat pain using electrical stimulation increased with the introduction of Melzack and Wall's gate theory in the 1960s [18,19]. Gate theory is the notion that non-painful inputs close nerve "gates" through the activation of Aβ fibers. Gate closure disrupts a painful input from traveling along signaling pathways to the central nervous system, a process that is the basis for spinal cord stimulation (SCS). SCS is currently approved by the U.S. Food and Drug Administration (FDA) to treat chronic pain of the trunk and limbs, intractable low back pain, leg pain, and pain from failed back surgery syndrome. In Europe, SCS is also approved for refractory angina pectoris and peripheral limb ischemia [20]. Success using SCS suggests that stimulation of other targets within the central nervous system may also modulate pain signaling. Positive results demonstrated by cortical stimulation support this. A recent pooled effect from 12 trials found motor cortex stimulation improves pain by 65.1% in postradicular plexopathy, 46.5% in trigeminal neuropathy, 35.2% after stroke, 34.1% in phantom limbs, and 29.8% in plexus avulsion [21]. Motor cortex stimulation works by affecting the activity in the thalamic nuclei and somatosensory regions. It modulates a vast network of structures, including the cerebellum, striatum, ventral posterolateral nucleus, and other thalamic areas. A more targeted approach is highly favorable to decrease the negative side effects associated with electrically stimulating all of these structures.

Whereas the path from Melzack and Wall's gate theory to present-day SCS is well defined, the path of DBS through the late 1900s meanders. After the disappointing results of septal DBS, studies continued on a wide array of potential anatomical brain targets in rodents and humans throughout the mid-to-late 1900s [22–28]. When studies translated from animals to human studies, they varied in electrode numbers, stimulation parameters, and anatomical targets, leading to inconsistent conclusions [17]. The FDA requested industry intervention to provide further data on safety and efficacy [14,29]. The first Medtronic study failed to show that half the patients had at least 50% pain relief [17]. The second trial failed because of a lack of enrollment (further details provided in Section 2). In 1989, the FDA rejected using DBS for chronic pain treatment [29].

To design safe and effective targeted therapies, such as DBS, it is critical to understand more about the circuits involved in pain processing in time and space and the potentially distributed nature of pain encoding in the human brain. The peripheral and spinal circuitry involved in pain is well characterized [30]. Here, we instead focus on the cerebral localization of pain networks, with an eye towards the development of targeted neurostimulation therapies for chronic pain [17]. The structures discussed in this review—such as the somatosensory cortex, thalamus, insula, and the ACC—consistently correlate with painful stimuli [17,31–34]. Neuroimaging studies routinely demonstrate activation in these areas, as shown in Figure 1 [35]. Therefore, we discuss the processing of conscious perception of pain in the cerebrum, the historical electrical stimulation of these regions, if pertinent, and the future application of DBS to modulate this activity.

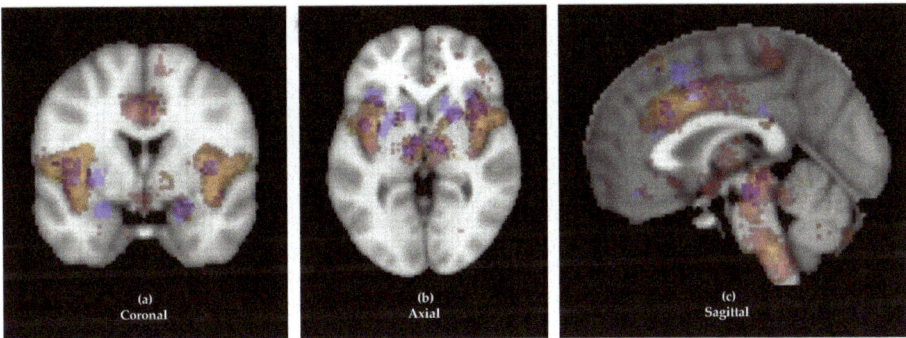

Figure 1. Overlay of three color-coded pain-related terms. "Chronic pain" is blue, "painful" is yellow, and "pain" is red. Functional magnetic resonance imaging (fMRI) studies of these terms are visualized in coronal (**a**), axial (**b**), and sagittal (**c**) axes from the Neurosynth database (neurosynth.org), showing consistent activation of the anterior cingulate cortex (ACC), thalamus, insula, and brainstem.

2. Anatomical Background

2.1. Somatosensory System and Relevant Inputs

Pain-sensing neurons, nociceptors, are pseudounipolar cells with somata, located in the dorsal root ganglion within the dorsal root of spinal nerves. Nociceptors were first described by Sherrington in 1906 [36]. Their afferent processes, either unmyelinated C fibers or myelinated Aδ fibers, project to peripheral tissues and typically end with free nerve endings capable of sensing painful mechanical or thermal stimuli. The efferent processes project to the thalamus, hypothalamus, and several midbrain areas, mainly via the contralateral anterolateral spinal cord. The disruption of information transmission along this tract via either surgical transection (first described by Spiller and Martin in 1912 [37]) or electrical stimulation has shown notable success in ameliorating some forms of chronic pain [38].

The descending pain modulatory pathway travels from the cerebrum to the ventrolateral periaqueductal gray (PAG) matter and rostral ventromedial medulla [39], and it projects to the dorsal horn of the spinal cord, as shown in Figure 2. The PAG matter in the brainstem contains bidirectional nociceptive pathways from medullary nuclei, allowing for modulation through both projections. As with other medullary nuclei, analgesia occurs via inhibitory serotonergic, enkephalin, mu-opioid, and GABA projections to the dorsal horn through descending pain control pathways. The other efferent nuclei from the medulla and pons appear to have a similar mechanism of analgesia. These are the same pathways thought to underlie opiate-induced analgesia [30]. Other notable efferents from the dorsal horn include the parabrachial nuclei, which project directly to the amygdala. The Kölliker-Fuse nucleus is found within the parabrachial nucleus and demonstrates noradrenergic descending inhibition [40]. Therefore, the parabrachial nuclei may be involved with salience or affective elements of pain [41,42].

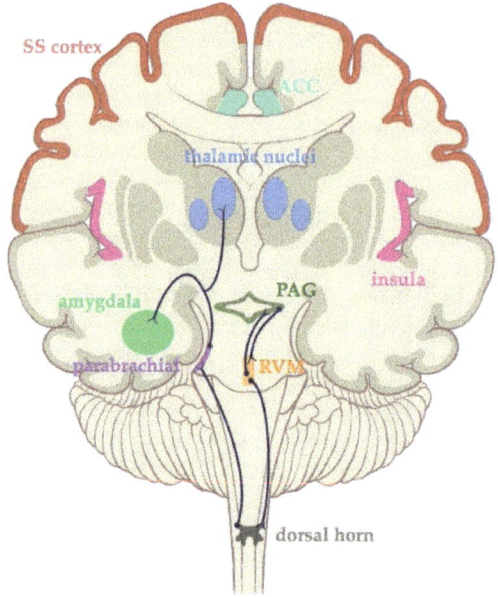

Figure 2. Descending pain modulatory pathway. The pathway originates in the cerebrum and descends to the periaqueductal gray (PAG) matter, rostral ventromedial medulla, and projects to the dorsal horn of the spinal cord. Bidirectional nociceptive pathways through the medullary nuclei are shown. The efferent pathway from the dorsal horn goes through the parabrachial nucleus, amygdala, and thalamic nuclei.

Nociceptive projections ascend through the PAG and then project to the thalamic nuclei, which have medial and lateral nuclear groups [43]. The lateral group, consisting of ventroposterior nuclei, has small receptive fields and projects to the somatosensory cortex. Circuits involving these nuclei are therefore likely responsible for the conscious identification and localization of painful stimuli. The medial group consists of the central lateral nucleus and intralaminar complex, which have widespread projections to the basal ganglia and cortex, and therefore likely mediate the arousal response to pain.

Following the disappointing results of septal stimulation in the 1960s, electrical stimulation of the PAG was tried in humans in the 1970s [16,17]. In one of the earliest studies on PAG stimulation, Richardson and Akil [26] reported on 30 patients with electrodes implanted for patient-controlled self-stimulation. Two thirds of the patients reported good outcomes (reduction in pain of >50%). Periventricular stimulation showed similar promise around the same time, with Hosobuchi et al. [28] showing pain relief in five of six patients. Young et al. [44] showed that stimulation of the Kölliker-Fuse subnucleus alone or in combination with stimulation in the PAG matter or the somatosensory thalamic nuclei provided self-reported "excellent" pain relief in three of six patients with intractable pain. Following these, and other promising early studies, were two negative randomized controlled trials involving Medtronic devices. One trial, based on the Model 3380 electrode, was discontinued after the first-generation production. The other trial involved the Model 3387 electrode. This clinical trial was stopped because of slow enrollment, high attrition, and low efficacy [29].

2.2. Thalamus

While the thalamus is like a relay station for nociceptive information, it also likely performs important computations on afferent nociceptive information. The most obvious way this could occur is by regulating cortical excitability via its activity or connectivity. Thalamic lesions in experimental animals seem to support this role, causing moderate changes in pain aversion behavior [45]. Correlative data from human subjects appear to accord with this role. Subjects with neuropathic pain had decreased blood oxygenation level–dependent activity and gray matter volume in the contralateral thalamus [46]. Furthermore, thalamic connectivity to the cortex is also reduced in patients with chronic pain, which may result in the reduced cortical gray matter [47,48].

A series of important papers on how human thalamic neurons are involved with pain were carried out by Lenz et al. in the 1980s and 1990s [49–54]. These included recording neuronal activity in the human principal sensory nucleus of the thalamus and microstimulating ventral thalamic neurons in patients undergoing implantation of DBS electrodes. Microstimulating [55,56] the human thalamic nucleus ventralis caudalis (Vc) in these patients caused acute thermal pain [51]. Neurons in the Vc also respond to specific types of painful stimuli in a graded fashion [50], which provides strong evidence that that pain information is organized somatotopically and by the type of nociceptor.

Even more importantly, some of these recordings were in patients experiencing chronic pain. The thalamic neurons in a patient with post-amputation deafferentation pain demonstrated bursting activity. Bipolar microstimulation of these neurons at 0.3 mA caused a burning pain, similar to the qualitative aspects of patients' chronic pain, although the location was different [49]. No sensations were describable at currents of 1.0 mA. Brief periods of stimulation with implanted chronic macroelectrodes caused a burning or tingling sensation with effective pain control for at least two years. Comparing thalamic recordings from multiple patients with amputations and control patients who were undergoing DBS for movement disorders showed a much larger thalamic homunculus than the corresponding region in these control patients. The same area also exhibited altered excitability [52]. These results further support the role of the thalamus in modulating excitability in the cortical pain network. Thalamic excitability and organization are related to chronic pain [53].

2.3. Insula

The insula has a cytoarchitectonically diverse organization based on posterior (*granular*), intermediate (*dysgranular*), and anterior (*agranular*) subdivisions. It is thought to encode sensation of the physiological condition for the entire body, which is known as interoception [31,57]. Craig et al. [31] showed the existence of 15 distinct cortical areas within the insula of long-tailed macaque monkeys (Macaca fascicularis) [31]. The architectonic map of the macaque insula is an important step towards understanding the connections and function of the insular cortex subareas. Recent models suggest interoceptive afferents are received in the posterior insula, processed by the intermediate insula, and then integrated for efferent autonomic regulation in the anterior insula [58].

A recent functional magnetic resonance imaging (fMRI) study suggested that the anterior insula, skin conductance, and pupil size encode a predictive model of pain. The anterior insula reflected the summed pain expectation and prediction errors from unexpected pain, while the posterior insula encoded pain intensity [59]. In subjects estimating pain intensity, fMRI activity during pain magnitude ratings was matched to that during visual magnitude ratings, to examine how pain perception is an assessment of stimulus intensity [60]. Posterior insular activity correlated with both the magnitude of the visual stimulus used in the task and pain intensity. Modality-specific pain estimation was located further anteriorly. The authors suggested this means pain perception within the insula results from the transformation of nociceptive information into subjective intensity assessment.

The insula is consistently included in circuits whose activity is correlated with pain perception. Some lesions of the insula result in a syndrome called pain asymbolia. In this condition, first described by Schilder in the 1930s, pain perception is intact, yet a patient's emotional response to pain is inappropriate [61]. Even though both the ACC and insula show elevated activity when viewing painful versus non-painful images [62], the symptoms resulting from insular lesions suggest the insula is more specifically involved in pain empathy. The organization of the insula lends itself to having both affective and somatosensory components. The ACC (discussed next) is likely more involved with affective processing, while the somatosensory cortex is more involved with sensory processing.

Widespread damage to the insula, obliterating its function, appears to increase experiential noxious pain perception and somatosensory activation ipsilateral to the lesion [63]. The insula may, therefore, help to suppress pain perception via specific inhibition of the somatosensory cortex.

Interestingly, the insula and the ACC both contain the highest concentrations of von Economo cells in the human brain. These are specialized cells with large cell bodies and axons that project to homeostatic regions in midbrain PAG and the parabrachial nucleus [64]. These cells are thought to mediate rapid social or behavioral inhibition, based on social or cognitive interoception. A recent study using patch clamp recordings of von Economo neurons demonstrated that they are regionally specific excitatory neurons [65]. The loss of these neurons is implicated in many neurological disorders and diseases. The insula and ACC are likely implicated in integrating general interoceptive information, among which pain information is distributed [32].

Direct electrical stimulation of the insula, as in epilepsy mapping, produces a variety of responses, including somatosensory, olfactory, thermal, auditory, and gustatory percepts [66]. Although early investigators, such as Penfield, failed to identify any evoked pain percepts by insular stimulation [33], more recent studies show pain responses from the insula at about 10% of sites. Systematic investigation may clarify the role of the insula in pain processing.

2.4. Anterior Cingulate Cortex

The ACC shows activation with pain, anxiety, and cognitive control, suggesting a role in responding to insults that are either corporeal or cognitive [67]. The ACC generally acts as a monitor that signals needed behavioral adjustments in response to corporeal or cognitive challenges [67,68]. In the late 1940s, frontal lobotomies were used to treat intractable pain and addiction with some success [69–71]. In the 1960s, Foltz and White [34] reported their experience performing cingulotomies (typically bilaterally) on 16 patients, for whom the affective components of chronic pain were particularly pronounced. The results were poor in only two of the 16 patients, although this was an early study lacking objective pain metrics. Intriguingly, the authors report that signs of opiate withdrawal were also lessened in these patients (14 of whom were "addicted") after cingulotomy. In 1988, Smith et al. [72] performed surgical cingulotomies on Sprague-Dawley rats, to investigate the role of the cingulate in stress-induced plasma beta-endorphin and morphine withdrawal. Beta-endorphin levels did not significantly increase after cingulotomy or postoperative induced stress, when each was tested independently. However, rat cingulotomy with postoperative induced stress caused a significant increase in plasma beta-endorphin concentrations. These findings suggested cingulum involvement in the regulation of the stress hormone response of beta-endorphin. More so, cingulotomy might be the cause of opiate withdrawal. A series of case reports and case series in humans followed this promising early work. A total of 13 case reports on cingulotomy were published prior to 2008—the majority before 1980 [73]. Results showed variable pain and opiate withdrawal improvements [73–75].

In the 1950s, attempts were made to electrically stimulate the ACC to treat chronic pain. Few effects were seen, most of which were adverse—such as speech arrest, vomiting, and tonic muscle contractions [76]. More recent studies using DBS with contemporary electrodes showed improved efficacy and reduced adverse effects [77,78]. For example, in the most extensive study to date using DBS to treat pain, Boccard et al. [79] found a significant 43% improvement on a numeric pain rating scale after six months. Improvements were also seen in other quality-of-life metrics, and on a general health scale. The cognitive and affective elements of chronic pain in these studies showed the most significant improvements, suggesting that ACC DBS may improve these aspects of chronic pain [80].

In comparison, a positive emission tomography (PET) study demonstrated that the ACC is activated during thalamic DBS in patients with chronic pain [55]. Together, these effects strongly implicate the dorsal ACC in processing affective components of pain; however, results about the directionality of cingulate effects are few and mixed. Recent studies have reported the essential nature of examining the temporal dynamics with which the ACC tracks internal cognitive state and induces cognitive control [74,81]. Improved understanding of the temporal dynamics of cingulate function relative to pain may be an important missing piece in understanding the cerebral localization of pain networks.

2.5. Beyond the Thalamus, Insula, and ACC

Other recent studies suggested that entirely different brain networks, engaged by the ACC, are responsible for pain regulation. Pain is understood to be a complex experience with sensory, cognitive, and emotional components [82]. Woo et al. [75] indicated that self-regulation of pain and the brain areas responsible for painful experiences are controlled by another circuit. The circuit consists of the genual and subgenual cingulate cortexes, the projections of the nucleus accumbens (NAc, involved in aversion, motivation, and reward valuation), and projections to the ventromedial prefrontal cortex. The suggested involvement of the cingulate is in the valuation of pain or weighting the context of painful stimuli, which preferentially projects to the NAc. A recent rodent study appears to support this mechanism of pain regulation [83]. In this study, the authors suggested that pain relief is associated with learning and motivation to seek environments associated with a relieved state. Endogenous opioid signaling in the rodent cingulate alters dopamine release in the NAc and pain avoidance behavior. Baliki et al. [84] also suggested a role for the NAc in pain valuation and analgesic potential. In this study, NAc activity in response to acute noxious thermal stimuli was compared in control and chronic back pain patients. At the acute noxious stimulus, normal subjects had positive phasic NAc activation, while chronic back pain patients demonstrated negative polarity phasic activity. The authors suggested the onset of acute pain relieved the chronic back pain, which was confirmed psychophysically. Mallory et al. [85] reported on sustained pain relief in a 72-year-old woman with a large right hemisphere infarct, who developed refractory left hemibody pain. Neither the NAc nor the PVG was successful in relieving pain when stimulated in isolation. The combined stimulation reduced the patient's pain from 10 to 0 at 11 months after surgery. The patient's post-stroke depression also stayed in remission. These results suggest the emotional aspects of pain can be treated quite well when stimulation involves the NAc.

Such a distributed organization of pain information makes large-scale electrical disruption of gray matter, such as that employed in cingulate DBS or cingulotomy, theoretically unlikely to provide the specificity required to disrupt pain without unintended side effects. These considerations motivate the use of white matter DBS of particular pain-associated tracts, such as the ventral internal capsule, along with the aggregates of grey matter involved in pain processing. It is also important to study the temporal dynamics of pain to determine whether there are temporal or frequency components unique to the development of chronic pain and various pain syndromes. This information may be used to determine when is the best time to modulate information processing in these areas to most effectively improve centralized chronic pain.

3. Temporal Dynamics of Pain

Studying the dynamic properties of pain perception is important for disentangling the neural correlates from the described anatomical areas that display a myriad of functions [86]. Few imaging studies have correlated fMRI signals with the temporal properties of pain [86–88]. An important consideration in studying the temporal dynamics of pain is that the time constants and activation functions of the various types of peripheral pain fibers are well characterized. The aforementioned unmyelinated C fibers transmit nociceptive information more slowly than myelinated Aδ fibers. These differences in conduction may resonate throughout the system in meaningful ways. As a psychophysical example, the discrimination of different painful sources (i.e., thermal, mechanical, chemical) becomes impossible with the loss of the rapidly conducting myelinated pain fibers. While these peripheral biophysics suggest that temporal dynamics may be necessary for understanding pain perception, studies have yet to use temporal properties of signals to study pain discrimination.

It is not clear to what extent, if any, temporal dynamics derived from the biophysics of peripheral sensors apply to chronic pain.

Electroencephalography (EEG) and magnetoencephalography (MEG) are the most readily available noninvasive methodologies to study high-temporal-resolution activity in the brain. EEG has been used to study acute responses to painful stimuli, mostly thermal pain evoked by lasers [89–92]. Laser-evoked pain has become the dominant psychophysical method for studying pain, because of safety, spatial precision, and how rapidly lasers turn on and off. The source localization of these responses also implicated the dorsal ACC and the insula [93,94]. It is not clear, however, to what extent these studies address the mechanisms underlying chronic pain. Studying chronic pain, per se, is fraught with numerous difficulties. Not only does chronic pain have various causes, but the expression of chronic pain in humans is heterogeneous. It is associated with varied bodily locations, triggers, and unpredictable responses to those triggers. Within chronic pain research, these complications are often simplified in animal models or very specific study populations. This limits the general applicability of results [95].

There have been few and mixed results of EEG studies of chronic pain. A recent meta-analysis of chronic pain EEG studies involved recording subjects during rest, sensory stimulation, and cognitive tasks and showed that subjects with chronic pain have elevated power in various regions across a range of frequencies [96]. Chronic pain was also associated with decreased evoked response amplitudes during cognitive tasks and sensory stimulation [96]. The dominant resting frequencies were typically lower than in healthy controls; however, the specific regions with power and the frequency changes were not consistent across studies. Increased resting frontal theta power was the most reproducible result in these studies. In one study, pathologically high theta power was localized to the insula, although this region is difficult to record with EEG [97]. Theta oscillations are associated with thalamocortical loops, so studies have attributed these oscillations to pathological integration of painful experience into normal circuits. As described, such pathological integration could be due to the regulation of excitability via tonic and burst firing modes in the thalamus. Altered dynamic ranges of frontal theta levels could represent chronic changes in thalamocortical networks.

Several studies have attempted to simulate chronic pain in the laboratory by elongating the duration of painful stimuli. Rhythmic or oscillatory responses to painful stimuli lasting up to tens of minutes in duration are consistently characterized by suppression of alpha- and beta-range power and increases in gamma power [98]. Perturbations of both the bottom-up (i.e., sensory) context and the top-down (i.e., attentional or cognitive) contexts consistently alter pain perception [99,100]. Furthermore, the oscillatory context is important for pain perception, as somatosensory alpha is negatively correlated with pain perception [101,102].

In one notable EEG study, painful tonic stimuli (10-min exposure) correlated with persistent frontocentral gamma power. The source localized to the dorsal ACC [98]. However, the reduction in beta oscillations that other studies have found was more posterior and determined to be correlated with the judgement of stimulus intensity. Such studies using long-duration painful stimuli suggest that the neural representation of pain changes with the duration of the painful experience. Apkarian et al. [103] showed that acute pain stimuli generally activate the somatosensory, insular, and cingulate cortical regions. Patients with chronic back pain had brain activity that localized to the medial prefrontal cortex and into the ACC, which was unique to the chronic pain patients. As the duration of the painful experience increases, fewer somatosensory regions are activated and there is more recruitment from limbic/affective/motivational regions. Their interpretation was that transient nociceptive activity, at some point, is converted into sustained emotional suffering. This result highlights the dynamic nature of chronic pain in time. How these dynamics evolve from the seconds–minutes domain of acute pain to the months and years of chronic pain is unknown, and they are important factors for delineating and treatment.

Finally, intracranial electrophysiological responses to acute painful stimuli in patients implanted with grid electrodes reproduced the changes in delta through beta power described in EEG studies [92,104]. Causal interactions were determined from local field potentials recorded during the response to a painful cutaneous laser stimulus. Cognitive pain control was related to information transfer between the ACC and somatosensory cortices [56,92]. These studies were only carried out in three patients and examined responses to brief thermal pain. Recording broadband high-frequency (e.g., high-gamma; ~70–200 Hz) local field potentials, which correlate with neuronal activity [105,106], yields an intriguing possibility of correlating pain network activity to neuronal populations with high temporal precision. Furthermore, the possibility of altering pain perception with brain stimulation could be highly informative for the development of DBS for chronic pain.

4. Pain Illusion Suggests Distinct Roles for the ACC and Insula in Chronic Pain

The "gate control theory" of pain was first described by Melzack and Wall in 1965 [21]; it implicated the relative activation and inhibition of areas in the ascending pain pathway [18]. This theory was sustained in part by studies using the thermal grill illusion (TGI). In the TGI, first discovered by Thunberg in 1896 [107], closely spaced alternating hot and cold stimuli—themselves non-painful—are perceived as painful when felt simultaneously. A three-dimensional rendering of a thermal grill interface constructed by our group is shown in Figure 3a. Each bar on the interface is programmable to a range of temperatures. Images captured with an infrared camera, shown in Figure 3b, demonstrate examples of the temperature arrangements acquired with our thermal grill interface. Since the 1890s, many explanations have been investigated to understand the physiological basis for perceived pain [107,108].

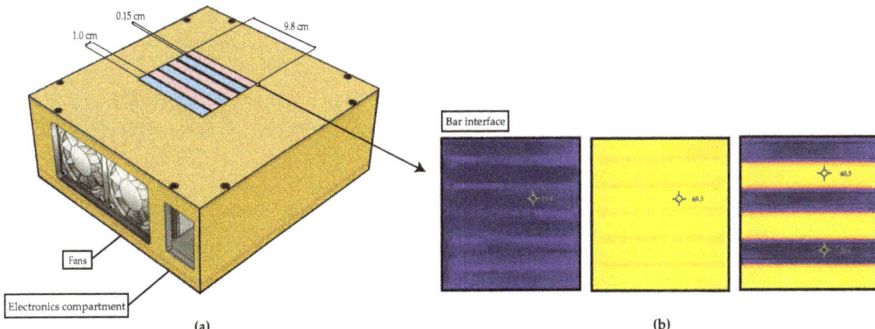

Figure 3. Rendering of a thermal grill interface and infrared images demonstrating patterns of warm and cool temperatures. Drawing (**a**) is representative of the interface that our group constructed. The top of the interface consists of six copper bars. Each bar is 1.0 cm in length and the bars are spaced 0.15 cm apart. The width of the six-bar interface is 9.8 cm. The electronic components fit inside the labeled compartment next to the fans, which allow for necessary air flow. Each bar is connected to a Peltier device, allowing for programmable temperature control (pink and blue coloring represents bars programmed to warm and cool temperatures, respectively). Infrared images acquired using the device are shown in (**b**). Left (**b**) shows all bars set to a cool temperature close to 20.0 °C. Middle (**b**) shows all bars set to a warm temperature close 40.0 °C. Right (**b**) shows one bar set at 20.0 °C and another bar near 40.0 °C. The alternating temperature setting is used to produce the pain illusion.

In 1994, Craig and Bushnell suggested that the integration of pain and temperature is the basis of cold-evoked, burning pain [107]. Although the mechanisms remain unclear, the underlying thermal stimuli are thought to inhibit each other, making way for summated nociceptive information without its accompanying somatosensory identity. A recent study in mice showed that the concurrent inhibition and excitation of polymodal channels provides the sensory code for warm perception [108].

Over time, the thermal grill has increased in popularity as a model for studying pain, because it induces neural activity that is perceived as burning pain without actually causing physical harm [109,110].

Clinical studies using the thermal grill have varied from evaluating perceived pain with surveys [111] to using fMRI [112] and PET [113] to evaluate structural involvement. Neuroimaging used in TGI studies suggests that hot or cold stimuli alone activate the insula and somatosensory cortex. Illusory pain from the TGI additionally activates the ACC [113]. The TGI produces a conscious perception of pain, perhaps unique to the ACC. Isolated thermal stimuli (either hot or cold) activate the insula and somatosensory cortex, demonstrating a dissociation between these regions and the cingulate. This further suggests separate roles for the areas involved in pain perception. Bouhassira et al. [114] and others [115,116] have reported that a subset of volunteers in thermal grill experiments are classified as poor or nonresponders. Bouhassira et al. defined these subjects based on not reporting at least one paradoxical painful sensation. There are a variety of reasons someone could be a nonresponder, such as anatomical differences due to calluses, prior injury, or variations in pain tolerance. Including poor-responding subjects in thermal grill experiments during intracranial recording will provide greater understanding of individual variations in pain processing.

Future studies using the thermal grill and neurophysiological data acquired with electroencephalography (ECoG) or stereoelectroencephalography (SEEG) will help to substantiate the temporal dynamics of pain perception. This experimental system may also provide data offering insight on the affective–motivational ("unpleasantness") and the discriminatory ("pain-intensity") aspects of pain [112]. Real-time acquisition from the thalamus, insula, and ACC may disentangle the complex relationship between these structures in pain processing. This groundwork will elucidate targets of electrical stimulation as a treatment for chronic pain.

5. Conclusions

Pain is a topic of great interest in the medical field because of the current opioid epidemic [6]. Medical providers in the 1990s trained with the establishment of "pain as the 5th vital sign" to improve the quality of patients' well-being [117]. Increasing pressure to treat pain was met with the availability to prescribe opioids. Although opioids interact with opioid receptors on nerves to block pain signaling, these drugs are problematic for a multitude of reasons, particularly tolerance and lethality. Future pain treatment modalities must be specific to pain but not as problematic for patients' quality of life as opioids have proven. We believe there is a viable target within the cerebrum based on the history of using DBS to treat pain; however, future work must systematically examine neural structures of interest, in space and time, to gain insight on how these networks interact.

We reviewed the evidence for the functional localization of the conscious perception of pain networks. Many of the gross anatomical correlates of pain are distributed and overlap with areas thought to be involved with interoception, affect, motivation, and cognition. This overlap motivates the need for novel approaches and techniques in understanding the neural mechanisms of pain [118]. The cerebral networks involved in pain are dynamic and distributed. Mapping these intracranial networks will require invasive neurosurgical techniques, such as ECoG and SEEG, to provide high-spatiotemporal-resolution recordings. We suggest that these techniques, in conjunction with the TGI, will provide information on the neurophysiological response of pain. Use of this system also allows for simultaneous qualitative pain evaluation. Further studies on pain intensity in conjunction with neural recordings in the insula, thalamus, and ACC will provide functional considerations for targeted electrical pain therapy in the future.

Author Contributions: Conceptualization, E.H.S., R.M.C., T.S.D., and J.D.R.; data acquisition (literature search and study selection), E.H.S. and R.M.C.; analysis and interpretation of data (literature), E.H.S. and R.M.C.; thermal grill construction, T.S.D. and R.M.C.; drafting of the manuscript, E.H.S. and R.M.C.; writing—review and editing the manuscript, R.M.C., E.H.S., T.S.D., and J.D.R. All authors have read and agreed to the published version of the manuscript.

Funding: Rolston receives NIH/NINDS K23 NS114178 funding. Smith is supported by a Young Investigator Grant from the "Brain and Behavior Research Foundation." The other authors have no personal, financial, or institutional interest in any of the drugs, materials, or devices described in this article.

Conflicts of Interest: The authors declare no conflict of interest.

References

1. Sandkühler, J. Models and Mechanisms of Hyperalgesia and Allodynia. *Physiol. Rev.* **2009**, *89*, 707–758. [CrossRef]
2. Jensen, T.S.; Finnerup, N. Allodynia and hyperalgesia in neuropathic pain: Clinical manifestations and mechanisms. *Lancet Neurol.* **2014**, *13*, 924–935. [CrossRef]
3. Gaskin, D.J.; Richard, P. The Economic Costs of Pain in the United States. *J. Pain* **2012**, *13*, 715–724. [CrossRef]
4. Institute of Medicine. *Relieving Pain in America: A Blueprint for Transforming Prevention, Care, Education, and Research*; The National Academies Press: Washington, DC, USA, 2011.
5. Unick, G.J.; Ciccarone, D. US regional and demographic differences in prescription opioid and heroin-related overdose hospitalizations. *Int. J. Drug Policy* **2017**, *46*, 112–119. [CrossRef]
6. Jones, M.R.; Viswanath, O.; Peck, J.; Kaye, A.D.; Gill, J.S.; Simopoulos, T.T. A Brief History of the Opioid Epidemic and Strategies for Pain Medicine. *Pain Ther.* **2018**, *7*, 13–21. [CrossRef]
7. Hariz, M.I.; Blomstedt, P.; Zrinzo, L. Deep brain stimulation between 1947 and 1987: The untold story. *Neurosurg. Focus* **2010**, *29*, E1. [CrossRef]
8. O'Neal, C.M.; Baker, C.M.; Glenn, C.A.; Conner, A.K.; Sughrue, M.E.; Robert, G. Heath: A controversial figure in the history of deep brain stimulation. *Neurosurg. Focus* **2017**, *43*, E12. [CrossRef]
9. Heath, R.G. ELECTRICAL SELF-STIMULATION OF THE BRAIN IN MAN. *Am. J. Psychiatry* **1963**, *120*, 571–577. [CrossRef]
10. Bishop, M.P.; Elder, S.T.; Heath, R.G.; Gottlieb, G. Intracranial Self-Stimulation in Man. *Science* **1963**, *140*, 394–396. [CrossRef]
11. Heath, R.G. Developments Toward New Physiologica Treatments in Psychiatry. *J. Neuropsychiatry* **1964**.
12. Heath, R.G. BRAIN FUNCTION AND BEHAVIOR. *J. Nerv. Ment. Dis.* **1975**, *160*, 159–175. [CrossRef]
13. Heath, R.G.; John, S.B.; Fontana, C.J. Stereotaxic Implantation of Electrodes in the Human Brain: A Method for Long-Term Study and Treatment. *IEEE Trans. Biomed. Eng.* **1976**, 296–304. [CrossRef]
14. Keifer, O.P.; Riley, J.P.; Boulis, N. Deep Brain Stimulation for Chronic Pain. *Neurosurg. Clin. N. Am.* **2014**, *25*, 671–692. [CrossRef]
15. Olds, J.; Milner, P.; James, O.; Peter, M. Positive reinforcement produced by electrical stimulation of septal area and other regions of rat brain. *J. Comp. Physiol. Psychol.* **1954**, *47*, 419–427. [CrossRef]
16. Gol, A. Relief of pain by electrical stimulation of the septal area. *J. Neurol. Sci.* **1967**, *5*, 115–120. [CrossRef]
17. Farrell, S.M.; Green, A.L.; Aziz, T.Z. The Current State of Deep Brain Stimulation for Chronic Pain and Its Context in Other Forms of Neuromodulation. *Brain Sci.* **2018**, *8*, 158. [CrossRef]
18. The gate control theory of pain. *BMJ* **1978**, *2*, 586–587. [CrossRef]
19. Melzack, R.; Wall, P.D. Pain Mechanisms: A New Theory. *Science* **1965**, *150*, 971–978. [CrossRef]
20. Song, J.J.; Popescu, A.; Bell, R.L. Present and potential use of spinal cord stimulation to control chronic pain. *Pain Physician* **2014**, *17*, 235–246.
21. Mo, J.-J.; Hu, W.-H.; Zhang, C.; Wang, X.; Liu, C.; Zhao, B.-T.; Zhou, J.-J.; Zhang, K. Motor cortex stimulation: A systematic literature-based analysis of effectiveness and case series experience. *BMC Neurol.* **2019**, *19*, 48. [CrossRef]
22. Mazars, G.; Mérienne, L.; Ciolocca, C. [Intermittent analgesic thalamic stimulation. Preliminary note]. *Rev. Neurol.* **1973**, *128*, 273–279. [PubMed]
23. Mark, V.H.; Ervin, F.R.; Hackett, T.P. Clinical Aspects of Stereotactic Thalamotomy in the Human. *Arch. Neurol.* **1960**, *3*, 351. [CrossRef]
24. Richardson, D.E.; Akil, H. Pain reduction by electrical brain stimulation in man. II. *J. Neurosurg.* **1977**, *47*, 184–194. [CrossRef]
25. Richardson, D.E.; Akil, H. Pain reduction by electrical brain stimulation in man. I. *J. Neurosurg.* **1977**, *47*, 178–183. [CrossRef] [PubMed]
26. E Richardson, D.; Akil, H. Long term results of periventricular gray self-stimulation. *Neurosurgery* **1977**, *1*, 199. [CrossRef] [PubMed]
27. Mayer, D.J.; Wolfle, T.L.; Akil, H.; Carder, B.; Liebeskind, J.C. Analgesia from Electrical Stimulation in the Brainstem of the Rat. *Science* **1971**, *174*, 1351–1354. [CrossRef] [PubMed]
28. Hosobuchi, Y.; Adams, J.; Linchitz, R. Pain relief by electrical stimulation of the central gray matter in humans and its reversal by naloxone. *Science* **1977**, *197*, 183–186. [CrossRef] [PubMed]

29. Coffey, R.J. Deep Brain Stimulation for Chronic Pain: Results of Two Multicenter Trials and a Structured Review. *Pain Med.* **2001**, *2*, 183–192. [CrossRef] [PubMed]
30. Kandel, E.; Schwartz, J.; Jessell, T.; Siegelbaum, S.; Hudspeth, A. *Principles of Neural Science*, 5th ed.; McGraw-Hill Ed: New York, NY, USA, 2013.
31. Evrard, H.C.; Logothetis, N.K.; Craig, A. (Bud) Modular architectonic organization of the insula in the macaque monkey. *J. Comp. Neurol.* **2013**, *522*, 64–97. [CrossRef]
32. Evrard, H.C.; Forro, T.; Logothetis, N.K. Von Economo Neurons in the Anterior Insula of the Macaque Monkey. *Neuron* **2012**, *74*, 482–489. [CrossRef]
33. Penfield, W.; Faulk, M.E. THE INSULA. *Brain* **1955**, *78*, 445–470. [CrossRef] [PubMed]
34. Foltz, E.L.; White, L.E. Pain "Relief" by Frontal Cingulumotomy. *J. Neurosurg.* **1962**, *19*, 89–100. [CrossRef] [PubMed]
35. Yarkoni, T. Neurosynth. Available online: http://neurosynth.org/ (accessed on 11 March 2020).
36. Freeman, R.B.F.N. The Integrative Action of the Nervous System. *J. Philos. Psychol. Sci. Methods* **1907**, *4*, 301. [CrossRef]
37. Spiller, W.G. The treatment of persistent pain of organic origin in the lower part of the body by division of the anterolateral column of the spinal cord. *J. Am. Med Assoc.* **1912**, 1489–1490. [CrossRef]
38. Vallejo, R.; Bradley, K.; Kapural, L. Spinal Cord Stimulation in Chronic Pain. *Spine* **2017**, *42*, S53–S60. [CrossRef] [PubMed]
39. Lueptow, L.; Fakira, A.; Bobeck, E. The Contribution of the Descending Pain Modulatory Pathway in Opioid Tolerance. *Front. Mol. Neurosci.* **2018**, *12*, 886. [CrossRef]
40. Hodge, C.J.; Apkarian, A.V.; Stevens, R.T. Inhibition of dorsal-horn cell responses by stimulation of the Kölliker-Fuse nucleus. *J. Neurosurg.* **1986**, *65*, 825–833. [CrossRef]
41. Palmiter, R. The Parabrachial Nucleus: CGRP Neurons Function as a General Alarm. *Trends Neurosci.* **2018**, *41*, 280–293. [CrossRef] [PubMed]
42. Roeder, Z.; Chen, Q.; Davis, S.; Carlson, J.D.; Tupone, D.; Heinricher, M.M. Parabrachial complex links pain transmission to descending pain modulation. *Pain* **2016**, *157*, 2697–2708. [CrossRef] [PubMed]
43. Craig, A.D.; Bushnell, M.C.; Zhang, E.-T.; Blomqvist, A. A thalamic nucleus specific for pain and temperature sensation. *Nature* **1994**, *372*, 770–773. [CrossRef] [PubMed]
44. Young, R.F.; Rinaldi, P.C. Chronic Stimulation of the Koelliker-Fuse Nucleus Region for Relief of Intractable Pain in Humans. *J. Neurosurg.* **1992**, *76*, 979–985. [CrossRef]
45. Yen, C.-T.; Lu, P.-L. Thalamus and pain. *Acta Anaesthesiol. Taiwanica* **2013**, *51*, 73–80. [CrossRef]
46. Gustin, S.; Peck, C.C.; Wilcox, S.L.; Nash, P.G.; Murray, G.M.; Henderson, L.A. Different Pain, Different Brain: Thalamic Anatomy in Neuropathic and Non-Neuropathic Chronic Pain Syndromes. *J. Neurosci.* **2011**, *31*, 5956–5964. [CrossRef] [PubMed]
47. Apkarian, A.V.; Sosa, Y.; Sonty, S.; Levy, R.M.; Harden, R.N.; Parrish, T.B.; Gitelman, D. Chronic Back Pain Is Associated with Decreased Prefrontal and Thalamic Gray Matter Density. *J. Neurosci.* **2004**, *24*, 10410–10415. [CrossRef] [PubMed]
48. DaSilva, A.F.; Becerra, L.; Pendse, G.; Chizh, B.; Tully, S.; Borsook, D. Colocalized Structural and Functional Changes in the Cortex of Patients with Trigeminal Neuropathic Pain. *PLoS ONE* **2008**, *3*, e3396. [CrossRef] [PubMed]
49. Lenz, F.A.; Tasker, R.R.; Dostrovsky, J.O.; Kwan, H.C.; Gorecki, J.; Hirayama, T.; Murphy, J.T. Abnormal single-unit activity recorded in the somatosensory thalamus of a quadriplegic patient with central pain. *Pain* **1987**, *31*, 225–236. [CrossRef]
50. Lenz, F.A.; Gracely, R.H.; Rowland, L.H.; Dougherty, P.M. A population of cells in the human thalamic principal sensory nucleus respond to painful mechanical stimuli. *Neurosci. Lett.* **1994**, *180*, 46–50. [CrossRef]
51. Lenz, F.A.; Seike, M.; Lin, Y.; Baker, F.; Rowland, L.; Gracely, R.; Richardson, R. Neurons in the area of human thalamic nucleus ventralis caudalis respond to painful heat stimuli. *Brain Res.* **1993**, *623*, 235–240. [CrossRef]
52. Lenz, F.; Garonzik, I.; Zirh, T.; Dougherty, P.M. Neuronal activity in the region of the thalamic principal sensory nucleus (ventralis caudalis) in patients with pain following amputations. *Neuroscience* **1998**, *86*, 1065–1081. [CrossRef]
53. Lenz, F.A.; Kwan, H.C.; Dostrovsky, J.O.; Tasker, R.R. Characteristics of the bursting pattern of action potentials that occurs in the thalamus of patients with central pain. *Brain Res.* **1989**, *496*, 357–360. [CrossRef]

54. Lenz, F.; Gracely, R.; Romanoski, A.; Hope, E.; Rowland, L.; Dougherty, P.M. Stimulation in the human somatosensory thalamus can reproduce both the affective and sensory dimensions of previously experienced pain. *Nat. Med.* **1995**, *1*, 910–913. [CrossRef] [PubMed]
55. Davis, K.D.; Taub, E.; Duffner, F.; Lozano, A.M.; Tasker, R.R.; Houle, S.; Dostrovsky, J.O. Activation of the anterior cingulate cortex by thalamic stimulation in patients with chronic pain: A positron emission tomography study. *J. Neurosurg.* **2000**, *92*, 64–69. [CrossRef] [PubMed]
56. Ohara, S.; Crone, N.E.; Weiss, N.; Lenz, F.A. Analysis of synchrony demonstrates 'pain networks' defined by rapidly switching, task-specific, functional connectivity between pain-related cortical structures. *Pain* **2006**, *123*, 244–253. [CrossRef] [PubMed]
57. Craig, A.D. How do you feel? Interoception: The sense of the physiological condition of the body. *Nat. Rev. Neuroscience* **2002**, *3*, 655–666. [CrossRef]
58. Evrard, H.C. The Organization of the Primate Insular Cortex. *Front. Neuroanat.* **2019**, *13*, 43. [CrossRef]
59. Geuter, S.; Boll, S.; Eippert, F.; Büchel, C. Functional dissociation of stimulus intensity encoding and predictive coding of pain in the insula. *eLife* **2017**, *6*. [CrossRef]
60. Baliki, M.N.; Geha, P.Y.; Apkarian, A.V. Parsing Pain Perception Between Nociceptive Representation and Magnitude Estimation. *J. Neurophysiol.* **2009**, *101*, 875–887. [CrossRef]
61. Schilder, P. Notes on The Psychopathology of Pain in Neuroses and Psychoses. *Psychoanal. Rev.* **1931**, *18*, 1–22.
62. Gu, X.; Liu, X.; Guise, K.G.; Naidich, T.P.; Hof, P.R.; Fan, J. Functional dissociation of the frontoinsular and anterior cingulate cortices in empathy for pain. *J. Neurosci.* **2010**, *30*, 3739–3744. [CrossRef]
63. Starr, C.J.; Sawaki, L.; Wittenberg, G.F.; Burdette, J.H.; Oshiro, Y.; Quevedo, A.; Coghill, R.C. Roles of the insular cortex in the modulation of pain: Insights from brain lesions. *J. Neurosci.* **2009**, *29*, 2684–2694. [CrossRef]
64. Saleh, T.; Logothetis, N.; Evrard, H. Insular projections to brainstem homeostatic centers in the macaque monkey. *Front. Mol. Neurosci.* **2017**, *11*, 11. [CrossRef]
65. Hodge, R.D.; Miller, J.A.; Novotny, M.; Kalmbach, B.E.; Ting, J.T.; Bakken, T.E.; Aevermann, B.D.; Barkan, E.R.; Berkowitz-Cerasano, M.L.; Cobbs, C.; et al. Transcriptomic evidence that von Economo neurons are regionally specialized extratelencephalic-projecting excitatory neurons. *Nat. Commun.* **2020**, *11*, 1172. [CrossRef] [PubMed]
66. Mazzola, L.; Lopez, C.; Faillenot, I.; Chouchou, F.; Mauguière, F.; Isnard, J. Vestibular responses to direct stimulation of the human insular cortex. *Ann. Neurol.* **2014**, *76*, 609–619. [CrossRef]
67. Cavanagh, J.F.; Shackman, A.J. Frontal midline theta reflects anxiety and cognitive control: Meta-analytic evidence. *J. Physiol.* **2014**, *109*, 3–15. [CrossRef] [PubMed]
68. Shenhav, A.; Botvinick, M.M.; Cohen, J.D. The expected value of control: An integrative theory of anterior cingulate cortex function. *Neuron* **2013**, *79*, 217–240. [CrossRef]
69. Lewin, W. OBSERVATIONS ON SELECTIVE LEUCOTOMY. *J. Neurol. Neurosurg. Psychiatry* **1961**, *24*, 37–44. [CrossRef]
70. E Scarff, J. Unilateral prefrontal lobotomy for the relief of intractable pain and termination of narcotic addiction. *Surgery, Gynecol. Obstet.* **1949**, *89*, 385–392.
71. Watts, J.W.; Freeman, W. Frontal lobotomy in the treatment of unbearable pain. *Res. Publ. Assoc. Res. Nerv. Ment. Dis.* **1949**, *27*, 715–722.
72. Smith, G.C.; Willis, G.L.; Copolow, A.L.; Recher, H.; Roller, L. Cingulotomy in the rat fails to block opiate withdrawal effects but elevates stress-induced plasma beta-endorphin. *Prog. Neuro-Psychopharmacol. Boil. Psychiatry* **1988**, *12*, 683–688. [CrossRef]
73. Cetas, J.S.; Saedi, T.; Burchiel, K.J. Destructive procedures for the treatment of nonmalignant pain: A structured literature review. *J. Neurosurg.* **2008**, *109*, 389–404. [CrossRef] [PubMed]
74. Smith, E.H.; Banks, G.; Mikell, C.B.; Cash, S.S.; Patel, S.R.; Eskandar, E.N.; Sheth, S.A. Frequency-Dependent Representation of Reinforcement-Related Information in the Human Medial and Lateral Prefrontal Cortex. *J. Neurosci.* **2015**, *35*, 15827–15836. [CrossRef] [PubMed]
75. Woo, C.-W.; Roy, M.; Buhle, J.T.; Wager, T.D. Distinct Brain Systems Mediate the Effects of Nociceptive Input and Self-Regulation on Pain. *PLoS Boil.* **2015**, *13*, e1002036. [CrossRef] [PubMed]
76. Lewin, W.; Whitty, C.W.M. Effects of anterior cingulate stimulation in conscious human subjects. *J. Neurophysiol.* **1960**, *23*, 445–447. [CrossRef] [PubMed]

77. Boccard-Binet, S.; Pereira, E.; Moir, L.; Van Hartevelt, T.; Kringelbach, M.L.; Fitzgerald, J.J.; Baker, I.W.; Green, A.L.; Aziz, T.Z. Deep brain stimulation of the anterior cingulate cortex. *NeuroReport* **2014**, *25*, 83–88. [CrossRef]
78. Spooner, J.; Yu, H.; Kao, C.; Sillay, K.; Konrad, P. Neuromodulation of the cingulum for neuropathic pain after spinal cord injury. *J. Neurosurg.* **2007**, *107*, 169–172. [CrossRef]
79. Boccard-Binet, S.; Prangnell, S.J.; Pycroft, L.; Cheeran, B.; Moir, L.; Pereira, E.; Fitzgerald, J.J.; Green, A.L.; Aziz, T.Z. Long-Term Results of Deep Brain Stimulation of the Anterior Cingulate Cortex for Neuropathic Pain. *World Neurosurg.* **2017**, *106*, 625–637. [CrossRef]
80. Russo, J.F.; Sheth, S.A. Deep brain stimulation of the dorsal anterior cingulate cortex for the treatment of chronic neuropathic pain. *Neurosurg. Focus* **2015**, *38*, E11. [CrossRef]
81. Smith, E.H.; Horga, G.; Yates, M.J.; Mikell, C.B.; Banks, G.P.; Pathak, Y.J.; Schevon, C.A.; McKhann, G.M.; Hayden, B.Y.; Botvinick, M.M.; et al. Widespread temporal coding of cognitive control in the human prefrontal cortex. *Nat. Neurosci.* **2019**, *22*, 1883–1891. [CrossRef]
82. Oluigbo, C.O.; Salma, A.; Rezai, A.R. Targeting the affective and cognitive aspects of chronic neuropathic pain using basal forebrain neuromodulation: Rationale, review and proposal. *J. Clin. Neurosci.* **2012**, *19*, 1216–1221. [CrossRef]
83. Navratilova, E.; Xie, J.Y.; Meske, D.; Qu, C.; Morimura, K.; Okun, A.; Arakawa, N.; Ossipov, M.; Fields, H.L.; Porreca, F. Endogenous opioid activity in the anterior cingulate cortex is required for relief of pain. *J. Neurosci.* **2015**, *35*, 7264–7271. [CrossRef]
84. Baliki, M.N.; Geha, P.Y.; Fields, H.L.; Apkarian, A.V. Predicting Value of Pain and Analgesia: Nucleus Accumbens Response to Noxious Stimuli Changes in the Presence of Chronic Pain. *Neuron* **2010**, *66*, 149–160. [CrossRef]
85. Mallory, G.W.; Abulseoud, O.; Hwang, S.-C.; Gorman, D.A.; Stead, S.M.; Klassen, B.T.; Sandroni, P.; Watson, J.C.; Lee, K.H. The Nucleus Accumbens as a Potential Target for Central Poststroke Pain. *Mayo Clin. Proc.* **2012**, *87*, 1025–1031. [CrossRef] [PubMed]
86. Davis, K.D.; Pope, G.; Crawley, A.; Mikulis, D. Neural correlates of prickle sensation: A percept-related fMRI study. *Nat. Neurosci.* **2002**, *5*, 1121–1122. [CrossRef]
87. Gao, C.; Gao, H.; Zhang, Q. Event-related brain potentials related to the identification of different types of signs. *NeuroReport* **2019**, *30*, 269–273. [CrossRef]
88. Porro, C.; Cettolo, V.; Francescato, M.P.; Baraldi, P. Temporal and intensity coding of pain in human cortex. *J. Neurophysiol.* **1998**, *80*, 3312–3320. [CrossRef] [PubMed]
89. Arendt-Nielsen, L.; Chen, A. Lasers and other thermal stimulators for activation of skin nociceptors in humans. *Neurophysiol. Clin. Neurophysiol.* **2003**, *33*, 259–268. [CrossRef] [PubMed]
90. Roberts, K.; Papadaki, A.; Gonçalves, C.; Tighe, M.; Atherton, D.; Shenoy, R.; McRobbie, D.W.; Anand, P. Contact heat evoked potentials using simultaneous EEG and fMRI and their correlation with evoked pain. *BMC Anesthesiol.* **2008**, *8*, 8. [CrossRef] [PubMed]
91. Liu, C.-C.; Ohara, S.; Franaszczuk, P.J.; Lenz, F.A. Attention to painful cutaneous laser stimuli evokes directed functional connectivity between activity recorded directly from human pain-related cortical structures. *Pain* **2011**, *152*, 664–675. [CrossRef] [PubMed]
92. Liu, C.-C.; Ohara, S.; Franaszczuk, P.J.; Crone, N.E.; Lenz, F.A. Attention to painful cutaneous laser stimuli evokes directed functional interactions between human sensory and modulatory pain-related cortical areas. *Pain* **2011**, *152*, 2781–2791. [CrossRef]
93. Garcia-Larrea, L.; Frot, M.; Valeriani, M. Brain generators of laser-evoked potentials: From dipoles to functional significance. *Neurophysiol. Clin. Neurophysiol.* **2003**, *33*, 279–292. [CrossRef]
94. Lorenz, J.; Garcia-Larrea, L. Contribution of attentional and cognitive factors to laser evoked brain potentials. *Neurophysiol. Clin. Neurophysiol.* **2003**, *33*, 293–301. [CrossRef]
95. Mao, J. Current challenges in translational pain research. *Trends Pharmacol. Sci.* **2012**, *33*, 568–573. [CrossRef]
96. Pinheiro, E.S.D.S.; De Queirós, F.C.; Montoya, P.; Santos, C.L.; Nascimento, M.A.D.; Ito, C.H.; Silva, M.; Santos, D.B.N.; Benevides, S.; Miranda, J.G.V.; et al. Electroencephalographic Patterns in Chronic Pain: A Systematic Review of the Literature. *PLoS ONE* **2016**, *11*, e0149085. [CrossRef]
97. Stern, C.; Passingham, R. The nucleus accumbens in monkeys (Macaca fascicularis). *Exp. Brain Res.* **1995**, *106*, 239–247. [CrossRef]

98. Schulz, E.; May, E.S.; Postorino, M.; Tiemann, L.; Nickel, M.; Witkovský, V.; Schmidt, P.; Gross, J.; Ploner, M. Prefrontal Gamma Oscillations Encode Tonic Pain in Humans. *Cereb. Cortex* **2015**, *25*, 4407–4414. [CrossRef] [PubMed]
99. Hauck, M.; Domnick, C.; Lorenz, J.; Gerloff, C.; Engel, A.K. Top-down and bottom-up modulation of pain-induced oscillations. *Front. Hum. Neurosci.* **2015**, *9*, 9. [CrossRef]
100. Ploner, M.; Gross, J.; Timmermann, L.; Pollok, B.; Schnitzler, A. Pain Suppresses Spontaneous Brain Rhythms. *Cereb. Cortex* **2005**, *16*, 537–540. [CrossRef] [PubMed]
101. Babiloni, C.; Brancucci, A.; Del Percio, C.; Capotosto, P.; Arendt-Nielsen, L.; Chen, A.C.; Rossini, P.M. Anticipatory Electroencephalography Alpha Rhythm Predicts Subjective Perception of Pain Intensity. *J. Pain* **2006**, *7*, 709–717. [CrossRef] [PubMed]
102. Tu, Y.; Zhang, Z.; Tan, A.; Peng, W.; Hung, Y.S.; Moayedi, M.; Iannetti, G.; Hu, L. Alpha and gamma oscillation amplitudes synergistically predict the perception of forthcoming nociceptive stimuli. *Hum. Brain Mapp.* **2015**, *37*, 501–514. [CrossRef]
103. Apkarian, A.V.; Hashmi, J.A.; Baliki, M.N. Pain and the brain: Specificity and plasticity of the brain in clinical chronic pain. *Pain* **2010**, *152*, S49–S64. [CrossRef]
104. Liu, C.C.; Franaszczuk, P.J.; Crone, N.E.; Jouny, C.; Lenz, F.A. Studies of properties of "Pain Networks" as predictors of targets of stimulation for treatment of pain. *Front. Integr. Neurosci.* **2011**, *5*. [CrossRef] [PubMed]
105. Manning, J.R.; Jacobs, J.; Fried, I.; Kahana, M.J. Broadband shifts in local field potential power spectra are correlated with single-neuron spiking in humans. *J. Neurosci.* **2009**, *29*, 13613–13620. [CrossRef] [PubMed]
106. Miller, K.J. Broadband spectral change: Evidence for a macroscale correlate of population firing rate? *J. Neurosci.* **2010**, *30*, 6477–6479. [CrossRef]
107. Craig, A.; Bushnell, M. The thermal grill illusion: Unmasking the burn of cold pain. *Science* **1994**, *265*, 252–255. [CrossRef] [PubMed]
108. Paricio-Montesinos, R.; Schwaller, F.; Udhayachandran, A.; Rau, F.; Walcher, J.; Evangelista, R.; Vriens, J.; Voets, T.; Poulet, J.F.; Lewin, G.R. The Sensory Coding of Warm Perception. *Neuron* **2020**, *106*, 830–841.e3. [CrossRef]
109. Fardo, F.; Beck, B.; Allen, M.; Finnerup, N.B. Beyond labeled lines: A population coding account of the thermal grill illusion. *Neurosci. Biobehav. Rev.* **2020**, *108*, 472–479. [CrossRef]
110. Kammers, M.; De Vignemont, F.; Haggard, P. Cooling the Thermal Grill Illusion through Self-Touch. *Curr. Boil.* **2010**, *20*, 1819–1822. [CrossRef]
111. Patwardhan, S.; Kawazoe, A.; Kerr, D.; Nakatani, M.; Visell, Y. Dynamics and Perception in the Thermal Grill Illusion. *IEEE Trans. Haptics* **2019**, *12*, 604–614. [CrossRef] [PubMed]
112. Lindstedt, F.; Johansson, B.; Martinsen, S.; Kosek, E.; Fransson, P.; Ingvar, M. Evidence for Thalamic Involvement in the Thermal Grill Illusion: An fMRI Study. *PLoS ONE* **2011**, *6*, e27075. [CrossRef]
113. Craig, A.; Reiman, E.M.; Evans, A.; Bushnell, M.C. Functional imaging of an illusion of pain. *Nature* **1996**, *384*, 258–260. [CrossRef]
114. Bouhassira, D.; Kern, D.; Rouaud, J.; Pelle-Lancien, E.; Morain, F. Investigation of the paradoxical painful sensation ('illusion of pain') produced by a thermal grill. *Pain* **2005**, *114*, 160–167. [CrossRef]
115. Adam, F.; Alfonsi, P.; Kern, D.; Bouhassira, D. Relationships between the paradoxical painful and nonpainful sensations induced by a thermal grill. *Pain* **2014**, *155*, 2612–2617. [CrossRef] [PubMed]
116. Hunter, J.; Dranga, R.; Van Wyk, M.; Dostrovsky, J. Unique influence of stimulus duration and stimulation site (glabrous vs. hairy skin) on the thermal grill-induced percept. *Eur. J. Pain* **2014**, *19*, 202–215. [CrossRef] [PubMed]
117. Levy, N.; Sturgess, J.; Mills, P. "Pain as the fifth vital sign" and dependence on the "numerical pain scale" is being abandoned in the US: Why? *Br. J. Anaesth.* **2018**, *120*, 435–438. [CrossRef] [PubMed]
118. Seymour, B. Pain: A Precision Signal for Reinforcement Learning and Control. *Neuron* **2019**, *101*, 1029–1041. [CrossRef] [PubMed]

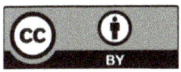 © 2020 by the authors. Licensee MDPI, Basel, Switzerland. This article is an open access article distributed under the terms and conditions of the Creative Commons Attribution (CC BY) license (http://creativecommons.org/licenses/by/4.0/).

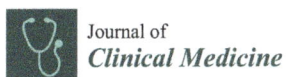

Review

A Deep Brain Stimulation Trial Period for Treating Chronic Pain

Prasad Shirvalkar [1,2,3,*], Kristin K. Sellers [2], Ashlyn Schmitgen [2], Jordan Prosky [1], Isabella Joseph [2], Philip A. Starr [2] and Edward F. Chang [2]

1. Department of Anesthesiology (Pain Management), University of California San Francisco, San Francisco, CA 94143, USA; Jordan.Prosky@ucsf.edu
2. Department of Neurological Surgery, University of California San Francisco, San Francisco, CA 94143, USA; Kristin.Sellers@ucsf.edu (K.K.S.); Ashlyn.Schmitgen@ucsf.edu (A.S.); Isabella.Joseph@ucsf.edu (I.J.); Philip.Starr@ucsf.edu (P.A.S.); Edward.Chang@ucsf.edu (E.F.C.)
3. Department of Neurology, University of California San Francisco, San Francisco, CA 94143, USA
* Correspondence: Prasad.Shirvalkar@ucsf.edu

Received: 1 September 2020; Accepted: 25 September 2020; Published: 29 September 2020

Abstract: Early studies of deep brain stimulation (DBS) for various neurological disorders involved a temporary trial period where implanted electrodes were externalized, in which the electrical contacts exiting the patient's brain are connected to external stimulation equipment, so that stimulation efficacy could be determined before permanent implant. As the optimal brain target sites for various diseases (i.e., Parkinson's disease, essential tremor) became better established, such trial periods have fallen out of favor. However, deep brain stimulation trial periods are experiencing a modern resurgence for at least two reasons: (1) studies of newer indications such as depression or chronic pain aim to identify new targets and (2) a growing interest in adaptive DBS tools necessitates neurophysiological recordings, which are often done in the peri-surgical period. In this review, we consider the possible approaches, benefits, and risks of such inpatient trial periods with a specific focus on developing new DBS therapies for chronic pain.

Keywords: deep brain stimulation; chronic pain; lead externalization; trial period; stereoEEG

1. Introduction

Deep brain stimulation (DBS), which involves the insertion of electrical leads into important cortical or subcortical structures to treat various neurological diseases, is often performed in a single surgery where the leads are subsequently connected to an implanted stimulator. Alternatively, DBS can be performed in a two-staged surgery where the leads (or electrodes) are first implanted, externalized (i.e., the non-neural side of the electrode exits the body), and connected to an external stimulator for a trial period to assess therapeutic benefit over 3–10 days. DBS trials with lead externalization have been used extensively over the last 50 years specifically for treating chronic pain [1–3]. Lead externalization permits inpatient testing of stimulation effects prior to permanent implantation, which is especially important for novel or unapproved DBS indications to ensure successful therapeutic response. This is especially important for diseases that encompass broad domains of symptoms spanning from neuropsychiatric to somatic, such as chronic pain syndromes. Because optimal brain targets for chronic pain are still unknown, such trials offer a key opportunity for the exploration and validation of both targets and pulse parameters that may modulate activity in multiple, relevant brain networks underlying various symptoms. Further, such a trial period allows the recording of neurophysiological activity from critical brain regions to further research and understand the mechanisms of action of stimulation. Modern recordings have aimed to uncover key biomarkers of chronic pain states toward the development of adaptive (or "closed-loop") control algorithms where stimulation delivery is adjusted in response to biomarkers to increase efficacy or avert the development of long-term tolerance.

Such trial periods that allow patients to "test drive" the neuromodulation therapy are used even when the general target regions are known, such as in spinal cord stimulation (SCS) [4]. A trial period is often necessary because of the large heterogeneity in patient response, to assess safety, and for the fine tuning of electrode position relative to the neural target so that patient benefit can be maximized before committing to an expensive therapy. It is worth pointing out that a short trial period to determine chronic brain stimulation targets assumes that an acute response to stimulation can be found (within minutes or hours of stimulation) and that these effects will translate to long-term efficacy. It remains to be determined whether this is the case for chronic pain.

The global burden of chronic pain is significant and growing alongside that of non-communicable diseases, which account for 78.6% of years lived with disability worldwide [5]. The economic impact of chronic neurological conditions such as chronic pain and epilepsy is greater than that of many other health conditions due to absenteeism, reduced levels of productivity, and increased risk of leaving labor markets, indicating that there is a significant indirect economic cost associated with these conditions [6]. Chronic pain also poses a significant cost to the healthcare system; analysis of a Canadian database indicates that the costs attributed to the healthcare of patients with painful neuropathic disorders were considerably higher than those in patients without chronic pain in the same age and sex demographics [6]. Perhaps most importantly, chronic neurological conditions have a significant debilitating effect on the overall quality of life of patients and are associated with some of the poorest quality-of-life indices, with the potential to impact social relationships, economic participation, and mental health. DBS for pain is still performed with a very limited trial period (off-label in the U.S.) resulting in highly variable success rates across patients.

In this review, we outline important considerations for DBS trial periods for chronic pain including possible brain targets for stimulating and recording. We then propose an argument for the use of stereoelectroencephalography (sEEG) in the trial and discuss possible trial related risks. An sEEG based approach is elaborated in the context of characterizing pain biomarkers and neurophysiological effects of stimulation. Finally, we offer practical advice for conducting a trial, including mitigating the placebo effect and rigorously ensuring therapeutic efficacy before permanent implantation.

2. Anatomical Targets/Considerations

Determining the optimal neural targets for stimulation-induced pain relief is a key goal of the DBS trial period. The trial period affords the opportunity to explore multiple pain-relevant brain regions based on pre-clinical and human experience to select the sites most appropriate for the pain syndrome and patient. In a survey of the current state of DBS for chronic pain, Farrell et al. focus on three prominent brain targets that have been tested most frequently: the ventral posterolateral/medial thalamus (VPL/VPM), the periventricular/periaqueductal grey (PVG/PAG), and the anterior cingulate cortex (ACC) across a wide variety of chronic pain syndromes [7]. Most studies highlighted in that review used a simple readout of somatic pain intensity (numeric or visual analog rating scale (NRS, VAS)); however, this approach fails to measure changes in the affective or cognitive domains of pain. Numerous other targets have been proposed such as motor cortex, ventral striatum, and insula. We will briefly discuss the most promising candidates below in the context of how these targets may offer pain relief across multiple dimensions of the pain experience. Importantly, the target efficacy for pain relief depends on the class of pain syndrome being treated and the unique qualities of the patient.

The motivation for treating intractable pain with brain surgery began with early results [8] demonstrating analgesia after thalamotomy and selective ablation. Following development by Mazars [9], Hosobuchi et al. used thalamic stimulation to produce successful masking of facial pain with electrically induced paresthesia in four of five patients, with pain relieving effects observed after a few minutes of stimulation [10]. Similar paresthesia-based analgesia for phantom limb pain has been reported previously [11]. Whereas VPL/VPM stimulation induces a phenomenon of purportedly "pleasant" paresthesia, PVG/PAG has been shown to induce a sense of warmth in painful areas. The pain relief following PAG/PVG stimulation has been attributed to the release of endogenous opioids as evidenced by abolished effect after naloxone [12]. In contrast, a study of 45 patients receiving chronic PAG or PVG stimulation for a wide variety of pain syndromes for one year demonstrated that despite the development of long-term tolerance to stimulation in twelve patients, there was no cross-tolerance with morphine [13]. This suggests that pain relief with PAG/PVG stimulation may not exclusively depend on an endogenous opioid mechanisms. Regardless, two large clinical trials evaluating combined VPL/PAG stimulation for chronic pain of various syndromes failed to meet therapeutic endpoints, though these studies were fraught with design and follow-up problems (see [14] for a discussion). Specifically, these trials targeted the same two brain regions across hundreds of patients with vastly different pain syndromes without placebo or randomized design. Notably, a significant portion of patients were lost to follow-up; the resulting patient attrition severely reduced power to detect a clinically meaningful effect and resulted in no significant benefit using an intention-to-treat analysis. These flaws highlight the need for individualized brain targeting based on etiology and the use of endpoints that measure multiple dimensions of pain.

Studies from Aziz and colleagues have ignited interest in targeting the affective dimension of pain by targeting the dorsal ACC. Patients suffering from a variety of chronic neuropathic pain syndromes were followed for up to 3 years, and significant benefit was found at the 6-month time point [2], though no significant effect was found on further follow-up. Further ACC stimulation at the wide pulse widths and high amplitudes required for analgesia was associated with de novo epilepsy in a handful of patients [15]. However, pain relief with ACC stimulation has been reported to have a long wash-in period (hours to 3 days), which may limit the ability to detect a beneficial effect in shorter timescales (however, see [16]). Nonetheless, the novelty of the ACC as a target has inspired a renewed interest in modulating the affective dimension of pain and basic research into pain-relevant mechanisms in the ACC. It is still unknown whether targeting other regions of the ACC may be beneficial for chronic pain despite functional imaging evidence that more anterior or posterior regions may be involved [16,17]; such alternative regions of the cingulate merit exploration for therapeutic DBS in a potential trial period.

Motor cortex stimulation (MCS) has also been studied for pain relief using both non-invasive [18] and direct cortical stimulation [19]. In a meta-analysis, 54% of 117 patients with central pain and 68% of 44 patients with trigeminal neuropathic pain experienced a greater than 40% reduction in pain scores, suggesting efficacy for neuropathic pain syndromes [20]. In contrast, double-blinded studies of MCS failed to show significant analgesia for the treatment of hemi-body post-stroke pain or post-herpetic neuralgia pain, while noting that patients suffering from facial pain and upper limb pain may obtain relief (e.g., see [21]). Potential mechanisms of analgesia resulting from MCS are still debated. Other targets such as the posterior insula have demonstrated increased thermal pain thresholds in epilepsy patients without chronic pain, though generalization to clinical pain states is unknown [22].

When selecting neural targets for deep brain stimulation trial periods, it is important to consider the specific type of chronic pain that the patient is suffering from. Certain types of pain such as facial and upper limb neuropathic pain may warrant targeting the contralateral motor cortex, while inflammatory pain syndromes may benefit relatively more from targeting the PAG. Stimulation of the ACC or insula are other potentially promising targets, though no systematic study has been able to demonstrate long-term pain relief through DBS, suggesting neural adaptation as a key obstacle. The only double-blind sham-controlled clinical trial for post-stroke pain targeted the ventral striatum/capsular region and aimed to mitigate the affective component of pain to improve pain-related disability [23]. At present, while there are numerous individual anecdotes of patients obtaining pain relief from the stimulation of various targets, there is a lack of clear evidence pointing to reliable targets for long-term pain relief. Advances in longitudinally stable pain biomarker detection will ideally inform next-generation closed-loop DBS therapy for chronic pain that may avert long-term tolerance [19,20,24].

The hope is that through individual "N-of-1" DBS trial periods, we may find brain targets that produce acute pain relief that further extends to longer time periods.

3. DBS Trial Period Safety and Risks

Trialing deep brain stimulation therapy in advance of a permanent implant can pose additional patient-specific and systemic risks both in relation to the surgery and potential success of this therapy as an option of last resort. Specifically, a DBS trial period may introduce the added risk of possible infection and additional costs of extended inpatient evaluation.

Beyond the risks from intracranial implantation, which can be mitigated with strict planning and surgical protocols, it is important to consider the costs of a temporary implant and inpatient trial period from a holistic perspective. For example, while we are studying the effects of DBS on pain, it is important to control for external factors, such as the effects of financial stress, social isolation, and physical restrictions that are associated with prolonged inpatient stay. However, by accounting for these effects, testing DBS in a temporary, resource-rich environment, and applying the predictive power of an inpatient trial, we may avoid the unnecessary financial and psychosocial burden of a long-term implant for unsuccessful trial patients. Thus, when assessing potential patients for DBS therapy for chronic pain, it is useful to consider the safety, appropriateness, fiscal neutrality, and effectiveness (SAFE) principles for neuromodulation therapies [25].

The SAFE (safety, appropriateness, fiscal neutrality, and effectiveness) principles can be used as an evidence-based algorithm to guide the selection of appropriate pain syndromes and DBS targets for individual patients. These principles further support using a minimally biased trial period to evaluate for benefit, similar to techniques used in SCS for chronic pain treatment. For example, studies using effective psychosocial screening for SCS trials produced a higher rate and longer duration of pain relief than studies in which no psychosocial screening was performed. Further, disregarding these psychosocial factors may increase the risk of injury to patients while creating unnecessary costs from ineffective therapeutic interventions. Thus, performing a well-designed, comprehensive inpatient trial in line with the SAFE principles, as described, can increase the chances of long-term success of DBS for chronic pain. By closely examining each of these guiding principles, as demonstrated below, both patients and researchers can perform a more thorough and personalized approach to trial DBS candidacy.

Safety: Reports of infection rates involved in temporary lead externalization have been mixed. An early single center, prospective analysis over a four-year period found an increased rate of infection when DBS for Parkinson's disease was performed using a staged procedure with externalization (15.3% vs. 4.2% for one-stage) [26]. However, in a two-stage surgical procedure, Rosa et al. found that lead externalization for 2–7 days did not increase post-operative infection risk following Stage I bilateral DBS lead implant when oral antibiotics were used for 5 days after Stage II lead extender and internal pulse generator (IPG) placement [27]. In this study of 105 patients, the rate of infection from this two-stage surgery (2.8%) was consistent with post-operative risk of infection in the literature. Bojanic et al. similarly observed no increased risk of infection when directly comparing externalized trial vs. one-stage DBS surgery [28]. Of 60 patients undergoing single-stage surgery, they observed 7 infections, while 86 patients undergoing an externalized trial resulted in 3 infections.

Appropriateness and efficacy: A temporary trial stage presents a measurable predictor of long-term clinical benefit. In order to ensure that the trial has realistic predictive value, however, it is critical to ensure a clinically meaningful benefit. Observation of a clinically significant benefit (a 12-point improvement on the 100-point visual analog scale [29]) relies on the consideration of intrinsic factors such as patient attentional biases, motivations, and study expectations. The expectation effects of pain or benefit from DBS can be understood through a motivation–decision model of pain, in which the threat of pain or promise of relief is a consequence of a computed decision to respond to or ignore this pain signal [30]. This is an especially important consideration when working with patients with chronic pain, who have been shown to bias expectations toward pain escape/avoidance and, thus, increase perceived pain intensity through top–down modulatory circuits. In fact, the patient's expectation of improvement at trial entry may be the single most robust predictor of reported pain reduction. Since anticipation of pain often becomes a self-fulfilling prophecy, addressing patient expectations should be incorporated into the trial plan. The trial stage presents an extended opportunity to use comprehensive psychosocial assessments, including the Structured Clinical Interview for DSM-5 (Diagnostic and Statistical Manual of Mental Disorders—Fifth Edition, SCID-5), Hamilton Depression Rating Scale, West Haven Yale Multidimensional Pain Inventory (WHYPI), Pain Catastrophizing Scale, Beck Depression Inventory, and Beck Anxiety Inventory, in addition to cognitive and behavioral testing to provide a more complete picture of patient outcomes.

Psychosocial components of pain, such as attention, culture, anxiety, and depression, similarly influence the perception of pain and the outcomes of therapies. Despite meeting all clinical criteria, sound surgical approaches, and even early signs of clinical benefit, a significant number of patients continue to fail neuromodulation therapy in the long term. This suggests that the inherent characteristics of patients are a strong factor in determining neuromodulation efficacy. Strict inclusion and exclusion criteria and extensive psychological evaluation are critical prior to trial enrollment [31]. Studies suggest that a comprehensive program consisting of pre-operative psychosocial assessment and consistent psychological and rehabilitative support throughout the trial phase and subsequent therapy are key elements for the success of neurostimulation.

Fiscal neutrality: Bojanic et al. found that despite the extra costs of seven additional inpatient days (up to £11,200), there were significant cost savings when compared to committing patients to a potentially ineffective implant (up to £147,000), particularly when the indication was chronic pain. At our institution, a similar DBS trial period of 7 days presents an actual cost of $34,000 including imaging, surgery, device, and inpatient costs ($150,000 billed to private insurance) versus a cost for a one-stage DBS implant of $90,000 ($203,000 billed to private insurance). With a trial to permanent implant conversion ratio of 50% (higher end), this represents a cost savings of up to $56,000 per every 2 patients ($53,000 when billed to private insurance). The concept of fiscal neutrality (maximizing the neuromodulation approach to be cost neutral in the long term), supports performing adequate trials for DBS for treating pain.

4. Motivation for a StereoEEG Trial in Patients with Chronic Pain

sEEG is most commonly used as a diagnostic tool for patients with refractory epilepsy. Localization of seizure onset zones is achieved using multi-contact depth electrodes, which are placed through burr holes targeting both cortical and deep structures of the brain. Continuous recording can provide a three-dimensional view of the origin and spread of epileptic seizures [32]. sEEG has been used to guide treatment of refractory epilepsy when non-invasive treatments such as pharmacology, diet, or other alternative therapeutic options are ineffectual. Similarly, we propose using sEEG in patients with chronic pain who have failed to achieve relief of symptoms with pharmacological interventions or spinal cord stimulators.

sEEG has been widely adopted internationally, with global studies generating extensive data in support of sEEG with potential synergistic applications in cognitive neurophysiology research. sEEG is an invasive monitoring technique, and a major concern is the potential for hemorrhagic complications, which can lead to neurological deficits or death. However, rates of clinically significant hemorrhage and other infections occur at much lower rates in sEEG compared to those in other neurophysiological surgical approaches (e.g., subdural strip and grid electrode implants). sEEG is often a highly efficacious and cost-efficient procedure with a low associated morbidity that has demonstrated success in network characterization for thousands of epilepsy patients worldwide.

sEEG is an appealing approach for neural circuit mapping and testing acute stimulation efficacy, which we propose can be used to identify optimal brain regions in candidate patients who are most likely to respond when a chronic DBS device is implanted. Specifically, for chronic pain, which engages multiple well-established nodes across a widespread pain network, an sEEG trial can be used to target multiple brain regions based on converging evidence from pre-clinical and human brain mapping studies (Figure 1, see Section 2, Anatomical Targets/Considerations). Similar prior efforts have been successful for epilepsy and even facilitated the development of new responsive brain stimulation therapy [33]. As sEEG is beneficial for intracranial investigations that require sampling from superficial and deep structures simultaneously across both hemispheres, we propose using sEEG as both a clinical tool and to advance research on the fundamental mechanisms of chronic pain processing in patients.

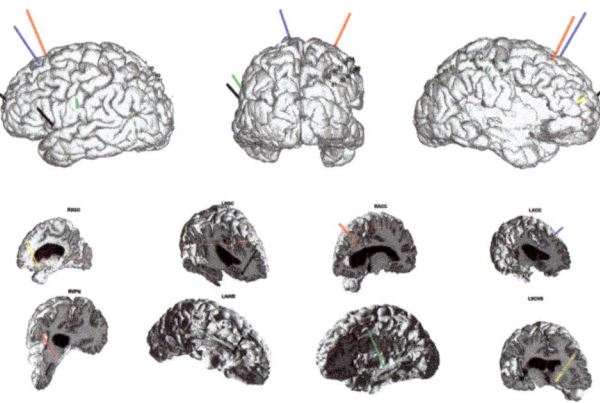

Figure 1. Stereoelectroencephalography (sEEG) targeting for deep brain stimulation (DBS) for chronic pain during the inpatient trial period. Top row depicts left lateral, posterior, and right lateral views in an example patient with post-stroke pain. Eight images across rows 2 and 3 depict individual electrode trajectories targeting labeled regions of interest. R/LSGC: right/left subgenual cingulate cortex, R/LACC: right/left anterior cingulate cortex, RVPN: right ventral posterior thalamic nucleus, LAINS: left anterior insula, LPINS: left posterior insula, LVCVS: left ventral capsule and ventral striatum.

The main benefit of sEEG over other approaches lies in the potential for focal stimulation combined with pain-related network discovery. Methods such as functional magnetic resonance imaging (fMRI) and magnetoencephalography (MEG) can be informative and useful in network discovery, potentially prior to a trial period, to discover optimal targets in each individual patient prior to electrode implantation. Regarding network discovery with other modalities, blood oxygen level dependent (BOLD) signals in fMRI can provide whole-brain localization and temporal tracking of neural activity correlated with pain states [34,35]. However, fMRI-based signals cannot be detected in the ambulatory setting, limiting their use in clinically relevant timescales for chronic pain therapy (however, see [36] for longitudinal fMRI). For example, due to the limitations of patient tolerance and equipment availability, fMRI cannot feasibly be used continuously over a period of hours, making it unrealistic for evaluating clinically relevant spontaneous pain fluctuations. Likewise, prior work has used simultaneous stimulation (with DBS or transcranial magnetic stimulation (TMS)) and recording with magnetoencephalography (MEG) [37] or scalp EEG [38] to identify predictive biomarkers of subjective pain experience without the associated risks of trial surgery. Studies evaluating network effects of DBS with EEG/MEG nonetheless require permanent DBS surgery, which poses greater risks than sEEG. Prior efforts to identify biomarkers of stimulation using TMS/EEG require averaging over larger volumes of tissue and can suffer more from stimulation artifact during simultaneous neural recording. Furthermore, TMS itself can be painful, confounding interpretation of any putative pain-relevant biomarkers. Non-invasive approaches remain an important complement to sEEG and, in theory, could even be used to identify key anatomical pain nodes in the future. For example, studies aiming to decode subjective pain intensity have been able to use MEG successfully to identify local field potential (LFP)-based biomarkers of pain, which are often reproducible within subjects [39];

such individualized MEG mapping may serve a useful pre-surgical step for target planning. While sEEG is limited by the number of electrodes and sampled regions per patient when compared to more global brain network approaches such as fMRI or MEG [40], it can better facilitate the characterization of biomarkers of clinical pain and stimulation with high spatiotemporal resolution.

5. Detecting Biomarkers of Chronic Pain and Stimulation-Related Pain Relief

While considerable effort has been devoted to identifying intracranial biomarkers of pain, the vast majority of studies to date have focused on experimental pain states in healthy individuals, which do not necessarily translate to altered brain dynamics seen in patients with chronic pain [34,41]. Rather than focusing exclusively on signatures of evoked pain, we suggest that studying the dynamics of spontaneous pain can be more informative. By further combining simultaneous recording and stimulation, it may be possible to dissociate neural correlates of the pain state from those of stimulation-related pain relief. Such converging evidence would help to develop practical approaches to personalized, adaptive neurostimulation.

5.1. Biomarkers of Chronic Pain and Network Discovery

Chronic pain is associated with both spontaneous and evoked pain, which are associated with distinct underlying brain activity. The chronic pain experience is almost certainly a network-wide phenomenon, but focusing on critical nodes of this network has pointed to brain regions that may harbor useful biomarkers [42]. fMRI studies provide evidence that brain activation patterns of sustained chronic pain states do not overlap with those of stimulus-evoked acute pain states in both patients and healthy subjects [43]. Baliki et al. found a double dissociation where sustained chronic low back pain in patients was associated with increased BOLD activity in the medial prefrontal cortex (mPFC) and rostral cingulate, while thermal experimental pain preferentially activated the insula both in patients and healthy controls. Further, the posterior thalamus and bilateral dorsolateral prefrontal cortex (DLPFC) exhibit atrophy over time in chronic pain [44]; pain-related activation of the DLPFC is also related to activity in the mPFC, but not in the insula [43]. The duration of experienced pain also influences brain representation of pain. Compared to patients experiencing subacute low back pain for only 2 months, patients with chronic back pain lasting >10 years show increased brain activity in the mPFC, orbitofrontal cortex, precuneus, and amygdala [45]. These authors and others have argued that the chronification of pain shifts brain representations from nociceptive to emotional circuits. Therefore, long-term chronic pain is associated with network-level changes in pain processing that cannot necessarily be inferred from solely studying evoked pain in healthy patients using experimental stimuli such as laser-evoked potentials or the thermal grill illusion. These data suggest that the sensory, cognitive, and emotional phenomenology of real-world chronic pain is distinct from that of experimentally induced pain. As such, the mPFC, rostral ACC, and DLPFC may be sensible targets to detect biomarkers of the chronic pain state.

Recordings of LFP from brain regions that are likely to harbor chronic-pain-relevant signals (e.g., mPFC, ACC, DLPFC) can be used to further understand mechanisms of pain and devise control strategies for closed-loop algorithms. Two brain stimulation devices with closed-loop functionality are current available: Neuropace® RNS (Neuropace, Mountain View, CA, USA) [46] and Medtronic® Percept (Medtronic, Minneapolis, MN, USA) (recently approved for sensing and stimulation [47] and full closed-loop functionality is anticipated soon). Theses device are capable of using neural power band-limited time series signals (e.g., alpha band power) as inputs to an embedded closed-loop controller that can modify stimulation parameters to optimize therapy. For this reason, we focus on band powers of interest that have previously been associated with predicting pain states.

Despite the limitations of interpreting biomarkers of acute/evoked pain state, there is an abundance of such data using sEEG, MEG, and EEG, which can provide a starting point. The most commonly reported neural features predictive of a high pain state have been a decrease in the central alpha band (8–12 Hz) power [48–50] and an increase in the parietal or prefrontal gamma band (>30 Hz) power [51,52]. Importantly, recent studies have distinguished neural correlates of painful stimuli from nonpainful stimuli, providing greater selectivity for pain states. Using sEEG, Liu et al. found significant evoked-pain-related cross-frequency coupling between theta (4–8 Hz) and gamma band activity in the amygdala and hippocampus, which can be tested for validity as a chronic pain biomarker [53]. While most studies of neural pain biomarkers seek to predict the pain VAS, it will be important for future research to identify what power bands may support different dimensions of pain (i.e., somatosensory, affective, cognitive) by analyzing alternative metrics (e.g., McGill Pain Questionnaire (MPQ) or pain unpleasantness). There remains a large gap in characterizing such power-band based biomarkers of naturalistic, spontaneous chronic pain; an sEEG trial can fill this gap. Ultimately, by combining recording with simultaneous stimulation in these areas, an sEEG trial period could inform adaptive DBS algorithms (for a thorough discussion of brain-based pain biomarkers see [42,54]).

5.2. Biomarkers of Stimulation-Induced Pain Relief

Beyond biomarkers that predict the chronic pain state, it is critical to characterize neural signals resulting from the electrical stimulation of various sites across many parameters. There are at least three strategies for detecting biomarkers of stimulation-induced pain relief. First, by recording LFPs from multiple brain regions either during or immediately after pain-relieving stimulation (see Section 6, Practical Considerations), spectral power within the frequency bands of interest can be compared to validate putative pain biomarkers that were detected in the absence of stimulation. For example, if ACC theta power was positively correlated with a high reported pain state, therapeutic stimulation would be expected to decrease ACC theta power if this biomarker was causal. Such a biomarker could be incorporated into a closed-loop algorithm using a simple threshold; for example, one algorithm could initiate stimulation when ACC theta power increased beyond some prespecified threshold power value. Second, neural activity in certain frequencies recorded at the site of stimulation may help predict whether and when stimulation may be beneficial. In a notable study, mechanistic evidence supporting the VPL/M as a target for both recording and stimulation was provided by Huang et al. in thirteen patients with chronic pain [55]. Distinct thalamic theta, alpha, high beta, and high gamma oscillations were correlated with pain relief and, thereby, suggested possible biomarkers by which one may identify individual patients who may benefit from VPL/M stimulation. Third, simultaneous recordings across multiple electrodes could provide a readout of functional connectivity in the pain network, which could be "pinged" by delivering intermittent single-pulse electrical stimulation (SPES) at various sites. SPES has previously been used to probe cortico-cortical connections and intra-areal plasticity by averaging LFP time-locked to the stimuli using sEEG in epilepsy patients [56]. The averaged LFP reflects cortico-cortical evoked potentials that can be recorded in adjacent and remote sites during periods of high and low pain states to provide a connectome representation of network changes related to chronic pain. Similar biomarkers of stimulation-induced pain relief can help to narrow down final candidate brain targets for permanent DBS implantation.

6. Practical Considerations for Chronic Pain DBS Trial Period

There are numerous factors to consider in the experimental design of a trial period: the duration of a trial period, how many patients to enroll, and outcome metrics of interest. Indeed, prior studies of DBS and chronic pain may have failed to reach primary endpoints because of nonrandomized design, heterogeneous patient populations, subjective assessment of patient outcomes, lack of measuring "meaningful" changes in symptoms, inconsistencies in sites stimulated, and other factors (see review [7]). Practical considerations should not be left to last minute planning. Common understanding of goals and procedures is needed across clinical specialties including neurological surgery, neurology, and pain management. The research team must work closely with neurosurgeons to map the targeting of electrodes for implantation; the administration of pain medications must be coordinated across pain providers, nursing staff, and research team so testing can be timed appropriately; patient care assistants and monitoring staff must be appraised of patient needs that differ from standard inpatient care on their unit; and research staff not accustomed to inpatient care must be oriented to the environment. We have found that participating in nursing staff meetings prior to patient implant is an effective way to coordinate activities and communicate DBS trial period goals between research staff, clinical personnel, and candidate patients.

The overall duration of implant for each patient should carefully weigh experimental need, insertional effect, patient tolerance, and infection risk (discussed further above). Experimental need can be broken down into multiple categories: resting-state biomarker discovery, stimulation efficacy, and modulation of task performance (task-based biomarker discovery/stimulation effects on task performance). Further, the insertional effect, or stun effect, which has been well-studied in Parkinson's disease patients undergoing trial periods for DBS, can often be described as a temporary improvement in disease symptoms in response to DBS lead placement [57]. The positive effect can often persist 6 months following surgical implantation and before the onset of stimulation. The insertional effect has been similarly described in chronic pain patients, in which some patients (43% of 21 patients) experience a substantial reduction in their pain immediately following lead implant [58]. While the cause and predisposing conditions of this insertional effect are not well understood, Hamani et al. found that a positive insertional effect was correlated with a successful stimulation period.

An emerging trend has been to use the inpatient DBS trial period to both test stimulation and record neural activity that may guide biomarker discovery toward developing closed-loop DBS algorithms. Resting-state biomarker discovery is best served by recording periods of brain activity during wakefulness in the absence of stimulation or tasks and across varying levels of reported pain metrics. Level of pain may be assessed using a collection of surveys or verbal reports that are repeatedly administered throughout the trial period. The dynamics of subjective pain experience varies widely across patients and pain subtypes [59]. As the timescale of pain predictability based on neural activity is relatively unknown, we opt to study brain activity for relatively long periods (e.g., 30 min) around each survey point to provide a starting point on studying individual dynamics/timescales. Each time a survey is administered translates to one data point; this should be repeated multiple times throughout the entire trial period. At least 10 data points, but preferably many more, are needed for a statistically valid association of neural activity with the symptom reports, necessitating a total trial duration of at least 3 days.

Evaluating for stimulation efficacy should involve testing at least two different stimulation locations and various parameters in order to identify putative therapeutic targets for permanent implant. Two critical factors should be considered during the design of stimulation efficacy testing: placebo effect and expected wash-in and wash-out durations. The placebo effect is an important confounder during DBS [60], and while it may be advantageous in the long-term treatment of chronic pain, care should be taken to control for short-term placebo effect during trial DBS. In order to account for this, double-blind, sham-controlled stimulation testing is needed. By design, when using clinically approved devices, the operator of the stimulator cannot be blinded to the stimulation condition. Thus, during double-blind stimulation testing, the individual operating the DBS stimulator should not interact with the patient in any way, and ideally should not be visible to the patient. All other people in the room (including the patient) should be blinded to the stimulation condition. Furthermore, it can be useful for all other people in the room and the patient to be naïve of stimulation (sham) onset and offset times. This may further mitigate expectation or anxiety associated with anticipated effects of stimulation, which may offer better predictive value of long-term success. Having a sham block paired with each verum stimulation block doubles testing time but provides more robust and interpretable results. If possible, having the patient self-administer surveys at cued times, with no researchers in the room, may also decrease Hawthorne effects [61]. This may not always be feasible due to safety considerations and the need for active monitoring of intracranial recordings during stimulation. The duration of stimulation and the wash-out period between testing sham/verum blocks or between stimulation locations should be determined as a function of expected wash-in and wash-out effects. While stimulation of some targets such as the VPL or PAG can produce rapid pain relief over seconds to minutes, the ACC or other sites may have much longer wash-in times over days. This remains an area of active investigation and varies as a function of disease duration and specific behavior/symptom assessed [16,62–64]. Longer wash-out periods provide more confidence that effects observed for subsequent stimulation parameters cannot be attributed to carryover effects from prior stimulation conditions. All candidate stimulation targets should be tested multiple times, so counterbalancing test order can also help mitigate carryover effects. Early in target discovery, it may be beneficial to stimulate different parameters within the same region (e.g., low vs. high pulse width or frequency) with shorter wash out; if a candidate brain region or parameter set for therapeutic efficacy is found, it is useful to retest it with longer wash out.

Recording neural activity during behavioral tasks, in the presence and absence of stimulation, can serve multiple purposes. Specifically, we propose using behavioral tasks that systematically assess various domains of the pain experience including somatic, affective, and cognitive ones. Tasks that are particularly relevant include quantitative sensory testing with thermal stimuli including pain thresholds [65] and mechanical pain thresholds with Von Frey filaments [66] (somatic); the emotional Stroop [67] and emotional facial recognition tasks (affective judgment and interference); and the oddball [68]; and Iowa gambling tasks [69] (cognitive attention and decision making). Task-based biomarkers can be used to track symptom status and treatment efficacy or identify brain regions that may be best targeted by stimulation for therapeutic benefit [70]. Machine learning methods can be applied to identify spectral properties that could serve as biomarkers for specific symptoms or induced states [71]. Variation in task performance may also more directly indicate the efficacy of stimulation. In order to make such conclusions, patients must be familiarized with tasks in order to prevent test–retest effects from skewing the results. Initial familiarization with tasks can be conducted prior to implant. Following implantation, tasks must be conducted multiple times (e.g., with and without stimulation) in order to determine baseline activity vs. potential changes induced by stimulation.

Not to be underestimated, patient tolerance and ability to actively participate during the trial period is critical for success. Detailed informed consent, ideally implementing teach-to-goal methods [72], should include clearly detailed information about what to expect during the trial period. In addition, we have found that having the patient complete questionnaire surveys (similar to those subsequently administered during the trial period) in his/her home environment prior to implant can decrease frustration with completing the same metric repeatedly. Continued clear communication with the patient and family members is vital. Having well-defined times when family members can visit or share a meal provides needed breaks in long days of testing. The depth of scientific discussion will need to be tailored to each patient's interest and level of understanding, but overall, we have found that patients are much more engaged when they clearly understand the need for each study and the role each test plays in the larger picture.

The selection of which metrics should be administered to assess pain and how often is again tied to both scientific need and patient tolerability. Patients experience survey fatigue in answering the same surveys repeatedly (e.g., upward of 50 times a day), which can hinder accurate communication of symptoms. Individual patents also differ in their adeptness of communicating pain through numeric ratings, free speech dialog, pain maps [73], or standardized surveys. Different methods of collecting information about pain symptoms also tap into different aspects of the pain experience [74], such as quantitative pain measures (e.g., numerical rating), pain experience (e.g., unpleasant sensory or emotional experience), and pain expression (e.g., qualitative words, pain narrative, and behavior to communicate pain, pain behavior). We found that a combination of metrics was the most useful, with short versions administered more frequently and long versions administered about three times per day.

When deciding how many people to enroll in a trial period, overall expense, and expected trial to permanent conversion ratio must be taken into consideration. Expense (both in time and money) impose a cap on the total number of patients who can be enrolled. A meta-analysis review of spinal cord stimulation showed a 41% conversion ratio from a trial period to a permanent implant [4]. While a higher conversion ratio may seem preferable, imposing increasingly strict inclusion criteria on a trial period may prevent testing in a broader population who could ultimately benefit from the therapy. Regardless, given the intensiveness of the trial period and subsequent management of patients with implanted devices, the size of DBS trials for chronic pain will likely remain small (<30 individuals) for the foreseeable future, until the therapy is sufficiently developed to obtain regulatory approval.

Lastly, we must balance the goal of full mechanistic understanding of neural circuitry underlying chronic pain vs. the identification of effective therapy. It is not practical to require the former as a prerequisite for providing treatment options for patients currently suffering from chronic pain. Rather, we recommend incorporating our current knowledge of pain circuits and using this as a starting point for where to implant electrodes for biomarker discovery. This approach has the benefit of not only being ready for implementation now but also being mechanistically informed according to current state of knowledge. Existing therapies, including spinal cord stimulation, have been shown to be effective at alleviating chronic pain in many individuals, but the mechanisms remain debated. Most important for clinical treatment is the efficacy of the therapy. While the number of patients implanted remains modest, it is likely more feasible to focus on a more individualized approach. Recording from implicated regions affords the relatively rare opportunity to identify correlative or causal factors that predict pain or pain relief in individual subjects. However, as the cohort of patients grow, looking for trends across patients will be incredibly valuable to determine whether patients share common biomarker features. This may be particularly fruitful to separate cohorts with different pain etiologies, pain dynamics, or even based on syndrome subtypes.

Author Contributions: Conceptualization P.S., E.F.C., and P.A.S.; writing—review and editing, P.S., K.K.S., A.S., J.P., I.J., E.F.C., and P.A.S.; funding acquisition, P.A.S., E.C., and P.S. All authors have read and agreed to the published version of the manuscript.

Funding: Research reported in this publication was supported by the National Institute of Neurological Disorders and Stroke of the National Institutes of Health under award number UH3NS115631. The content is solely the responsibility of the authors and does not necessarily represent the official views of the National Institutes of Health.

Conflicts of Interest: P.S., E.F.C., and P.A.S. have investigator-initiated clinical trial agreements with Medtronic Inc. and receive only equipment and supplies.

References

1. Ben-Haim, S.; Mirzadeh, Z.; Rosenberg, W.S. Deep brain stimulation for intractable neuropathic facial pain. *Neurosurg. Focus* **2018**, *45*, E15. [CrossRef]
2. Boccard, S.G.J.; Pereira, E.A.C.; Moir, L.; Aziz, T.Z.; Green, A.L. Long-term Outcomes of Deep Brain Stimulation for Neuropathic Pain. *Neurosurgery* **2013**, *72*, 221–231. [CrossRef]
3. Levy, R.M.; Lamb, S.; Adams, J.E. Treatment of chronic pain by deep brain stimulation: Long term follow-up and review of the literature. *Neurosurgery* **1987**, *21*, 885–893. [CrossRef]
4. Huang, K.T.; Martin, J.; Marky, A.; Chagoya, G.; Hatef, J.; Hazzard, M.A.; Thomas, S.M.; Lokhnygina, Y.; Lad, S.P. A National Survey of Spinal Cord Stimulation Trial-to-Permanent Conversion Rates. *Neuromodul. Technol. Neural Interface* **2015**, *18*, 133–140. [CrossRef]
5. Jackson, T.; Thomas, S.; Stabile, V.; Shotwell, M.; Han, X.; McQueen, K. A Systematic Review and Meta-Analysis of the Global Burden of Chronic Pain without Clear Etiology in Low- and Middle-Income Countries: Trends in Heterogeneous Data and a Proposal for New Assessment Methods. *Anesth. Analg.* **2016**, *123*, 739–748. [CrossRef]
6. Phillips, C.J. The Cost and Burden of Chronic Pain. *Rev. Pain* **2009**, *3*, 2–5. [CrossRef]
7. Farrell, S.; Green, A.; Aziz, T. The Current State of Deep Brain Stimulation for Chronic Pain and Its Context in Other Forms of Neuromodulation. *Brain Sci.* **2018**, *8*, 158. [CrossRef]
8. Pool, J.L. Psychosurgery in Older People. *J. Am. Geriatr. Soc.* **1954**, *2*, 456–466. [CrossRef]
9. Mazars, G.; Roge, R.; Mazars, Y. Results of the stimulation of the spinothalamic fasciculus and their bearing on the physiopathology of pain. *Rev. Neurol.* **1960**, *103*, 136–138.

10. Hosobuchi, Y.; Adams, J.E.; Rutkin, B. Chronic Thalamic Stimulation for the Control of Facial Anesthesia Dolorosa. *Arch. Neurol.* **1973**, *29*, 158–161. [CrossRef]
11. Nandi, D.; Yianni, J.; Humphreys, J.; Wang, S.; O'sullivan, V.; Shepstone, B.; Stein, J.F.; Aziz, T.Z. Phantom limb pain relieved with different modalities of central nervous system stimulation: A clinical and functional imaging case report of two patients. *Neuromodul. J. Int. Neuromodul. Soc.* **2004**, *7*, 176–183. [CrossRef]
12. Adams, J.E. Naloxone reversal of analgesia produced by brain stimulation in the human. *Pain* **1976**, *2*, 161–166. [CrossRef]
13. Young, R.F.; Chambi, V.I. Pain relief by electrical stimulation of the periaqueductal and periventricular gray matter: Evidence for a non-opioid mechanism. *J. Neurosurg.* **1987**, *66*, 364–371. [CrossRef]
14. Coffey, R.J. Deep brain stimulation for chronic pain: Results of two multicenter trials and a structured review. *Pain Med. Malden Mass* **2001**, *2*, 183–192. [CrossRef]
15. Maslen, H.; Cheeran, B.; Pugh, J.; Pycroft, L.; Boccard, S.; Prangnell, S.; Green, A.L.; FitzGerald, J.; Savulescu, J.; Aziz, T. Unexpected Complications of Novel Deep Brain Stimulation Treatments: Ethical Issues and Clinical Recommendations. *Neuromodul. Technol. Neural Interface* **2018**, *21*, 135–143. [CrossRef] [PubMed]
16. Bijanki, K.R.; Manns, J.R.; Inman, C.S.; Choi, K.S.; Harati, S.; Pedersen, N.P.; Drane, D.L.; Waters, A.C.; Fasano, R.E.; Mayberg, H.S.; et al. Cingulum stimulation enhances positive affect and anxiolysis to facilitate awake craniotomy. *J. Clin. Investig.* **2019**, *129*. [CrossRef] [PubMed]
17. Spisak, T.; Kincses, B.; Schlitt, F.; Zunhammer, M.; Schmidt-Wilcke, T.; Kincses, Z.T.; Bingel, U. Pain-free resting-state functional brain connectivity predicts individual pain sensitivity. *Nat. Commun.* **2020**, *11*, 187. [CrossRef]
18. Lefaucheur, J.-P.; Drouot, X.; Cunin, P.; Bruckert, R.; Lepetit, H.; Créange, A.; Wolkenstein, P.; Maison, P.; Keravel, Y.; Nguyen, J.-P. Motor cortex stimulation for the treatment of refractory peripheral neuropathic pain. *Brain* **2009**, *132*, 1463–1471. [CrossRef] [PubMed]
19. Nandi, D.; Smith, H.; Owen, S.; Joint, C.; Stein, J.; Aziz, T. Peri-ventricular grey stimulation versus motor cortex stimulation for post stroke neuropathic pain. *J. Clin. Neurosci.* **2002**, *9*, 557–561. [CrossRef]
20. Fontaine, D.; Hamani, C.; Lozano, A. Efficacy and safety of motor cortex stimulation for chronic neuropathic pain: Critical review of the literature: Clinical article. *J. Neurosurg.* **2009**, *110*, 251–256. [CrossRef]
21. Nguyen, J.-P.; Velasco, F.; Brugières, P.; Velasco, M.; Keravel, Y.; Boleaga, B.; Brito, F.; Lefaucheur, J.-P. Treatment of chronic neuropathic pain by motor cortex stimulation: Results of a bicentric controlled crossover trial. *Brain Stimulat.* **2008**, *1*, 89–96. [CrossRef] [PubMed]
22. Denis, D.J.; Marouf, R.; Rainville, P.; Bouthillier, A.; Nguyen, D.K. Effects of insular stimulation on thermal nociception. *Eur. J. Pain* **2016**, *20*, 800–810. [CrossRef] [PubMed]
23. Lempka, S.F.; Malone, D.A.; Hu, B.; Baker, K.B.; Wyant, A.; Ozinga, J.G.; Plow, E.B.; Pandya, M.; Kubu, C.S.; Ford, P.J.; et al. Randomized clinical trial of deep brain stimulation for poststroke pain. *Ann. Neurol.* **2017**, *81*, 653–663. [CrossRef] [PubMed]
24. Shirvalkar, P.; Veuthey, T.L.; Dawes, H.E.; Chang, E.F. Closed-Loop Deep Brain Stimulation for Refractory Chronic Pain. *Front. Comput. Neurosci.* **2018**, *12*. [CrossRef]
25. Krames, E.S.; Monis, S.; Poree, L.; Deer, T.; Levy, R. Using the SAFE principles when evaluating electrical stimulation therapies for the pain of failed back surgery syndrome. *Neuromodul. J. Int. Neuromodul. Soc.* **2011**, *14*, 299–311, discussion 311. [CrossRef]
26. Constantoyannis, C.; Berk, C.; Honey, C.R.; Mendez, I.; Brownstone, R.M. Reducing hardware-related complications of deep brain stimulation. *Can. J. Neurol. Sci. J. Can. Sci. Neurol.* **2005**, *32*, 194–200. [CrossRef]
27. Rosa, M.; Scelzo, E.; Locatelli, M.; Carrabba, G.; Levi, V.; Arlotti, M.; Barbieri, S.; Rampini, P.; Priori, A. Risk of Infection After Local Field Potential Recording from Externalized Deep Brain Stimulation Leads in Parkinson's Disease. *World Neurosurg.* **2017**, *97*, 64–69. [CrossRef]
28. Bojanic, S.; Sethi, H.; Hyam, J.; Yianni, J.; Nandi, D.; Joint, C.; Carter, H.; Gregory, R.; Bain, P.; Aziz, T.Z. Externalising deep brain electrodes: An increased risk of infection? *J. Clin. Neurosci.* **2004**, *11*, 732–734. [CrossRef]
29. Hawker, G.A.; Mian, S.; Kendzerska, T.; French, M. Measures of adult pain: Visual Analog Scale for Pain (VAS Pain), Numeric Rating Scale for Pain (NRS Pain), McGill Pain Questionnaire (MPQ), Short-Form McGill Pain Questionnaire (SF-MPQ), Chronic Pain Grade Scale (CPGS), Short Form-36 Bodily Pain Scale (SF-36 BPS), and Measure of Intermittent and Constant Osteoarthritis Pain (ICOAP). *Arthritis Care Res.* **2011**, *63*, S240–S252. [CrossRef]

30. Fields, H.L. How expectations influence pain. *Pain* **2018**, *159* (Suppl. 1), S3–S10. [CrossRef]
31. Beltrutti, D.; Lamberto, A.; Barolat, G.; Bruehl, S.P.; Doleys, D.; Krames, E.; Meglio, M.; North, R.; Olson, K.; Reig, E.; et al. The Psychological Assessment of Candidates for Spinal Cord Stimulation for Chronic Pain Management. *Pain Pract.* **2004**, *4*, 204–221. [CrossRef] [PubMed]
32. Almeida, A.N.; de Olivier, A.; Quesney, F.; Dubeau, F.; Savard, G.; Andermann, F. Efficacy of and morbidity associated with stereoelectroencephalography using computerized tomography—Or magnetic resonance imaging—Guided electrode implantation. *J. Neurosurg.* **2006**, *104*, 483–487. [CrossRef] [PubMed]
33. Kossoff, E.H.; Ritzl, E.K.; Politsky, J.M.; Murro, A.M.; Smith, J.R.; Duckrow, R.B.; Spencer, D.D.; Bergey, G.K. Effect of an external responsive neurostimulator on seizures and electrographic discharges during subdural electrode monitoring. *Epilepsia* **2004**, *45*, 1560–1567. [CrossRef] [PubMed]
34. Wager, T.D.; Atlas, L.Y.; Lindquist, M.A.; Roy, M.; Woo, C.-W.; Kross, E. An fMRI-Based Neurologic Signature of Physical Pain. *N. Engl. J. Med.* **2013**, *368*, 1388–1397. [CrossRef] [PubMed]
35. Rosa, M.J.; Seymour, B. Decoding the matrix: Benefits and limitations of applying machine learning algorithms to pain neuroimaging. *Pain* **2014**, *155*, 864–867. [CrossRef]
36. Apkarian, A.V.; Baliki, M.N.; Farmer, M.A. Predicting transition to chronic pain. *Curr. Opin. Neurol.* **2013**, *26*, 360–367. [CrossRef]
37. Gopalakrishnan, R.; Burgess, R.C.; Malone, D.A.; Lempka, S.F.; Gale, J.T.; Floden, D.P.; Baker, K.B.; Machado, A.G. Deep brain stimulation of the ventral striatal area for poststroke pain syndrome: A magnetoencephalography study. *J. Neurophysiol.* **2018**, *119*, 2118–2128. [CrossRef]
38. Lefaucheur, J.-P.; Jarry, G.; Drouot, X.; Ménard-Lefaucheur, I.; Keravel, Y.; Nguyen, J.-P. Motor cortex rTMS reduces acute pain provoked by laser stimulation in patients with chronic neuropathic pain. *Clin. Neurophysiol.* **2010**, *121*, 895–901. [CrossRef]
39. Gross, J.; Schnitzler, A.; Timmerman, L.; Ploner, M. Gamma oscillations in human primary somatosensory cortex reflect pain perception. *PLoS Biol.* **2007**, *5*. [CrossRef]
40. Bartolomei, F.; Lagarde, S.; Wendling, F.; McGonigal, A.; Jirsa, V.; Guye, M.; Benar, C. Defining epileptogenic networks: Contribution of SEEG and signal analysis. *Epilepsia* **2017**, *58*, 1131–1147. [CrossRef]
41. Coghill, R.C.; McHaffie, J.G.; Yen, Y.-F. Neural correlates of interindividual differences in the subjective experience of pain. *Proc. Natl. Acad. Sci. USA* **2003**, *100*, 8538–8542. [CrossRef] [PubMed]
42. Tracey, I.; Woolf, C.J.; Andrews, N.A. Composite Pain Biomarker Signatures for Objective Assessment and Effective Treatment. *Neuron* **2019**, *101*, 783–800. [CrossRef] [PubMed]
43. Baliki, M.N.; Chialvo, D.R.; Geha, P.Y.; Levy, R.M.; Harden, N.; Parrish, T.B.; Apkarian, A.V. Chronic Pain and the Emotional Brain: Specific Brain Activity Associated with Spontaneous Fluctuations of Intensity of Chronic Back Pain. *J. Neurosci.* **2006**, *26*, 12165–12173. [CrossRef] [PubMed]
44. Apkarian, A.V.; Sosa, Y.; Sonty, S.; Levy, R.M.; Harden, R.N.; Parrish, T.B.; Gitelman, D.R. Chronic Back Pain Is Associated with Decreased Prefrontal and Thalamic Gray Matter Density. *J. Neurosci.* **2004**, *24*, 10410–10415. [CrossRef] [PubMed]
45. Hashmi, J.A.; Baliki, M.A.; Huang, L.; Baria, A.T.; Torbey, S.; Hermann, K.M.; Schnitzer, T.J.; Apkarian, A.V. Shape shifting pain: Chronification of back pain shifts brain representation from nociceptive to emotional circuits. *Brain* **2013**, *136*, 2751–2768. [CrossRef]
46. Sun, F.T.; Morrell, M.J. The RNS System: Responsive cortical stimulation for the treatment of refractory partial epilepsy. *Expert Rev. Med. Devices* **2014**, *11*, 563–572. [CrossRef]
47. Medtronic FDA Approves Percept DBS Device. Available online: https://www.medtronic.com/us-en/about/news/fda-approval-percept.html (accessed on 20 September 2020).
48. Ploner, M.; Gross, J.; Timmermann, L.; Pollok, B.; Schnitzler, A. Oscillatory activity reflects the excitability of the human somatosensory system. *NeuroImage* **2006**, *32*, 1231–1236. [CrossRef]
49. Mouraux, A.; Guérit, J.M.; Plaghki, L. Non-phase locked electroencephalogram (EEG) responses to CO_2 laser skin stimulations may reflect central interactions between A partial partial differential- and C-fibre afferent volleys. *Clin. Neurophysiol. Off. J. Int. Fed. Clin. Neurophysiol.* **2003**, *114*, 710–722. [CrossRef]
50. Babiloni, C.; Brancucci, A.; Del Percio, C.; Capotosto, P.; Arendt-Nielsen, L.; Chen, A.C.N.; Rossini, P.M. Anticipatory electroencephalography alpha rhythm predicts subjective perception of pain intensity. *J. Pain Off. J. Am. Pain Soc.* **2006**, *7*, 709–717. [CrossRef]

51. Zhang, Z.G.; Hu, L.; Hung, Y.S.; Mouraux, A.; Iannetti, G.D. Gamma-Band Oscillations in the Primary Somatosensory Cortex—A Direct and Obligatory Correlate of Subjective Pain Intensity. *J. Neurosci.* **2012**, *32*, 7429–7438. [CrossRef]
52. Chien, J.H.; Liu, C.C.; Kim, J.H.; Markman, T.M.; Lenz, F.A. Painful cutaneous laser stimuli induce event-related oscillatory EEG activities that are different from those induced by nonpainful electrical stimuli. *J. Neurophysiol.* **2014**, *112*, 824–833. [CrossRef] [PubMed]
53. Liu, C.C.; Chien, J.H.; Kim, J.H.; Chuang, Y.F.; Cheng, D.T.; Anderson, W.; Lenz, F.A. Cross-frequency coupling in deep brain structures upon processing the painful sensory inputs. *Neuroscience* **2015**, *303*, 412–421. [CrossRef] [PubMed]
54. Davis, K.D.; Aghaeepour, N.; Ahn, A.H.; Angst, M.S.; Borsook, D.; Brenton, A.; Burczynski, M.E.; Crean, C.; Edwards, R.; Gaudilliere, B.; et al. Discovery and validation of biomarkers to aid the development of safe and effective pain therapeutics: Challenges and opportunities. *Nat. Rev. Neurol.* **2020**, *16*, 381. [CrossRef] [PubMed]
55. Huang, Y.; Green, A.L.; Hyam, J.; Fitzgerald, J.; Aziz, T.Z.; Wang, S. Oscillatory neural representations in the sensory thalamus predict neuropathic pain relief by deep brain stimulation. *Neurobiol. Dis.* **2018**, *109*, 117–126. [CrossRef]
56. Matsumoto, R.; Kunieda, T.; Nair, D. Single pulse electrical stimulation to probe functional and pathological connectivity in epilepsy. *Seizure Eur. J. Epilepsy* **2017**, *44*, 27–36. [CrossRef]
57. Mestre, T.A.; Lang, A.E.; Okun, M.S. Factors influencing the outcome of deep brain stimulation: Placebo, nocebo, lessebo, and lesion effects. *Mov. Disord.* **2016**, *31*, 290–298. [CrossRef]
58. Hamani, C.; Schwalb, J.M.; Rezai, A.R.; Dostrovsky, J.O.; Davis, K.D.; Lozano, A.M. Deep brain stimulation for chronic neuropathic pain: Long-term outcome and the incidence of insertional effect. *Pain* **2006**, *125*, 188–196. [CrossRef]
59. Foss, J.M.; Apkarian, A.V.; Chialvo, D.R. Dynamics of Pain: Fractal Dimension of Temporal Variability of Spontaneous Pain Differentiates Between Pain States. *J. Neurophysiol.* **2006**, *95*, 730–736. [CrossRef]
60. Mercado, R.; Constantoyannis, C.; Mandat, T.; Kumar, A.; Schulzer, M.; Stoessl, A.J.; Honey, C.R. Expectation and the placebo effect in Parkinson's disease patients with subthalamic nucleus deep brain stimulation. *Mov. Disord. Off. J. Mov. Disord. Soc.* **2006**, *21*, 1457–1461. [CrossRef]
61. McCambridge, J.; Witton, J.; Elbourne, D.R. Systematic review of the Hawthorne effect: New concepts are needed to study research participation effects. *J. Clin. Epidemiol.* **2014**, *67*, 267–277. [CrossRef]
62. Cooper, S.E.; McIntyre, C.C.; Fernandez, H.H.; Vitek, J.L. Association of Deep Brain Stimulation Washout Effects with Parkinson Disease Duration. *JAMA Neurol.* **2013**, *70*, 95–99. [CrossRef] [PubMed]
63. Cooper, S.E.; Driesslein, K.G.; Noecker, A.M.; McIntyre, C.C.; Machado, A.M.; Butson, C.R. Anatomical targets associated with abrupt versus gradual washout of subthalamic deep brain stimulation effects on bradykinesia. *PLoS ONE* **2014**, *9*, e99663. [CrossRef] [PubMed]
64. Perera, T.; Yohanandan, S.A.C.; Vogel, A.P.; McKay, C.M.; Jones, M.; Peppard, R.; McDermott, H.J. Deep brain stimulation wash-in and wash-out times for tremor and speech. *Brain Stimul. Basic Transl. Clin. Res. Neuromodul.* **2015**, *8*, 359. [CrossRef]
65. Rolke, R.; Magerl, W.; Campbell, K.A.; Schalber, C.; Caspari, S.; Birklein, F.; Treede, R.D. Quantitative sensory testing: A comprehensive protocol for clinical trials. *Eur. J. Pain* **2006**, *10*, 77–88. [CrossRef]
66. Dualé, C.; Daveau, J.; Cardot, J.-M.; Boyer-Grand, A.; Schoeffler, P.; Dubray, C. Cutaneous Amitriptyline in Human VolunteersDifferential Effects on the Components of Sensory Information. *Anesthesiol. J. Am. Soc. Anesthesiol.* **2008**, *108*, 714–721. [CrossRef]
67. Andersson, G.; Haldrup, D. Personalized pain words and Stroop interference in chronic pain patients. *Eur. J. Pain* **2003**, *7*, 431–438. [CrossRef]
68. Fichtenholtz, H.M.; Dean, H.L.; Dillon, D.G.; Yamasaki, H.; McCarthy, G.; LaBar, K.S. Emotion–attention network interactions during a visual oddball task. *Cogn. Brain Res.* **2004**, *20*, 67–80. [CrossRef]
69. Bechara, A.; Damasio, A.R.; Damasio, H.; Anderson, S.W. Insensitivity to future consequences following damage to human prefrontal cortex. *Cognition* **1994**, *50*, 7–15. [CrossRef]
70. Reckziegel, D.; Vachon-Presseau, E.; Petre, B.; Schnitzer, T.J.; Baliki, M.; Apkarian, A.V. Deconstructing biomarkers for chronic pain: Context and hypothesis dependent biomarker types in relation to chronic pain. *Pain* **2019**, *160*, S37–S48. [CrossRef]

71. Vijayakumar, V.; Case, M.; Shirinpour, S.; He, B. Quantifying and Characterizing Tonic Thermal Pain Across Subjects From EEG Data Using Random Forest Models. *IEEE Trans. Biomed. Eng.* **2017**, *64*, 2988–2996. [CrossRef]
72. Chiong, W.; Leonard, M.K.; Chang, E.F. Neurosurgical Patients as Human Research Subjects: Ethical Considerations in Intracranial Electrophysiology Research. *Neurosurgery* **2018**, *83*, 29–37. [CrossRef] [PubMed]
73. Andreassen Jaatun, E.A.; Hjermstad, M.J.; Gundersen, O.E.; Oldervoll, L.; Kaasa, S.; Haugen, D.F. Development and Testing of a Computerized Pain Body Map in Patients With Advanced Cancer. *J. Pain Symptom Manag.* **2014**, *47*, 45–56. [CrossRef] [PubMed]
74. Wideman, T.H.; Edwards, R.R.; Walton, D.M.; Martel, M.O.; Hudon, A.; Seminowicz, D.A. The Multimodal Assessment Model of Pain. *Clin. J. Pain* **2019**, *35*, 212–221. [CrossRef] [PubMed]

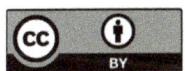

© 2020 by the authors. Licensee MDPI, Basel, Switzerland. This article is an open access article distributed under the terms and conditions of the Creative Commons Attribution (CC BY) license (http://creativecommons.org/licenses/by/4.0/).

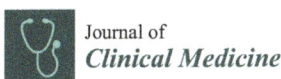

Article

Optimal Parameters of Deep Brain Stimulation in Essential Tremor: A Meta-Analysis and Novel Programming Strategy

I. Daria Bogdan [1,2], Teus van Laar [1,*], D.L. Marinus Oterdoom [2], Gea Drost [1,2], J. Marc C. van Dijk [2] and Martijn Beudel [3]

1. Department of Neurology, University Medical Center Groningen, University of Groningen, 9713 GZ Groningen, The Netherlands; i.d.bogdan@umcg.nl (I.D.B.); g.drost@umcg.nl (G.D.)
2. Department of Neurosurgery, University Medical Center Groningen, University of Groningen, 9713 GZ Groningen, The Netherlands; d.l.m.oterdoom@umcg.nl (D.L.M.O.); j.m.c.van.dijk@umcg.nl (J.M.C.v.D.)
3. Department of Neurology, Amsterdam Neuroscience Institute, Amsterdam University Medical Center, 1007 MB Amsterdam, The Netherlands; m.beudel@amsterdamumc.nl
* Correspondence: t.van.laar@umcg.nl

Received: 21 May 2020; Accepted: 9 June 2020; Published: 14 June 2020

Abstract: The programming of deep brain stimulation (DBS) parameters for tremor is laborious and empirical. Despite extensive efforts, the end-result is often suboptimal. One reason for this is the poorly understood relationship between the stimulation parameters' voltage, pulse width, and frequency. In this study, we aim to improve DBS programming for essential tremor (ET) by exploring a new strategy. At first, the role of the individual DBS parameters in tremor control was characterized using a meta-analysis documenting all the available parameters and tremor outcomes. In our novel programming strategy, we applied 10 random combinations of stimulation parameters in eight ET-DBS patients with suboptimal tremor control. Tremor severity was assessed using accelerometers and immediate and sustained patient-reported outcomes (PRO's), including the occurrence of side-effects. The meta-analysis showed no substantial relationship between individual DBS parameters and tremor suppression. Nevertheless, with our novel programming strategy, a significantly improved (accelerometer $p = 0.02$, PRO $p = 0.02$) and sustained ($p = 0.01$) tremor suppression compared to baseline was achieved. Less side-effects were encountered compared to baseline. Our pilot data show that with this novel approach, tremor control can be improved in ET patients with suboptimal tremor control on DBS. In addition, this approach proved to have a beneficial effect on stimulation-related complications.

Keywords: DBS; tremor; stimulation parameters; DBS programming algorithm; DBS side effects; thalamic nucleus; zona incerta

1. Introduction

Essential tremor (ET) is the most prevalent movement disorder, affecting up to 4% of the adult population [1]. Medical management of ET is limited and is often unsatisfactory [2]. For medically refractory cases, deep brain stimulation (DBS) may be considered. The long-term safety and efficacy of DBS are well-established [3], although it is not certain whether its initially reported superior tremor suppression is also achieved in successive cohorts [4]. Additionally, evidence shows that 33 out of 45 patients in one study (73.3%) reported waning tremor control at a mean time of 18.8 ± 15.1 months postoperatively [5].

The outcome of ET-DBS depends on several factors. Preoperative considerations include but are not limited to tremor characteristics [6] and the anatomical target of the intervention [7,8]. Postoperatively, optimal tremor reduction is achieved with time-consuming programming. The current strategy for symptom control starts with a standardized evaluation of several conventional stimulation parameters, representing the highest probability for success. Pulse widths with an estimated chronaxie (i.e., the minimum time for exciting a neural element using half the intensity to elicit a threshold response, for review see [9]) for myelinated axons in ET-DBS average 40–90 µs [10]. As far as frequency is concerned, it should be noted that during the first application of DBS, 50 Hz stimulation was considered as high-frequency stimulation [11]. Ever since, a broad range of stimulation frequencies up to 185 Hz has been explored, although there is no clear relation between the stimulation frequency and degree of tremor suppression. All parameters are further titrated in a 'trial and error' fashion, until satisfactory tremor suppression is achieved in the absence of side effects. In practice, this requires extensive programming sessions, in which patient fatigue may hamper achieving the desired results. Empirical titration becomes additionally challenging when conventional DBS parameters do not address individual requirements [12] or become subject to tremor habituation [13], requiring broader parameter searches than feasible. A clear understanding of the therapeutic role of the stimulation parameters is therefore essential. Unfortunately, the relation of any of the stimulation parameters and degree of tremor suppression remains insufficiently understood. A study exploring high-frequency stimulation as a putative cause for worsening balance in ET patients demonstrated that reducing stimulation frequency from 170–185 to 130 Hz after optimizing tremor control improved axial cerebellar signs [14]. In addition, therapeutic DBS intensity levels suppress tremor, while supra-therapeutic amplitudes and pulse-widths cause (gait) ataxia [15,16]. The deleterious effect of excessive stimulation translates thus into a narrow therapeutic window for tremor suppression.

Despite efforts to individualize and improve DBS programming [17,18], these are either not robust enough or are too technically challenging to be routinely applied in clinical practice. In the absence of an explicit, validated programming protocol, the process remains laborious and outcomes inconsistent, with average tremor reduction varying between 33 and 74% [2]. Outcomes may be improved with expert programming, shown to provide significant improvement in 37% of patients and partial improvement in 15% [12].

In this study, we aim to improve DBS programming protocols. We start by reviewing all documented DBS parameters and tremor outcomes in ET, with the aim to gain insight into the advancement of DBS programming over time, as well as to characterize the role of the DBS-parameters (voltage, pulse width, and frequency). Next, as a proof of concept, we introduce a novel approach for a timely and thorough exploration of the DBS parameter space in individual patients.

2. Methods

2.1. Meta-Analysis

2.1.1. Search Strategy and Selection Criteria

We conducted a PubMed search for DBS parameters in ET on 05/03/2018, using the following string: ("DBS" OR "Deep Brain Stimulation") AND ("essential tremor"). The search was conducted by two independent reviewers (DB and MO). Articles written in English, containing the key terms "DBS" or "stimulation" and "essential tremor" were included for full text screening. Animal studies, experiments in which patients had co-existing movement disorders (e.g., Parkinson's disease), as well as review articles were excluded from further analysis. For full text screening the following exclusion criteria were applied: (1) either stimulation parameters or outcomes were not reported; (2) interventions following failed DBS or thalamotomy (the latter might still exert therapeutic effects); (3) reports earlier than three months post-operatively (when the microlesion effect might influence tremor) or with unspecified follow-up moment; (4) cohorts already reported; (5) irretrievable articles; (6) pooled data of ET with Parkinson's patients; (7) IPG malfunctions. Review articles were checked for any relevant missing articles. The remaining articles were selected for data extraction.

2.1.2. Data Extraction

From each relevant study, the following data were extracted: publication year, size of patient sample, DBS target, average stimulation voltage, pulse width and frequency, tremor reduction, scale of tremor measurement, follow-up moment and side-effects. Side-effects were categorized as paresthesia, gait and balance problems, ataxia, dysarthria and diplopia or visual disturbances.

2.1.3. Data Synthesis

Data were recorded as mean ± standard deviation. For analysis, weighted values of the stimulation parameters and tremor outcomes were used. Reports of tremor suppression were heterogenous not only in terms of tremor scale, but also follow-up duration. Therefore, tremor outcomes were converted to percentages of tremor reduction and the primary outcome time point was used for each study. Given that the tremor measurements were performed at various follow-up durations, time might have possibly exerted an effect on the tremor outcomes owing to disease progression or tremor adaption. For this reason, follow-up durations were split into quartiles and the corresponding tremor outcomes were compared between the four groups.

2.1.4. Comparisons

To characterize the explored range of stimulation parameters and the evolution of tremor outcomes from the first application of DBS for tremor (1987) until the present, we correlated these values with time, i.e., corresponding publication year. Next, we explored the relationship between voltage, pulse width, frequency and tremor control. We also documented the encountered side-effects and correlated their frequency with the corresponding stimulation parameters.

2.2. Experimental DBS Programming

2.2.1. Patients

Eight consecutive patients treated with bilateral DBS for medically refractory ET participated in the study. Prior medical treatment included propranolol, primidone and topiramate, or a combination of the three. The efficacy of the treatment has been thoroughly reviewed before deeming the patient therapy-resistant and discussed multi-disciplinarily to establish the indication for DBS. All patients were implanted (Medtronic model 3387 lead, contacts 1.5 mm in length, spaced 3 mm center-to-center; Medtronic, Inc.) using the Leksell G frame (Elekta, Stockholm, Sweden). Accurate electrode positioning was tested using intra-operative macrostimulation (up to 5 V, with 60 µs pulses and a frequency of 185 Hz) and was confirmed by postoperative MRI (Philips Intera, Eindhoven, the Netherlands) and/or CT-scanning (Sensation 64, Siemens, Erlangen, Germany). The post-implantation CT images were fused with preoperative 3T-MRI images using BrainLAB software (BrainLAB, Heimstetten, Germany). The electrode configurations and stimulation parameters had been reviewed at length and optimized by using Medtronic's 8840 N'Vision Clinician Programmer (Medtronic, Inc., Northridge, CA, USA), according to the best current practice [19]. None of the patients were on any medication for tremor following DBS. Patients were recruited at the outpatient neurological department at the University Medical Centre Groningen (UMCG). The experimental procedure was approved by the medical ethical review board of the UMCG (registration number 2017406) and deemed "care as usual". Under these circumstances, written informed consent was not required.

2.2.2. Experimental Paradigm

The experimental paradigm started with a baseline tremor measurement, using the current stimulation parameters. Tremor was assessed in various arm postures and quantified by an in-house developed accelerometer (UMCG, Groningen, The Netherlands). For each posture, the total distance amplitude (TDamp) was calculated over 5 s by a custom-written script in LabVIEW (2014 SP1) and was used to assess tremor severity. This was done by calculating the second integral of the accelerometer signal. After the baseline measurement, the posture in which tremor was most severe, was used for the adjustment of DBS parameters.

In this posture, 10 random combinations of stimulation parameters (voltage, pulse width and frequency) were tested. These combinations were generated by a custom-written script in MATLAB (version R2014a, MathWorks, MA, USA), for each patient individually. The ranges from which the stimulation parameters were randomly extracted were as follows: voltage 1.5–4 V with intervals of 0.1 V; pulse width 60–240 µs with intervals of 10µs and frequency 60–185 Hz with intervals of 5 Hz. The script selected *at random* one voltage, one pulse width and one frequency, from a pool of 12,844 theoretical combinations. The process was repeated 10 times for every patient. For each experimental combination, a 5s accelerometer recording was performed once the effects of the previous settings disappeared. Patients also indicated whether stimulation felt better in terms of tremor control compared to baseline. If side-effects emerged, stimulation was not further increased (thus attaining a pseudorandom set of parameters). However, the transition between combinations was done systematically to maximize the chance of employing a given set of parameters. Namely, we identified the parameters that needed to be lowered or increased in the subsequent setting. Given that higher current charges are more likely to cause side-effects, the parameters were prioritized as follows: parameter requiring the greatest decrements, followed by eventual lesser decrements, least increments and greatest increments, respectively. Therefore, parameters requiring decreases were adjusted first. If the remaining parameters needed to be increased, the one requiring the smallest increase was adjusted first. If the remaining changes were to cause side-effects, increments would be stopped, and the final combination would be noted. By applying this system, the pseudo character of the random parameters was deemed by the patient safety and not by the clinician's bias.

In case the new stimulation parameters led to improved tremor control and/or less side-effects compared to the baseline settings, patients maintained these parameters. To evaluate whether the new empirical settings retained tremor control, patients were approached by telephone 6–17 weeks later. Patients indicated whether tremor control was similar, better or worse compared to baseline settings and whether side-effects had emerged.

2.2.3. Evaluation of the Experimental Settings

The combinations of stimulation parameters that led to the best tremor reduction were identified by the individual ratings of the patients (subjective) and the accelerometer signal (objective). The effect on tremor of the best subjective and objective random stimulation parameters was compared to that of the baseline settings. Medium-term efficacy (i.e., beyond the clinical setting) was determined by contrasting the patient-reported improvements to baseline tremor control. Next, the subjective and objective stimulation parameters were compared to baseline settings to determine whether tremor control was achieved with significantly different parameters or levels of total electrical energy delivered (TEED, [20]).

3. Statistical Analysis

Statistical analysis was performed using SPSS (SPSS IBM version 23.0, Armonk, NY, USA). Data normality was tested with the Kolmogorov–Smirnov test. For correlations, Pearson's correlation or Spearman's rank-order correlation were used accordingly and reported together with the percentage of explained variance (r^2). In the case of within-subject measurements, paired sample *t*-tests were used for normally distributed data and two-tailed Wilcoxon signed-rank tests for nonparametric distributions. For nonparametric, independent comparisons, the Kruskal–Wallis test was used. Significance was set at $p < 0.05$.

4. Results

4.1. Meta-Analysis

4.1.1. Study Inclusion and Data Characteristics

Our PubMed search yielded a total of 777 studies. Four duplicates were removed, leaving 773 studies for title and abstract screening. Here, 538 studies did not fulfil the inclusion criteria. The remainder of 235 full-text studies were assessed for eligibility. Four additional studies were identified through cross-reference screening and added to the eighty-three studies selected for data extraction, involving 1652 patients (Figure 1, Supplementary Table S1). Data exhibited a nonparametric distribution.

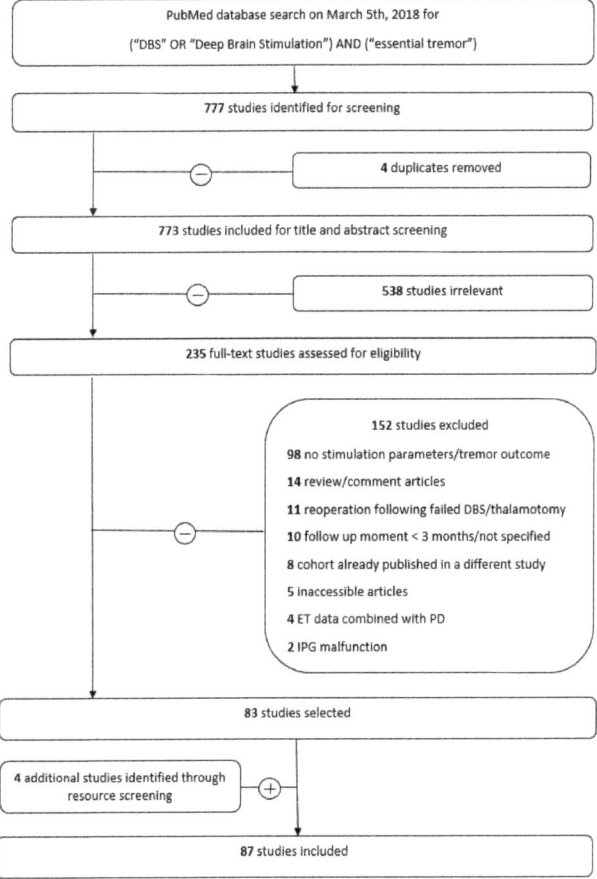

Figure 1. Preferred Reporting Items for Systematic Reviews and Meta-Analyses (PRISMA) flowchart.

4.1.2. DBS parameters and Tremor Outcomes

The correlation coefficients of the stimulation parameters with time were $r(1159) = -0.17$, $r^2 = 0.02$ (2.89%), $p < 0.001$ for voltage, $r(1312) = -0.17$, $r^2 = 0.02$ (2.89%) $p < 0.001$ for pulse width and $r(1258) = 0.08$, $r^2 = 0.006$ (0.6%) $p < 0.05$ for frequency. Overall, the average tremor suppression achieved by DBS was 62.98% ± 16%, $r(1466) = 0.16$, $r^2 = 0.02$ (2.56%), $p < 0.001$ (Supplementary Figure S1).

4.1.3. Correlation of Stimulation Parameters and Tremor Suppression

Follow-up times were split into quartiles, which yielded four groups of tremor outcomes corresponding to reports ranging from 3 to 6 months, 7 to 12 months, 13 to 30 months and 31 to 150 months, respectively. Although tremor outcomes differed significantly between the four groups ($\chi^2(3) = 186$, $p < 0.001$), the means did not exhibit a consistent downward trend ($M_1 = 57.42$, 95% CI: 55.78–59.08; $M_2 = 70.93$, 95% CI: 69.8–72.02; $M_3 = 62.25$, 95% CI: 60.47–64.14; $M_4 = 55.95$, 95% CI: 53.73–58.16). Thus, no correction for the variable follow-up times was applied. Regarding the interdependence of stimulation parameters and tremor, an inverse relationship is observed between voltage $r(1159) = -0.09$, $r^2 = 0.008$ (.81%), $p < 0.05$, and tremor. Although the same trend is observed for pulse width $r(1312) = -0.06$, $r^2 = 0.003$ (0.36%), $p = 0.05$, and frequency $r(1258) = -0.03$, $r^2 = 0.0009$ (0.09%), $p = 0.28$, these are not statistically significant.

4.1.4. Side Effects

Thirty-seven of the 87 included studies reported side effects (N = 785). Namely, 7.89% of patients complained of paresthesia (N = 62), 5.47% of gait and balance problems (N = 43), 2.03% of ataxia (N = 16), 15.28% of dysarthria (N = 120) and 0.12% of diplopia (N = 1). Only voltage exhibited a significant correlation, with dysarthria $r(118) = 0.43$, $r^2 = 0.43$ (18.49%), $p = 0.01$.

4.2. Experimental DBS Programming

4.2.1. Experimental Tremor Titration

The experiment was conducted in eight ET patients (Table 1, Supplementary Figure S2). None of the patients was on any tremor medication following DBS surgery. Baseline tremor control could not be documented in one patient (ET6) and was excluded from the corresponding statistical analysis. Given that subjective improvement was nevertheless achieved and sustained in the thr medium term, ET6 is still documented in Table 1. The experimental paradigm showed significant tremor reduction compared to baseline stimulation, according to both subjective ($t(6) = -2.95$, $p = 0.02$) and objective ($t(6) = -3.07$, $p = 0.02$) measurements (Figure 2). Notably, the tremor improvement perceived by the patients corresponded to the accelerometer measurements. On average, the results were achieved after 23.8 ± 8.03 min per patient. Upon follow-up, 45% of the patients reported medium-term tremor control superior to baseline ($p = 0.01$). None of the patients reported the new setting as being worse than the previous. As far as side effects are concerned, four patients (ET2, ET4, ET7, ET8) reported stimulation-induced ataxia and/or dysarthria at baseline. Following experimental re-titration, side-effects were resolved in all but one patient (ET4), who reported re-emergence of ataxia upon follow-up.

Table 1. Patient demographics and deep brain stimulation (DBS) parameters. Baseline tremor control was measured prior re-titration with the patients retaining their current DBS settings. Next, ten random combinations of stimulation parameters were tested in eight essential tremor (ET) patients. The random combinations affording the most tremor suppression according to both patient-reported outcomes (subjective) and accelerometer recordings (objective) are presented here. Tremor severity is expressed in arbitrary units (TDAmp) as returned by the accelerometer. "Since youth" implies that the patients were diagnosed before the age of 18 years old.

Patient	Age (Years)	Gender	Disease Duration (years)	DBS Duration	DBS Target	DBS Contacts	Baseline				Best-Subjective				Best-Objective			
							V	P	F	TDAmp	V	P	F	TDAmp	V	P	F	TDAmp
ET1	53	male	Since youth	2	Vim	−1	2	90	185	0.87	3.2	180	80	0.32	3.3	200	95	0.20
ET3	77	male	22	1	Vim	−10	3	90	185	1.03	3.5	180	145	0.27	3.9	150	160	0.24
ET4	73	male	33	20	Vim	−0	0.8	60	180	0.14	1.6	70	165	0.11	2.1	170	85	0.11
ET5	69	male	52	1	Vim	−1/2+	2.8	60	185	0.07	2.7	210	170	0.07	3.2	140	175	0.07
Average tremor improvement (%) compared to baseline for Vim-DBS according to subjective (53%) and objective (58%) measurements.																		
ET2	78	male	Since youth	3	ZI	−3	3.3	60	185	0.94	3.6	60	160	0.36	3.9	70	150	0.28
ET6	70	male	27	4	ZI	−9/10+	1.7	60	180	n.a.	1.5	90	155	0.43	1.5	90	155	0.43
ET7	72	female	Since youth	6	ZI	−1	1.8	90	180	1.07	2.2	140	140	0.20	2.2	140	140	0.20
ET8	51	female	48	6	ZI	−1/2+	1	90	185	1.81	2.2	160	180	0.11	1.5	220	180	0.06
Average tremor improvement (%) compared to baseline for ZI-DBS according to subjective (79%) and objective (82%) measurements.																		

Abbreviations: ET = essential tremor, F = frequency (Hz), TDAmp = arbitrary unit of measurement representing tremor severity, P = pulse width (μs), V = voltage (V), Vim = ventral intermediate thalamic nucleus, ZI = zona incerta.

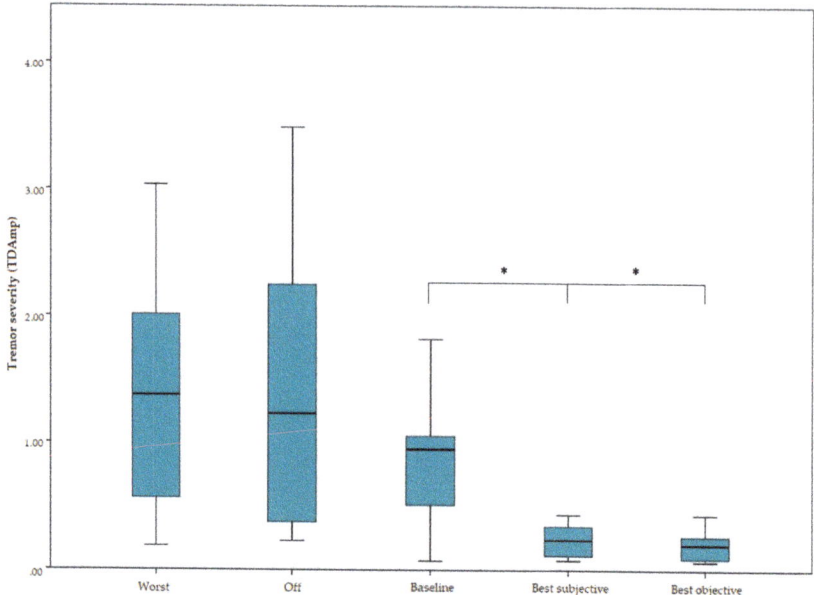

Figure 2. Experimental ET-DBS titration. Ten random combinations of stimulation parameters were tested and characterized subjectively (patient reported outcomes) and objectively (accelerometer measurements). The tremor outcomes during the experimental parameter exploration are categorized as follows: worst (least tremor reduction), off (stimulation turned off), baseline (initial settings), best subjective (best random settings according to the patient), best objective (best random settings according to accelerometer measurements). The novel programming strategy afforded significant tremor reduction ($t(6) = -2.95$, $p = 0.02$) in the absence of side-effects. (*) represents a statistically significant ($p < 0.05$) difference.

4.2.2. Random DBS Parameters

An example of the randomly generated parameters is given in Supplementary Figure S2. Parameter optimization was achieved with significantly broader pulse widths according to both subjective $Z = -2.37$, $p = 0.01$ and objective $Z = -2.52$, $p = 0.01$ measurements. Conversely, significantly lower frequencies proved superior to baseline settings in both subjective $Z = -2.53$, $p = 0.01$ and objective ratings $Z = -2.52$, $p = 0.01$. No significant difference was detected for either subjective $Z = -1.12$, $p = 0.26$ or objective $Z = -1.54$, $p = 0.12$ ratings of voltage. More optimal tremor reduction was achieved with higher levels of TEED, in both subjective $t(7) = -2.12$, $p = 0.07$ and objective $t(7) = -3.08$, $p = 0.01$ measurements.

5. Discussion

5.1. Meta-Analysis

Our meta-analysis shows that, in more than 30 years, the outcome of ET-DBS improved only modestly. Given that there was no relevant change in the studied DBS parameters, the observed improvement might possibly be attributed to improved patient selection [6], DBS targeting [7,21] and stereotactic planning [22]. Although beneficial, these developments are efficient mostly in the short-term. Provided that tremor outcomes significantly decline over time [23], with habituation of the stimulation settings accounting for more than 10% of the decrease in outcome [24], more efforts should be focused on programming. In line with this, there is evidence for alternating stimulation settings to reduce habituation. However, side-effects remain a great limiting factor.

From the available literature, there appears to be no substantial relationship between DBS parameters and tremor suppression or side-effects. Given that several follow-up reports extend up to 150 months, it raises the concern that tremor outcomes might be affected by either disease progression or tremor adaption. Although tremor outcomes differed significantly in the four time-groups (follow-up-duration quartiles), no downward trend suggesting declining outcomes was observed. As such, the observed differences stem more likely from patient heterogeneity, rather than being the effect of time. In line with these results, we introduced random combinations of stimulation parameters for conducting comprehensive and time-saving parameter searches in individual patients. We show that this novel programming strategy is effective in optimizing individual tremor control and resolving side effects.

Despite that DBS parameters remain relatively constant over time, the corresponding tremor outcomes show large variations. Although voltage is the only parameter to show a significant correlation with tremor suppression and dysarthria, the low value of the explained variation falls short to explain this observation (significance in this case reflects the large N rather than a clinical significance) These findings confirm the inconsistent results from DBS-parameter explorations reported elsewhere [25–27]. Such discrepancies suggest that uniform parameters might not exist, and that programming should particularly address the individual anatomy [7] and tremor characteristics [25].

The Rationale behind Conventional Stimulation Parameters

Conventional stimulation parameters have originally been extrapolated from structure–effect relationships to address the anatomical target and tremor characteristics [10,28]. However, they consistently appear to fall short of the mark, with room for improving clinical outcomes. Despite increasing evidence that better individualizing the DBS dose is key to maximizing symptom control [17,27], conventional parameters have remained the mainstay. However, as long as the precise spatiotemporal coordinates of the neuroanatomical substrate required for clinical benefits remain insufficiently understood, finding the optimal DBS parameters will remain challenging.

Firstly, the complexity of stimulating neural tissue stems from multiple determinants, e.g., the interaction with different neuronal elements and relative distance to the electrode [29,30], as well as the direction of propagation of the action potentials [31,32]. This is consistent with the difficulty of modeling electric field predictions [33,34]. Secondly, this spatial component of DBS is further raveled by the yet unknown mechanism of action. Several hypotheses have been proposed [35,36], illustrating the wide-ranging effects of DBS. Elucidating the precise effects that determine the clinical outcome will be key to refining the electric field predictions to address both the local and global dynamics of the targeted circuitopathies. Lastly, the third obstacle in finding optimal DBS parameters are the temporal adjustments of stimulation. Refining DBS to be delivered only in response to pathological biomarkers (adaptive DBS; aDBS) appears promising for both ameliorating symptoms and reducing side-effects [37,38].

Attempts to understand the stimulation parameters have yielded inconsistent results. Most commonly, the effect of varying one DBS-parameter is documented, while the remaining parameters are maintained at constant [39]. The limitation of such an approach is that the constant parameters determine the therapeutic window of the parameter of interest [16]. This generates irreproducible results due to inter-patient variability. In this study, we emphasize how insufficiently understood the interdependence of the stimulation parameters is, i.e., unexpected stimulation parameters can be clinically meaningful only when provided with the right interaction of these three parameters. Given that (1) the stimulation substrate exhibits a highly complex, dynamic and individualized spatiotemporal fabric and that (2) individual stimulation parameters cannot be considered for titration alone, future studies should allow for mutual dynamism to be exercised between the two. Therefore, programming strategies should be as robust as possible.

5.2. Experimental DBS Programming

Increasing understanding of the complexity of the stimulation substrate, as well as that of the interdependence of the stimulation parameters, has increasingly discouraged the use of conventional parameters. However, the infeasibility of clinically exploring the range of DBS parameters, to a greater extent, has precluded this transition. Testing ten random combinations of stimulation parameters results in a thorough, time-saving exploration, which allows for ET-DBS optimization in individual patients. Safety is ensured by gradually transitioning between combinations and having the patient report the emergence of side effects, beyond which stimulation is not further increased. Notably, the most optimal parameters are selected by patient intrinsic factors, e.g., anatomopathological substrate [40–42] and lead positioning [16,43]. The fact that significantly lower frequencies have been favored in this assumption-free trial is in line with the observed deleterious effects of supra-threshold frequency [14]. It is also tempting to attribute the resolution of side-effects in three of our four patients to this. This pilot approach raises thus great interest by opening the gate towards more individualized, comprehensive, and faster DBS titration.

The foremost limitations of the meta-analysis are publication bias [4] and perhaps overly enthusiastic early reports [44]. Additionally, the analysis of the relationship between DBS parameters and tremor outcomes could have benefited from objective tremor measurements (e.g., accelerometry). Nevertheless, validated tremor scales have been used [45]. Regarding the experiment, one limitation might be using shorter (between 1–2 min) wash-out periods than usual [18] in some patients. However, it has been shown that Vim-DBS for ET provides tremor suppression over seconds [2]. Additionally, the sustained tremor suppression upon follow-up excluded that the therapeutic benefit of the definitive experimental settings was confounded by phase-resetting or carryover effects. In addition, it would have been desirable to also provide tremor scores. However, the value of tremor scales would have been limited in this case, given that only one posture of one limb was assessed and tremor scales cannot detect subtle differences due to their ordinal character. Ideally, medium-term tremor reports should have been supplemented by accelerometer measurements. Another limitation might be using pre-determined electrode configurations. This was done because the electrode configurations with the largest therapeutic windows had already been determined in previous programming sessions and we wanted to limit patient fatigue to a minimum. However, it would be interesting, in a future study, to explore the role of random stimulation parameters in determining the therapeutic window. Lastly, there is no evidence that, after ten trials of random parameters, convergence is reached. However, we started with a pragmatic approach that could be tested during a regular outpatient visit. In future studies, we will explore whether testing more parameters brings further improvements.

6. Conclusions

DBS programming provides options beyond conventional parameter selection. Access to these parameters is particularly important for addressing ET that does not respond to conventional DBS parameters [12] or develops habituation [13,24]. Deep-learning modalities might be able to further refine this approach to avoid supra-therapeutic stimulation, minimize battery consumption, and enable the titration of more complex devices [46,47]. The role of the individual DBS parameters in tremor control remains elusive. Our proof of concept underscores the interdependence of voltage, pulse width, and frequency, warranting further research.

Supplementary Materials: The following are available online at http://www.mdpi.com/2077-0383/9/6/1855/s1, Figure S1: Overall tremor outcomes; Figure S2. Experimental Set-up, Table S1. Characteristics of studies included in the meta-analysis.

Author Contributions: M.B., I.D.B., J.M.C.v.D. and T.v.L. designed the study. M.B. and I.D.B. collected the data. M.B., I.D.B., G.D., T.v.L. and D.L.M.O. analyzed and interpreted the data. M.B. and I.D.B. conducted the statistical analysis. I.D.B. drafted the article. M.B., J.M.C.v.D., G.D., T.v.L. and D.L.M.O. critically revised the article and reviewed the submitted version of the manuscript. M.B. supervised the study. The final version of the manuscript was approved by all authors. All authors have read and agreed to the published version of the manuscript.

Funding: Universitair Medisch Centrum Groningen: 2017-1.

Acknowledgments: This work was supported by the Healthy Aging Pilot funding (2017-1) from the University Medical Center Groningen.

Conflicts of Interest: None of the authors has any conflict of interest to disclose.

References

1. Louis, E.D. Treatment of essential tremor: Are there issues we are overlooking? *Front. Neurol.* **2011**, *2*, 91. [PubMed]
2. Flora, E.D.; Perera, C.L.; Cameron, A.L.; Maddern, G.J. Deep brain stimulation for essential tremor: A systematic review. *Mov. Disord.* **2010**, *25*, 1550–1559. [CrossRef] [PubMed]
3. Baizabal-Carvallo, J.F.; Kagnoff, M.N.; Jimenez-shahed, J.; Fekete, R.; Jankovic, J. The safety and efficacy of thalamic deep brain stimulation in essential tremor: 10 years and beyond. *J. Neurol. Neurosurg. Psychiatry* **2014**, *85*, 567–572. [CrossRef] [PubMed]
4. Tyrer, P.; Kendall, T. The spurious advance of antipsychotic drug therapy. *Lancet* **2009**, *373*, 4–5. [CrossRef]
5. Fasano, A.; Helmich, R.C. Tremor habituation to deep brain stimulation: Underlying mechanisms and solutions. *Mov. Disord.* **2019**, *34*, 1761–1773. [CrossRef]
6. Sandoe, C.; Krishna, V.; Basha, D.; Sammartino, F.; Tatsch, J.; Picillo, M.; di Biase, L.; Poon, Y.; Hamani, C.; Reddy, D.; et al. Predictors of deep brain stimulation outcome in tremor patients. *Brain Stimul.* **2018**, *11*, 592–599. [CrossRef]
7. Schlaier, J.; Anthofer, J.; Steib, K.; Fellner, C.; Rothenfusser, E.; Brawanski, A.; Lange, M. Deep brain stimulation for essential tremor: Targeting the dentato-rubro-thalamic tract? *Neuromodulation* **2015**, *18*, 105–112. [CrossRef]
8. Coenen, V.A.; Varkuti, B.; Parpaley, Y.; Skodda, S.; Prokop, T.; Urbach, H.; Li, M.; Reinacher, P. Postoperative neuroimaging analysis of DRT deep brain stimulation revision surgery for complicated essential tremor. *Acta Neurochir.* **2017**, *159*, 779–787. [CrossRef]
9. Kringelbach, M.L.; Jenkinson, N.; Owen, S.L.; Aziz, T.Z. Translational principles of deep brain stimulation. *Nat. Rev. Neurosci.* **2007**, *8*, 623–635. [CrossRef]
10. Holsheimer, J.; Dijkstra, E.A.; Demeulemeester, H.; Nuttin, B. Chronaxie calculated from current-duration and voltage-duration data. *J. Neurosci. Methods* **2000**, *97*, 45–50. [CrossRef]
11. Hassler, R.; Riechert, T.; Mundinger, F.; Umbach, W.; Ganglberger, J.A. Physiological observations in stereotaxic operations in extrapyramidal motor disturbances. *Brain* **1960**, *83*, 337–350. [CrossRef] [PubMed]
12. Okun, M.S. Management of referred deep brain stimulation failures: A retrospective analysis from 2 movement disorders centers. *Arch. Neurol.* **2005**, *62*, 1250–1255. [CrossRef] [PubMed]
13. Barbe, M.T.; Liebhart, L.; Runge, M.; Pauls KA, M.; Wojtecki, L.; Schnitzler, A.; Allert, N.; Fink, G.; Sturm, V.; Maarouf, M.; et al. Deep brain stimulation in the nucleus ventralis intermedius in patients with essential tremor: Habituation of tremor suppression. *J. Neurol.* **2011**, *258*, 434–439. [CrossRef] [PubMed]
14. Ramirez-Zamora, A.; Boggs, H.; Pilitsis, J.G. Reduction in DBS frequency improves balance difficulties after thalamic DBS for essential tremor. *J. Neurol. Sci.* **2016**, *367*, 122–127. [CrossRef]
15. Fasano, A.; Herzog, J.; Raethjen, J.; Rose, F.E.; Muthuraman, M.; Volkmann, J.; Falk, D.; Elble, R.; Deuschl, G. Gait ataxia in essential tremor is differentially modulated by thalamic stimulation. *Brain* **2010**, *133*, 3635–3648. [CrossRef]
16. Groppa, S.; Herzog, J.; Falk, D.; Riedel, C.; Deuschl, G.; Volkmann, J. Physiological and anatomical decomposition of subthalamic neurostimulation effects in essential tremor. *Brain* **2014**, *137*, 109–121. [CrossRef]
17. Cagnan, H.; Brittain, J.S.; Little, S.; Foltynie, T.; Limousin, P.; Zrinzo, L.; Hariz, M.; Joint, C.; Fitzgerald, J.; Green, A.; et al. Phase dependent modulation of tremor amplitude in essential tremor through thalamic stimulation. *Brain* **2013**, *136*, 3062–3075. [CrossRef]
18. Akbar, U.; Raike, R.S.; Hack, N.; Hess, C.W.; Skinner, J.; Martinez-Ramirez, D.; DeJesus, S.; Okun, M.S. Randomized, blinded pilot testing of nonconventional stimulation patterns and shapes in parkinson's disease and essential tremor: Evidence for further evaluating narrow and biphasic pulses. *Neuromodulation Technol. Neural Interface* **2016**, *19*, 343–356. [CrossRef]

19. Picillo, M.; Lozano, A.M.; Kou, N.; Puppi munhoz, R.; Fasano, A. Programming deep brain stimulation for parkinson's disease: The toronto western hospital algorithms. *Brain Stimul.* **2016**, *9*, 425–437. [CrossRef]
20. Koss, A.M.; Alterman, R.L.; Tagliati, M.; Shils, J.L. Calculating total electrical energy delivered by deep brain stimulation systems. *Ann. Neurol.* **2005**, *58*, 168. [CrossRef]
21. Sandvik, U.; Koskinen, L.O.; Lundquist, A.; Blomstedt, P. Thalamic and subthalamic deep brain stimulation for essential tremor: Where is the optimal target? *Neurosurgery* **2012**, *70*, 840–845. [CrossRef] [PubMed]
22. Calabrese, E. Diffusion tractography in deep brain stimulation surgery: A review. *Front. Neuroanat.* **2016**, *10*, 45. [CrossRef] [PubMed]
23. Paschen, S.; Forstenpointner, J.; Becktepe, J.; Heinzel, S.; Hellriegel, H.; Witt, K.; Helmers, A.K.; Deuschl, G. Long-term efficacy of deep brain stimulation for essential tremor: An observer-blinded study. *Neurology* **2019**, *92*, e1378–e1386. [CrossRef] [PubMed]
24. Seier, M.; Hiller, A.; Quinn, J.; Murchison, C.; Brodsky, M.; Anderson, S. Alternating thalamic deep brain stimulation for essential tremor: A trial to reduce habituation. *Mov. Disord. Clin. Pract.* **2018**, *5*, 620–626. [CrossRef] [PubMed]
25. Cagnan, H.; Pedrosa, D.; Little, S.; Pogosyan, A.; Cheeran, B.; Aziz, T.; Green, A.; Fitzgerald, J.; Foltynie, T.; Limousin, P.; et al. Stimulating at the right time: Phase-specific deep brain stimulation. *Brain* **2017**, *140*, 132–145.
26. Gildenberg, P.L. Evolution of neuromodulation. *Stereotact Funct. Neurosurg.* **2005**, *83*, 71–79. [CrossRef]
27. Huang, H.; Watts, R.L.; Montgomery, E.B. Effects of deep brain stimulation frequency on bradykinesia of Parkinson's disease. *Mov. Disord.* **2014**, *29*, 203–206. [CrossRef]
28. Blomstedt, P.; Hariz, G.M.; Hariz, M.I.; Koskinen, L.O. Thalamic deep brain stimulation in the treatment of essential tremor: A long-term follow-up. *Br. J. Neurosurg.* **2007**, *21*, 504–509. [CrossRef]
29. Histed, M.H.; Bonin, V.; Reid, R.C. Direct activation of sparse, distributed populations of cortical neurons by electrical microstimulation. *Neuron* **2009**, *63*, 508–522. [CrossRef]
30. Pastor, J.; Vega-zelaya, L. A new potential specifically marks the sensory thalamus in anaesthetised patients. *Clin. Neurophysiol.* **2019**, *130*, 1926–1936. [CrossRef]
31. Montgomery, E.B. *Deep Brain Stimulation Programming: Principles and Practice*; Oxford University Press: Oxford, UK, 2010.
32. Hartmann, C.J.; Hirschmann, J.; Vesper, J.; Wojtecki, L.; Butz, M.; Schnitzler, A. Distinct cortical responses evoked by electrical stimulation of the thalamic ventral intermediate nucleus and of the subthalamic nucleus. *NeuroImage Clin.* **2018**, *20*, 1246–1254. [CrossRef] [PubMed]
33. Chaturvedi, A.; Butson, C.R.; Lempka, S.F.; Cooper, S.E.; Mcintyre, C.C. Patient-specific models of deep brain stimulation: Influence of field model complexity on neural activation predictions. *Brain Stimul.* **2010**, *3*, 65–67. [CrossRef] [PubMed]
34. Howell, B.; Mcintyre, C.C. Analyzing the tradeoff between electrical complexity and accuracy in patient-specific computational models of deep brain stimulation. *J. Neural Eng.* **2016**, *13*, 036023. [CrossRef] [PubMed]
35. Chiken, S.; Nambu, A. Mechanism of deep brain stimulation: Inhibition, excitation, or disruption? *Neuroscientist* **2016**, *22*, 313–322. [CrossRef]
36. Jakobs, M.; Fomenko, A.; Lozano, A.M.; Kiening, K.L. Cellular, molecular, and clinical mechanisms of action of deep brain stimulation-a systematic review on established indications and outlook on future developments. *EMBO Mol. Med.* **2019**, *11*, e9575. [CrossRef]
37. Little, S.; Beudel, M.; Zrinzo, L.; Foltynie, T.; Limousin, P.; Hariz, M.; Neal, S.; Cheeran, B.; Cagnan, H.; Gratwicke, J.; et al. Bilateral adaptive deep brain stimulation is effective in Parkinson's disease. *J. Neurol. Neurosurg. Psychiatry* **2016**, *87*, 717–721. [CrossRef]
38. Beudel, M.; Sadnicka, A.; Edwards, M.; De jong, B.M. Linking pathological oscillations with altered temporal processing in parkinsons disease: Neurophysiological mechanisms and implications for neuromodulation. *Front. Neurol.* **2019**, *10*, 462. [CrossRef]
39. Cooper, S.E.; Kuncel, A.M.; Wolgamuth, B.R.; Rezai, A.R.; Grill, W.M. A model predicting optimal parameters for deep brain stimulation in essential tremor. *J. Clin. Neurophysiol.* **2008**, *25*, 265–273. [CrossRef]

40. Bhatia, K.P.; Bain, P.; Bajaj, N.; Elble, R.J.; Hallett, M.; Loui, E.D.; Raethjen, J.; Stamelou, M.; Testa, C.M.; Deuschl, G. Tremor Task Force of the International Parkinson and Movement Disorder Society Consensus statement on the classification of tremors. From the task force on tremor of the international parkinson and movement disorder society. *Mov. Disord.* **2018**, *33*, 75–87. [CrossRef]
41. Deuschl, G.; Bergman, H. Pathophysiology of nonparkinsonian tremors. *Mov. Disord.* **2002**, *17*, 41–48. [CrossRef]
42. Middlebrooks, E.H.; Holanda, V.M.; Tuna, I.S.; Deshpande, H.D.; Bredel, M.; Almeida, L.; Walker, H.C.; Guthrie, B.L.; Foote, K.D.; Okun, M.S. A method for pre-operative single-subject thalamic segmentation based on probabilistic tractography for essential tremor deep brain stimulation. *Neuroradiology* **2018**, *60*, 303–309. [CrossRef] [PubMed]
43. Pedrosa, D.J.; Reck, C.; Florin, E.; Pauls, M.; Maarouf, M.; Wojtecki, L.; Dafsari, S.H.; Sturm, V.; Schnitzler, A.; Fink, G.R.; et al. Essential tremor and tremor in Parkinson's disease are associated with distinct 'tremor clusters' in the ventral thalamus. *Exp. Neurol.* **2012**, *237*, 435–443. [CrossRef] [PubMed]
44. Walsh, V.Q. Ethics and social risks in brain stimulation. *Brain Stimul.* **2013**, *6*, 715–717. [CrossRef] [PubMed]
45. Elble, R.; Bain, P.; Forjaz, M.J.; Haubenberger, D.; Testa, C.; Goetz, C.G.; Leentjens, A.F.G.; Martinez-Martin, P.; Pavy-Le Traon, A.; Post, B.; et al. Task force report: Scales for screening and evaluating tremor: Critique and recommendations. *Mov. Disord.* **2013**, *28*, 1793–1800. [CrossRef]
46. Willsie, A.; Dorval, A. Fabrication and initial testing of the DBS: A novel deep brain stimulation electrode with thousands of individually controllable contacts. *Biomed. Microdevices* **2015**, *17*, 56. [CrossRef]
47. Timmermann, L.; Jain, R.; Chen, L.; Maarouf, M.; Barbe, M.T.; Allert, N.; Brucke, T.; Kaiser, I.; Beirer, S.; Sejio, F.; et al. 134 VANTAGE trial: Three-year outcomes of a prospective, multicenter trial evaluating deep brain stimulation with a new multiple-source, constant-current rechargeable system in parkinson disease. *Neurosurgery* **2016**, *63*, 155. [CrossRef]

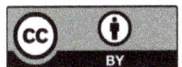

© 2020 by the authors. Licensee MDPI, Basel, Switzerland. This article is an open access article distributed under the terms and conditions of the Creative Commons Attribution (CC BY) license (http://creativecommons.org/licenses/by/4.0/).

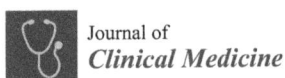

Review

Bilateral Subthalamic Nucleus Deep Brain Stimulation under General Anesthesia: Literature Review and Single Center Experience

Hye Ran Park [1], Yong Hoon Lim [2], Eun Jin Song [2], Jae Meen Lee [3], Kawngwoo Park [4], Kwang Hyon Park [5], Woong-Woo Lee [6], Han-Joon Kim [7], Beomseok Jeon [7] and Sun Ha Paek [2,*]

1. Department of Neurosurgery, Soonchunhyang University Seoul Hospital, Seoul 04401, Korea; c99867@schmc.ac.kr
2. Department of Neurosurgery, Seoul National University Hospital, Seoul 03080, Korea; lim.yh@daum.net (Y.H.L.); moineun@daum.net (E.J.S.)
3. Department of Neurosurgery, Pusan National University Hospital, Busan 49241, Korea; geosung1@naver.com
4. Department of Neurosurgery, Gachon University Gil Medical Center, Incheon 21565, Korea; medicwoo@gmail.com
5. Department of Neurosurgery, Chuungnam National University Sejong Hospital, Sejong 30099, Korea; tooez4me@naver.com
6. Department of Neurology, Nowon Eulji Medical Center, Eulji University, Seoul 01830, Korea; w2pooh@hanmail.net
7. Department of Neurology, Seoul National University Hospital, Seoul 03080, Korea; movement@snu.ac.kr (H.-J.K.); brain@snu.ac.kr (B.J.)
* Correspondence: paeksh@snu.ac.kr; Tel.: +82-22-072-2876

Received: 31 August 2020; Accepted: 17 September 2020; Published: 21 September 2020

Abstract: Bilateral subthalamic nucleus (STN) Deep brain stimulation (DBS) is a well-established treatment in patients with Parkinson's disease (PD). Traditionally, STN DBS for PD is performed by using microelectrode recording (MER) and/or intraoperative macrostimulation under local anesthesia (LA). However, many patients cannot tolerate the long operation time under LA without medication. In addition, it cannot be even be performed on PD patients with poor physical and neurological condition. Recently, it has been reported that STN DBS under general anesthesia (GA) can be successfully performed due to the feasible MER under GA, as well as the technical advancement in direct targeting and intraoperative imaging. The authors reviewed the previously published literature on STN DBS under GA using intraoperative imaging and MER, focused on discussing the technique, clinical outcome, and the complication, as well as introducing our single-center experience. Based on the reports of previously published studies and ours, GA did not interfere with the MER signal from STN. STN DBS under GA without intraoperative stimulation shows similar or better clinical outcome without any additional complication compared to STN DBS under LA. Long-term follow-up with a large number of the patients would be necessary to validate the safety and efficacy of STN DBS under GA.

Keywords: general anesthesia; intraoperative computed tomography; intraoperative magnetic resonance imaging; local anesthesia; microelectrode recording; Parkinson's disease; subthalamic nucleus; deep brain stimulation

1. Introduction

Parkinson's disease (PD) is the second most common neurodegenerative disease following Alzheimer's disease, characterized by bradykinesia, rigidity, resting tremor and postural instability [1]. The long-term use of anti-Parkinsonian drugs has been found to be associated with dyskinesia and symptom fluctuation. Since the introduction of deep brain stimulation (DBS) in 1980s, DBS has been accepted as a preferred surgical treatment for PD [2]. Internal globus pallidus (GPi) and subthalamic nucleus (STN) are the main stimulation targets [3]. In particular, bilateral STN DBS is known to significantly improve not only primary motor symptoms, but also non-motor symptoms, such as sensory symptoms and sleep disturbances [4,5].

Traditionally, DBS surgery is performed under local anesthesia (LA) and conscious sedation to evaluate clinical benefit and side effects by localizing electrophysiological target using microelectrode recording (MER) and/or intraoperative test stimulation while the patient is awake [6–15]. STN DBS has several advantages when implemented under LA. The spike features of MER can be analyzed, and symptom relief or side effects by stimulation can be evaluated with intraoperative macrostimulation. In addition, by using electrophysiological targeting using MER, it is possible to compensate for errors from planning based on preoperative imaging, which is caused by brain shift due to cerebrospinal fluid (CSF) leakage after dura opening. However, MER under LA requires PD patients to withstand surgical procedure with approximately 18 h of antiparkinsonian medication discontinued. Most PD patients are old age and have severe multiple neuro-skeleto-muscular symptoms due to comorbidity, such as spinal stenosis and herniated intervertebral disc. Moreover, patients have to wear a frame on their head during the entire procedure and undergo surgery with the frame fixed to the operation table; thus, the patients may suffer from intolerable pain and psychological sequelae. The risk of hemorrhage risk also increases if an unintended large motion occurs due to cough or tremor during surgery. Patient cooperation is one of the factors that may influence the outcome after surgery.

Because of these concerns, many authors have consistently tried STN DBS under GA and reported that the clinical outcome is not inferior compared to under LA. However, there have been no randomized trials comparing DBS surgery under LA and GA due to logistical concerns. Only class II evidence has been compared through retrospective data analysis [16]. Here, we aimed to review previously published literature on STN DBS under GA as an alternative to STN DBS under LA. The technique and clinical outcome using intraoperative imaging and MER in DBS under GA are thoroughly reviewed along with the introduction of single-center experience of our institution.

2. STN DBS Using Intraoperative Imaging or Microelectrode Recording Under GA

The DBS surgical procedure can be divided into two stages: the intracranial implantation of DBS electrodes and the implantation of implantable pulse generator (IPG). In the case of IPG implantation, GA is generally preferred because tunneling is required subcutaneously. For intracranial electrode implantation, the STN DBS procedure under LA and GA are similar, but the specific details are different. The main difference between the STN DBS surgical procedure under LA and GA is the intraoperative verification method for the intended target acquisition, i.e., test stimulation or intraoperative imaging with or without MER. An accurate electrode location is a key factor to determine the postoperative prognosis after STN DBS surgery [17–20]. Image verification of the lead position is an important step, whether intra- or postoperatively [21]. For STN DBS under GA, some centers perform intraoperative verification using MER even under GA, and other centers use intraoperative imaging without MER. We reviewed each method of STN DBS under GA using intraoperative imaging or MER, respectively (Table 1).

Table 1. Summary data of published literature presenting clinical outcome effect of after subthalamic nucleus deep brain stimulation under general anesthesia in patients with Parkinson's disease.

Author	Year	No. of Patients	Age (yrs)	Disease Duration (yrs)	Follow-Up Months	UPDRS III Medication Off				LEDD			
						Baseline	Follow-Up *	% Change	p-Value	Baseline	Follow-Up *	% Change	p-Value
					Interventional MRI								
Starr et al. [22]	2010	29	58 ± 8.1	NR	9	49 ± 13	19 ± 14	60%	0.0001	NR	NR	NR	NR
Foltynie et al. [23]	2011	79	58.9 ± 7.7	11.5 ± 7	14	51.5 ± 14.9	23.8 ± 11.2	52%	0.0001	NR	NR	NR	NR
Nakajima et al. [24]	2011	14	56.1 ± 6.5	13.8 ± 8.1	12 ± 6.1	57.9 ± 16.6	27.3 ± 11.8	53%	0.0001	1505 ± 764	764 ± 435	49.20%	<0.01
Ostrem et al. [25]	2013	17	59.8	11.1	6	44.5 ± NA	22.5	49.44%	0.001	1337 ± 482	NR	24.70%	0.003
Saleh et al. [26]	2015	14	64 ± 11.9	10.9 ± 3.8	5.86 ± 1.15	NR	NR	NR	NR	NR	NR	49.27%	0.0031
Ostrem et al. [27]	2016	20	63.2 ± 6.8	10.8 ± 2.9	12	40.75 ± 10.9	24.35 ± 8.8	40.20%	0.001	1072.5 ± 382	828.25 ± 492	21.13%	0.046
Sidiropoulous et al. [28]	2016	12	64.7 ± 5.9	11.9 ± 3.7	13.5 ± 3.7	37.2	20.2	46.2%	0.03	1458 ± 653	1337 ± 733	8.3%	0.7
Chircop et al. [29]	2018	26	60.2 ± 9.3	8.8 ± 2.7	12	45.9 ± 14.3	26.7 ± 11.5	41.70%	<0.001	863 ± 211	599 ± 273	30.60%	<0.001
Matias et al. [30]	2018	33	67.2 ± 6.4	12.7 ± 6.9	9.1	52.8 ± 14.9	28.6 ± 11.9	45.8%	<0.001	NR	NR	NR	NR
					Intraoperative CT								
Mirzadeh et al. [31]	2016	35	61.1	10.7	6	48.4 ± 13.8	28.9 ± 12.5	40.30%	<0.0001	1207 ± 733	1035 ± 478	14%	0.004
					Microelectrode recording								
Hertel et al. [32]	2006	9	70.7 ± 3.6	13.6 ± 6.0	3	43.0 ± NR	19 ± NR	55.80%	NR	NR	NR	NR	NR
Lefaucheur et al. [33]	2008	30	57.7 ± 11.1	14.0 ± 4.0	12	47.9 ± 13.6	48.6 ± 19.0	69.10%	0.87	1470.8 ± 729.5	NR	66.4 ± 17.2	NR
Lin et al. [34]	2008	10	58.9 ± 9.9	8.8 ± 3.7	6	50.2 ± 12.9	25.6 ± 11.68	48.85%	<0.05	NR	NR	NR	NR
Fluchere et al. [35]	2014	188	61 ± 7	12 ± 4	12	33.6 ± 13.3	13.2 ± 9.1	61.00%	<0.001	1173 ± 495	636 ± 376	46.00%	<0.001
This study	2020	90	57.43 ± 7.85	11.67 ± 4.75	6	38.11 ± 13.96	21.48 ± 12.33	43.60%	<0.001	1448.0 ± 546.93	483.99 ± 330.42	66.60%	<0.001

Data are presented as: mean ± standard deviation UPDRS, Unified Parkinson's Disease Rating Scale; LEDD, Levodopa equivalent daily dose; NR, Not reported. * On stimulation.

2.1. Using Intraoperative Imaging

With the development of the quality of magnetic resonance imaging (MRI) over the past decades, it has become feasible to identify the STN boundary can to easily implement DBS under GA using direct targeting using advanced imaging [36]. The combination of direct targeting based on MRI visualization of anatomical structures and intraoperative imaging used to confirm accurate lead placement enables surgeons to accurately identify STN targets. It may allow STN DBS procedure to be performed in an asleep state under general anesthesia (GA) without neurophysiological test [37–39].

Successful clinical results on the intraoperative imaging to verify the accuracy of STN lead position instead of electrophysiological structure mapping or stimulation tests during DBS surgery have been reported [23,29,31,37,40–44]. In recent studies on the advancement of intraoperative imaging, no significant clinical results were found when compared to awake DBS [16,30,37,45,46]. However, most of these studies are retrospective analyses with a small number of patients and significant heterogeneity in anesthesia and surgical techniques. In addition, most of the studies were conducted in highly specialized centers with considerable experience in intraoperative imaging. Although these results may not be generalized to all DBS centers for these reasons, current results of STN DBS under GA are promising.

2.1.1. Intraoperative CT

In some centers, intraoperative computed tomography (iCT) during surgery is used to verify the accuracy of lead placement (Table 1). This is achieved through fusion of iCT scans and preoperative MRI scans after intracranial electrode implantation [31,37,41,44,47]. In awake DBS surgery with MER guidance, iCT provides useful information, such as hemorrhage and a general idea of electrode location when fused with preoperative MRI [21]. According to a study about the accuracy of microelectrode trajectory in patients receiving MER-guided awake DBS using iCT, median (IQR) radial error 0.59 (0.64) mm, and median (IQR) absolute x and y coordinate errors were 0.29 (0.52) and 0.38 (0.44) mm, respectively [21]. Burchiel et al. fused and compared iCT and trajectory planning images after electrode implantation for various targets [37]. The mean vector error and mean deviation of trajectory was 1.59 ± 1.11 mm and 1.24 ± 0.87 mm, respectively, and the intraoperative replacement was performed on one electrode with a vector error of more than 3 mm. There was a significant correlation between the distance from the ventricle and the error. Kremer et al. stated that the mean difference between lead tips was 0.98 ± 0.49 mm, and the upper confidence interval did not exceed the non-inferiority margin described when comparing postoperative MRI with iCT [48].

Some centers use MER without test stimulation but with intraoperative imaging to verify the intended target acquisition in STN DBS surgery under GA [32,49–58]. A recent study compared the mean errors of MER-guided electrode implantation in DBS surgery under LA and those of iCT scan-guided intracranial electrode implantation in STN DBS surgery under GA [42]. When targeting STN, mean radial errors of the LA and GA group was about 0.9 ± 0.3 mm without significant difference ($P = 0.70$). The average number of brain penetration for electrode implantation in DBS surgery under LA and GA was similar (1.1 ± 0.2 and 1.1 ± 0.3 penetrations, $p = 0.97$). Brodsky et al. compared 6-months of the clinical outcomes between the group of LA and GA with iCT [59]. There was no significant difference in the improvement in UPDRS III and II, but the improvement in summary index ($p = 0.004$), subscores for cognition ($p = 0.011$), communication ($p < 0.001$), and speech outcome (category, $p = 0.0012$; phonemic fluency, $p = 0.038$) was found better in the GA group.

A few authors have published the results of a study using the intraoperative O-arm. Sharma et al. performed STN DBS surgery under GA using intraoperative O-arm without MER for various targets, and no significant targeting error due to incorporation of iCT images into preoperative CT or MRI was observed [60]. Carlson et al. also reported that intraoperative O-arm images provided a higher accuracy in determining the location of STN DBS electrodes than postoperative CT and MRI images [61].

2.1.2. Intraoperative MRI

Other centers use intraoperative (interventional) MRI (iMRI) to guide DBS electrode placement to the STN (Table 1) [23–29,44,62–64]. For example, the UCSF group reported their experience about bilateral STN DBS in PD patients using a first-generation MRI system (Nexframe, high-field interventional MR-imaging) [25] and ClearPoint system (ClearPoint interventional MRI) [27]. There have been few published studies on the use of intraoperative MRI [23,24,26–28,44,62–67]. One of the reported advantages of iMRI is that it provides a real-time image acquisition to prospectively guided both trajectory planning and intended target verification prior to electrode placement [66]. Therefore, iMRI is one of the most useful methods for DBS targeting that allows precise validation of the real location of electrodes relative to the intended targets [66].

Researches using iMRI with or without stereotactic frame have shown that an accuracy of less than 1 mm can be achieved with mean error close to 0.7 ± 0.3 mm [22,23,25,27,64,66]. The main advantage of electrode implantation using iMRI is that electrode trajectory can be accurately implanted and adjusted before final placement by visualizing the intended target [66]. The error after correcting the electrode location using iMRI under GA without MER was similar to the error of using MER [30]. When comparing the electrode location on both sides, the error was smaller in the second insertion side than in the first insertion side, which is presumed to be due to the correction based on the iMRI result after the first insertion. Sidiropoulos et al. performed STN and GPi DBS surgery in advanced PD patients using the ClearPoint system and found that the mean radial error was 1.2 ± 0.7 mm in the STN group and 0.8 ± 0.3 mm in the GPi group [28]. Starr et al. et al. demonstrated a significantly lower rate of radial error compared to when inserted using the traditional frame-based stereotaxy (3.1 ± 1.41 mm) in the iMRI-guided placement group (1.2 ± 0.65 mm) through burr hole-mounted trajectory guide [22]. They explained that the possibility of brain shift-related errors was reduced because iMRI was performed after burr hole creation and intracranial air flow. Clinically, the UPDRS III "off" medication score and LEDD improved one year after surgery with iMRI [27].

2.1.3. Targeting Accuracy

The theoretical assumption of STN DBS under GA surgery is that the accuracy in targeting STN is not less and the results are better than STN DBS surgery under LA using MER. Kochanski et al. analyzed MER trajectories after STN DBS using 227 iCTs and found that 1.2 ± 0.2mm of radial error occurred in comparison with the location of the intended targets [68]. These errors may be related to the mechanical errors related with the frame, arc, guide tube, and frame, which can lead to lead deviation [69]. In a large-scale study of DBS patients who underwent surgery using iCT, there were greater Euclidean error and greater medial deviation in the trajectory targeting Vim. The authors found that there are systematic tendencies in stereotactic error that differ with respect to the structure targeted [70]. In the study analyzing stereotactic accuracy of iMRI, the DBS lead placement using iMRI guidance showed a radial targeting error of 0.6–1.2 mm, while the error using iCT was 0.8–1.24 mm [22,25,27,28,31,37,71]. STN DBS surgery under GA using confirmatory iCT is based on the assumption that CT-MRI merge was performed correctly, but there may be some errors in the fusion of imaging modality, which may lead to suboptimal targeting [38,72,73]. The advantage of STN DBS surgery with iMRI guidance is that it has less dependence on image fusion and can reflect brain shift after dura opening. Analysis of the iMRI study revealed that the deep brain structure moves about 2 mm after opening the dura [74].

2.2. Using Microelectrode Recording

2.2.1. Is MER Mandatory for STN DBS Surgery?

In the standard STN DBS procedure under LA, MER is used during surgery to obtain a signal to identify the deep structure [75]. The final site of electrode implantation is determined by considering both MER and intraoperative test stimulation [7–9,11,13–15]. Sedative drugs, such as propofol, dexmedetomidine, and remifentanil, are given to patients when it is not necessary for them to be awake [76,77]. The goal of using MER in STN DBS surgery is to obtain high accuracy in radiographic and neurophysiological targeting. Theoretically, the ideal target should be one and the same, but several important factors can lead to errors in targeting, resulting in inconsistency between optimal radiographic and neurophysiological targets. In the report on awake STN DBS, about 25% (38/150) of the electrodes were found very accurately located on the intended target very accurately with an error of less than 1mm, but electrophysiological recording did not match with the target in MER and/or intraoperative stimulation, or showed an unacceptably low side-effect threshold by stimulation [68]. Although these findings may be explained by brain shifts, these cases indicate that MER is essential for target confirmation during DBS surgery. Even small merge error combined with brain shift can lead to discrepancies between optimal radiographic and neurophysiological targets [38,72,74,78–80]. The advantage of this method is that it is possible to observe the changes in MER related to passive motion during surgery, and immediately evaluate the effects and side effects through test stimulation [9,81]. By reflecting this result and modifying the electrode position, the effect can be maximized while the complications of stimulation can be minimized.

MER signals may be mixed with many noises which may be caused by snoring or movements of the patient. The reliability and usefulness of MER during STN DBS surgery under LA are still being investigated. However, awake surgery may not be possible for some patients with severe anxiety, fear, reduced cooperation, severe pain, respiration difficulties and so on.

MER may increase the risk of intracranial hemorrhage and cognitive decline [82]. Binder et al. reported a bleeding rate of 3.3% and a risk of permanent defects 0.6% [83]. The number of MER trajectory was found slightly higher in patients with hemorrhage without statistical significance than the patients without hemorrhage [84]. Some researchers have also questioned whether MER has a real significant impact on target refinement [8]. They argued that a short MER-determined STN length alone cannot predict the occurrence of stimulation-related side effect [18]. Moreover, the MER procedure increases both surgical time and the cost [8,85].

Macrostimulation test cannot be performed if the patients are asleep during the operation. There is also controversy about whether intraoperative stimulation is needed during DBS surgery. Some researchers believe that it is necessary to confirm the effectiveness of the stimulus. On the other hand, some argued that discontinuation of the drug in LA makes the results less reliable, especially if it is not located in the correct position within the STN, the effect can be easily observed and difficult to distinguish from the lesion effect [86].

Due to the improved image quality of preoperative imaging, determining the final electrode location by imaging alone without MER does not negatively affect motor improvement and LEDD, and does not aggravate surgical complications [24,26,29,42,87]. The UPDRS III reduction rate at postoperative 3 months was higher in the group of STN DBS under LA with MER cohort ($p = 0.006$), but there was no significant difference at 1 year ($p = 0.18$), as well as in dysarthria, capsular, oculomotor, and sensory side effects [87]. Chen et al. also reported that there was no difference in the UPDRS III reduction rate and score 6 months after STN DBS surgery between the MER group and the non-MER group [42]. In addition to frequently used imaging sequences, direct targeting can be used with quantitative susceptibility mapping (QSM) and diffusion tensor imaging (DTI) [68].

2.2.2. Is MER Possible Under GA?

STN DBS under GA has traditionally been used in patients who are unable to tolerate awake surgery including pediatric patients, or in patients who do not require clinical testing, such as obsessive-compulsive disorder or epilepsy. The biggest concern with STN DBS surgery under GA for movement disorder is the possibility of diminution of MER signals. A few small-sized retrospective studies have reported that MER obtained from STN, GPi, substantia nigra in STN DBS surgery under GA with both volatile and intravenous anesthetics in PD and dystonia patients showed no significant difference compared with patients awake during the procedure [54,88–91]. Notably, the neural activity of typical burst pattern disappeared when higher anesthetic doses were used. However, the results of these studies are controversial given the small sample size and heterogeneity of the anesthetic used. A prospective, double-blinded study is needed to compare the effects of anesthetic agents on MER quality in patients undergoing STN DBS surgery under GA.

The next concern is that since intraoperative stimulation cannot be performed under GA, immediate response of clinical effects and adverse effects associated with stimulation cannot be assessed during the STN DBS surgery. Several trials of MER in deep sedation have been performed without intraoperative stimulation [32,33,89]. In these studies, propofol or remifentanil tended to interfere with the electrophysiological signal, but there were no significant differences in terms of exact targeting, clinical effectiveness, and adverse event profiles. Other authors also reported that although there was significant MER signal attenuation in deep sedation with propofol, it did not interfere with the optimal approach to the target [32,33,92,93].

Although a few studies have previously investigated the effects of anesthetics on MER over the past 20 years, the exact effect has not been fully elucidated. Most studies were retrospective analyses with heterogeneity in the anesthesia protocol used and the patient population, and thus, no definitive conclusions could be drawn [77]. Therefore, most of the knowledge revealed to date is derived from the case reports or small case series. During MER, background neuronal discharges and spike activity patterns are an important part of the precise localization of the target nucleus. Anesthetics have been shown to affect background activity and neuronal spike activity in a dose-dependent manner, primarily through activation of γ-aminobutyric acid (GABA) receptors. In addition, anesthetics do not have the same effect on neuronal activity in various target nucleus. Since most anesthetics enhance the inhibitory action of GABA, this difference in GABA-input of the target nucleus plays an important role [94,95].

MER from STN in PD patients was successfully obtained under sedation with low-dose anesthetics. The anesthesia techniques used during MER ranged from conscious sedation with propofol, dexmedetomidine with no airway manipulation to GA with intravenous or inhalation anesthetics. Although anesthetics have been shown to reduce the spike activity, localization of the target areas was proven possible in most studies. Nevertheless, most studies did not mention the exact effect on the background activity, degree of suppression of spike activity, and the number of trajectories used for localization [34,58,80,89].

Under desflurane inhalation, Lin et al. observed that MER could be performed with a typical neuronal firing pattern and motion-related firing of STN, and the clinical results were similar in both groups [34,96].

Our group performed MER and implantation by administering propofol and fentanyl for sedation under LA, and reported the effects of propofol and fentanyl on MER and the clinical outcome. The locations of all electrodes were positioned within the STN. The postoperative 6-months UPDRS II and III, total "off" scores, Hoehn and Yahr (H&Y) scale, Schwab-England ADL scale scores, and LEDD have been greatly improved [92,93].

Although the effects of short-acting opioid receptor agonists, such as remifentanil, on MER are not well known, some data suggest that GABAergic neurons may play a central role [76,77,97]. A few reports showed that anesthesia using propofol reduces the firing rate of basal ganglia in a few reports [95,98], while one study showed no significant difference in firing rate compared to LA when administered with propofol and fentanyl [92]. Monitored anesthesia using propofol appears to be a safe technique for DBS procedure [99]. In some studies, MER was properly performed without affecting the surgical outcome only when remifentanil administration was discontinued and propofol was carefully monitored [32,54,100]. However, the spontaneous firing patterns of STN and substantia nigra remained similar to those under LA [14,100]. Chen et al. also reported that there was no significant difference between the GA and LA groups in terms of MER trajectory, recorded STN depths, postoperative coordinates, and overall incidence of stimulation-related side effect [55]. Under remifentanil or ketamine anesthesia, no significant differences were found in number of spikes detected, mean firing rate, pause index, and burst index compared to LA [57]. However, Moll et al. observed a long interburst between abnormally long group discharges under propofol and remifentanil [89].

Benzodiazepines are direct GABA-agonists, which can completely eliminate MER and cause dyskinesia. Dexmedetomidine may be a better alternative for anxiety relief. The effect of dexmedetomidine on neural activity has not been fully elucidated, but it seems to be a reasonable option due to the non-GABA-mediated mechanism of action. Several studies to date have shown minimal effects of low-dose dexmedetomidine on MER in STN and GPi [101–104]. Some authors reported that low doses of dexmedetomidine (<0.5 µg/kg/h) did not significantly affect the quality of MER in STN or GPi [76,99,103]. Although dexmedetomidine may affect the MER result, it does not affect target localization [50].

2.2.3. Clinical Experiences of STN DBS Using MER under GA

Some authors performed STN DBS surgery on PD patients under GA and reported favorable clinical outcomes (Table 1). Hertel et al. reported that patients' daily off phases decreased from 50% to 17%, while the Unified Parkinson's Disease Rating Scale (UPDRS) III score was reduced from 43 (preoperative; medication off) to 19 (stimulation on; medication off) and 12 (stimulation on; medication on) [32]. Yamada et al. also reported that UPDRS II, III, IV on and off scores were significantly lower in the LA and GA groups at 3 months postoperatively, and the activities of daily living(ADL)s and motor symptoms, such as bradykinesia, tremor, rigidity, and axial symptoms, have improved significantly [54]. In this study, a reduction in dyskinesia duration ($p < 0.001$), disability ($p = 0.009$) and off period duration, and improvement of sleep disorders were observed. Other authors also reported significant improvement in off-medication UPDRS, levodopa-equivalent daily dose (LEDD), and quality of life [29,35]. Harries et al. reported a long-term clinical outcome of more than 5 years [49]. In their study, not only the UPDRS II and III off score, but also the total UPDRS off scores at postoperative 1 year improved significantly, and the total UPDRS score continued to improve for up to 7 years.

Previously, authors have suggested the use of bispectral analysis (BIS) of the electroencephalogram in STN DBS surgery under GA using MER. An appropriate MER signal can be easily obtained by adjusting the anesthesia depth using BIS [100,105]. BIS of 65–85 and 40–65 is recommended for sedation and GA, respectively [106]. In the case of sedation using dexmedetomidine, it has been reported that the MER signal does not differ from the nonsedated state if the BIS value is maintained below 80 [80].

2.3. Intraoperative Imaging vs. MER in STN DBS under GA

Recent meta-analysis reported that no significant difference was found in the improvement of UPDRS III score or LEDD between LA and GA cohort (Tables 2–4) [16,33,46,54,55,107]. Lefaucheur et al. reported that the rate of reduction in UPDRS III axial, gait, postural stability, and rigidity subscores tended to be greater when performed under LA compared to GA, but the difference was not statistically significant [33]. On the other hand, Chen et al. reported that the LA cohort showed greater improvement in posture and walking than the GA cohort ($p = 0.054$), while the GA cohort showed a significant decrease in cognitive function ($p = 0.017$) [55].

Some studies have used MER in STN DBS surgery under GA (mean 1.92 ± 0.68) and LA cohort (mean 2.27 ± 1.31) with respect to the maximum error of each read ($p = 0.557$) despite the varying targets [33,52,55]. Ho et al. reported that there was no significant difference between GA (mean 1.92 ± 0.68) and LA cohort (mean 2.27 ± 1.31) with respect to the maximum error of each lead ($p = 0.557$), but their study included a variety of targets [16]. The number of lead passes and the incidence of intracranial hemorrhage and infection were lower in STN DBS under GA, but treatment-related side effects based on the UPDRS IV "off" score were lower in DBS under LA (LA cohort 78.4% vs GA cohort 59.7%, $p = 0.022$) [16,35]. However, other studies showed no difference in the UPDRS IV subscore between the GA and LA groups [24,107]. As for LEDD, some studies reported that the 6-months postoperative LEDD reduction was significantly greater in the LA group, while others showed statistically similar reductions (LA cohort 38.27%, GA cohort 49.27%, $p = 0.4447$) [26,107]. Tsai et al. reported that symptoms of the patients with PD improved after DTN DBS in both LA and GA cohorts without significant differences in LEDD and UPDRS IV scores [52].

When the long-term outcome was investigated, the authors found that the probability of side effects by stimulation and lead revision was higher in the GA cohort without MER and test stimulation [68]. On the other hand, no difference was observed in UPDRS III score, LEDD, stimulation parameters, coordination of targeting, STN recording length, and side effects in the two groups [108].

STN DBS surgery can be safely performed with a low complication rate in both LA and GA cohort, and the results of the studies to date show that there is no significant difference in complication rates between the two groups. Some authors reported that overall DBS-related complications, such as intracranial hemorrhage (GA 0.3% vs LA 1.1%) and infection (GA 0.7% vs LA 1.4%), were significantly lower in GA cohort ($p < 0.001$) [16,35]. Martin et al. reported the incidence of hardware infection is due to electrode implantation after 10 years of MRI-guided STN DBS surgery [109]. In the study, the overall infection rate of 164 iMRI-guided surgeries with 272 electrodes implanted was 3.6%, which was similar to that reported in the previous STN DBS surgery under LA. The results of a systematic review on the incidence of complications, hospitalization time, and readmission rate of patients who underwent awake and asleep STN DBS surgery were recently published, and there was no statistical difference in the complication rate, length of hospitalization, and readmission rate of LA and GA cohort [110].

The mean total cost of STN DBS surgery under GA and LA was similar at \$38,850 ± \$4830 in GA and \$40,052 ± \$6604 in LA, respectively, but the standard deviation in DBS under GA was significantly lower [111]. This indicates that there is no difference in the total cost of DBS surgery under GA and LA, but the cost fluctuation is lower due to the lower incidence of unexpected variables in DBS surgery under GA. However, there are limitations to generalizing such result, since it is a single-center experience.

Table 2. Summary data of published literature comparing clinical outcome effect of after subthalamic nucleus deep brain stimulation under general anesthesia and local anesthesia in patients with Parkinson's disease: Baseline patient characteristics

Author	Year	Study Type	Number of Patients		Age (yrs)		Disease Duration (yrs)		Follow-Up (Months)
			GA	LA	GA	LA	GA	LA	
Maltete et al. [58]	2004	Clinical	15	15	59.8 8.0	58.0 6.1	13.4 3.7	13.5 2.6	6
Yamada et al. [54]	2007	Clinical	15	10	65.2 7.0	65.6 8.6	11.1 5.0	6.8 2.4	3
Saleh et al. [26]	2015	Clinical	14	23	64.0 ± 11.9	60.6 ± 7.0	10.9 ± 3.8	11.3 ± 4.9	6
Tsai et al. [52]	2016	Clinical	8	8	49.6 ± 7.1 *	41.1 ± 10.2 *	9.3 ± 2.4	12.4 ± 9.2	6
Brodsky et al. [59]	2017	Clinical	27 (20 GPi, 7 STN)	34 (20 GPi, 14 STN)	63.7 ± 9.79	63.1 ± 7.61	NR	NR	6
Lefranc et al. [112]	2017	Clinical	13	10	62.80 ± 7.1	63.1 ± 10	12.60 ± 3.6	12.10 ± 3.5	12
Blasberg et al. [87]	2018	Clinical	48	48	65.75 ± 1.18	65.52 ± 1.13	11.65 ± 0.81	10.87 ± 0.78	6
Chen et al. [42]	2018	Clinical	41	14	64.6 ± 8.25	63.1 ± 10.1	7.5 ± 3.4	8.6 ± 4.6	6
Ho et al. [16]	2018	Meta-analysis	663	6441	58.3 ± 6.8	59.4 ± 5.2	11.0 ± 1.5	12.3 ± 2.1	12
Liu et al. [113]	2019	Meta-analysis	967	556	NR	NR	NR	NR	NR
Tsai et al. [108]	2019	Clinical	22	9	57.7 ± 7.4	49.4 ± 12.2	57.7 ± 7.4	49.4 ± 12.2	60
This study	2020	Clinical	90	56	57.43 ± 7.85	58.91 ± 8.65	11.67 ± 4.75	10.55 ± 4.89	6

Data are presented as: mean ± standard deviation GA, general anesthesia; LA, local anesthesia; GPi, Internal globus pallidus; STN, subthalamic nucleus; NR, Not reported * Age of Onset.

Table 3. Summary data of published literature comparing clinical outcome effect of after subthalamic nucleus deep brain stimulation under general anesthesia and local anesthesia in patients with Parkinson's disease: Baseline and Follow-up Unified Parkinson's Disease Rating Scale (UPDRS) III score and Levodopa equivalent daily dose (LEDD).

Author	Baseline UPDRS III GA	Baseline UPDRS III LA	Follow-Up UPDRS III * GA	Follow-Up UPDRS III * LA	%UPDRS III Change GA	%UPDRS III Change LA	p Value	Baseline LEDD GA	Baseline LEDD LA	Follow-Up LEDD GA	Follow-Up LEDD LA	%LEDD reduction GA	%LEDD reduction LA	p Value
Maltete et al.	47.1 ± 15.4	39.9 ± 13.9	17.0 ± 8.6	10.9 ± 7.2	63.9%	72.7%	0.07	1449 ± 398	1507 ± 465	310 ± 350	392 ± 440	78.6%	74.0%	0.06
Yamada et al.	52.4 ± 19.0	45.9 ± 17.7	14.3 ± 15.4	7.1 ± 7.0	72.7%	82.5%	No significant difference	375.7 ± 195.6	425.0 ± 171.8	303.3 ± 164.7	261.1 ± 164.0	16.6%	38.2%	NR
Saleh et al.	NR	NR	NR	NR	NR	NR	NR	NR	NR	NR	NR	NR	NR	NR
Tsai et al.	41.7 ± 29.4	39.9 ± 16.3	NR	NR	65.7%	45.8 ± 26.2%	NR	2134.9 ± 1175.8	1702.7 ± 876.0	NR	NR	49.27%	38.27%	0.4447
Brodsky et al.	42.2 ± 10.6	41.7 ± 12.5	14.8 ± 8.9 **	17.6 ± 12.26 **	35%%	42.2%%	0.19	NR	NR	NR	NR	NR	NR	NR
Lefranc et al.	35.92 ± 11.15	33.10 ± 5.38	18.0 ± 7.2	20.0 ± 10.47	49%	40.30%	0.336	1585.10 ± 496.40	1247.70 ± 579.80	519.17 ± 282.71	716.80 ± 320.14	Significantly greater in the GA than in the LA		0.03
Blasberg et al.	38.47 ± 1.94	34.79 ± 1.61	NR	NR	48.8%	40.3%	0.18	NR	NR	NR	NR	NR	NR	0.008
Chen et al.	53.8 ± 16.4	53.7 ± 17.0	18.0 ± 7.2	21.6 ± 7.3	51.1 ± 16.6% (n = 510)	46.7 ± 27.4 ± (n = 4931)	0.20	1070.72 ± 49.67	972.23 ± 55.15	NR	NR	NR	NR	0.49
Ho et al.	NR	NR	NR	NR	NR	NR	0.494	NR	NR	NR	NR	45 ± 12.8% (n = 444)	47 ± 26.6% (n = 3893)	0.752
Liu et al.	46.3 ± 14.4	28.6 ± 9.3	NR	24.6 ± 7.8	43.2 ± 14.1%	46.8 ± 13.8%	0.60	NR	NR	NR	NR	NR	NR	0.23
Tsai et al.		42.9 ± 17.4				NR	0.45	1448.0 ± 546.93	1031.63 ± 451.08	483.99 ± 330.42	461.3 ± 284.65	47.56 ± 18.98%	51.37 ± 31.73%	0.51
This study	38.11 ± 13.96	40.42 ± 15.30	21.48 ± 12.33	24.68 ± 12.51	43.6%	38.9%	0.136					66.6%	55.3%	<0.0001

Data are presented as: mean ± standard deviation. UPDRS, Unified Parkinson's Disease Rating Scale; LEDD, Levodopa equivalent daily dose; GA, general anesthesia; LA, local anesthesia; GPi, Internal globus pallidus; STN, subthalamic nucleus; NR, Not reported * off medication, on stimulation ** recorded as reduced score.

Table 4. Summary data of published literature comparing clinical outcome effect of after subthalamic nucleus deep brain stimulation under general anesthesia and local anesthesia in patients with Parkinson's disease: Perioperative complications.

Author	Number of MER Tracks	Overall Adverse Effects	Hemorrhage	Infection	Operation Time
Maltete et al.	NR	No adverse reaction to the use of propofol, 1 pulmonary atelectasia	NR	NR	NR
Yamada et al.	NR	NR	NR	NR	NR
Saleh et al.	NR	No significant differences	NR	NR	GA 424 ± 12 vs LA 307 ± 80 p = 0.0026
Tsai et al.	NR	No significant differences	NR	NR	NR
Brodsky et al.	NR	NR	1 small venous hemorrhage in LA, 1 small nonhemorrhagic infarct in GA	1 in GA	NR
Lefranc et al.	NR	No significant differences p = 0.39	NR	NR	0.31
Blasberg et al.	NR	No significant differences	1.00	1.00	GA 266.0 ± 60.6 vs LA 260.9 ± 57.6 p = 0.78
Chen et al.	NR	NR	NR	NR	GA 253.7 ± 82.3 vs LA 272.4 ± 92.5 p = 0.748
Ho et al.	GA 1.4 ± 0.44 vs LA 2.1 ± 0.69 p = 0.006	NR	%ICH/lead: GA 0.3 ± 0.0 vs LA 1.1 ± 0.3, p < 0.001	%infection/lead GA 0.7 ± 0.0 vs LA 1.4 ± 0.0, p < 0.001	NR
Liu et al.	NR	0.94	0.64	NR	0.47
Tsai et al.	Significantly less in GA p = 0.04	Similar adverse effects	NR	NR	NR
This study		1 required revision due to inappropriate lead position in LA		1 IPG site infection treated by antibiotics in LA	

MER, microelectrode recording; NR, not recorded; GA, general anesthesia; LA, local anesthesia; IPG, implantable pulse generator.

Table 6. Cont.

	Medication	Anesthesia	Baseline	6 Month *	p Value **	p Value ***
Dyskinesia Disability		General	2.72 ± 1.31	1.04 ± 1.27	<0.001	0.062
		Local	2.21 ± 1.39	0.79 ± 1.21	<0.001	
LEDD (mg/day)		General	1448.00 ± 546.93	483.99 ± 330.42	<0.001	0.000
		Local	1031.63 ± 451.08	461.3 ± 284.65	<0.001	
MMSE		General	27.61 ± 2.52	27.23 ± 2.33	0.314	0.621
		Local	26.53 ± 2.76	25.78 ± 3.71	0.493	
BDI		General	17.72 ± 10.28	16.57 ± 10.56	0.473	0.277
		Local	19 ± 10.82	19.78 ± 9.68	0.524	
SF-36 Physical health		General	156.25 ± 72.58	203.14 ± 90.03	<0.001	0.600
		Local	132.86 ± 61.09	188.34 ± 74.5	<0.001	
SF-36 Mental health		General	177.62 ± 80.37	206.88 ± 84.62	0.021	0.988
		Local	150.39 ± 72.59	181.44 ± 80.95	0.076	

* DBS on, ** between baseline and follow-up, *** between two groups: general and local anesthesia.

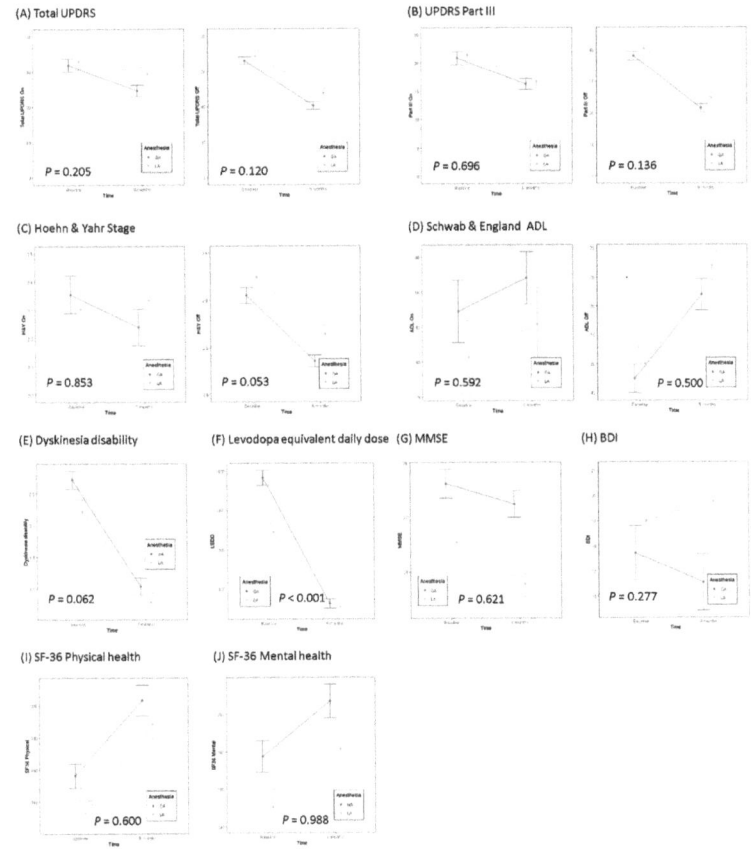

Figure 1. Comparison of clinical outcomes between baseline and 6 months after STN Deep brain stimulation (DBS) under local anesthesia (LA) and general anesthesia (GA) each cohort. (**A**) Total Unified Parkinson's Disease Rating Scale (UPDRS) and (**B**) UPDRS part III showed significant improvement after 6 months compared to baseline, except for LA cohort medication on state, there was no statistically significant difference between LA and GA cohort. (**C**) Hoehn & Yahr stage and (**D**) Schwab & England

activities of daily living (ADL) showed no significant change in the medication on state in both LA and GA cohort, and no significant difference between two cohorts. (**E**) Dyskinesia disability and (**F**) Levodopa equivalent daily dose (LEDD) were significantly decreased in both LA and GA cohort. Only LEDD showed a significant difference in the change between LA and GA cohort. (**G**) Mini Mental State Examination (MMSE) and (**H**) Beck's Depression Inventory (BDI), showed no statistically significant decrease in both LA and GA cohort. (**I**) Short form -36 (SF-36) physical health and (**J**) Short form -36 (SF-36) mental health showed no statistically significant increase in both LA and GA cohort.

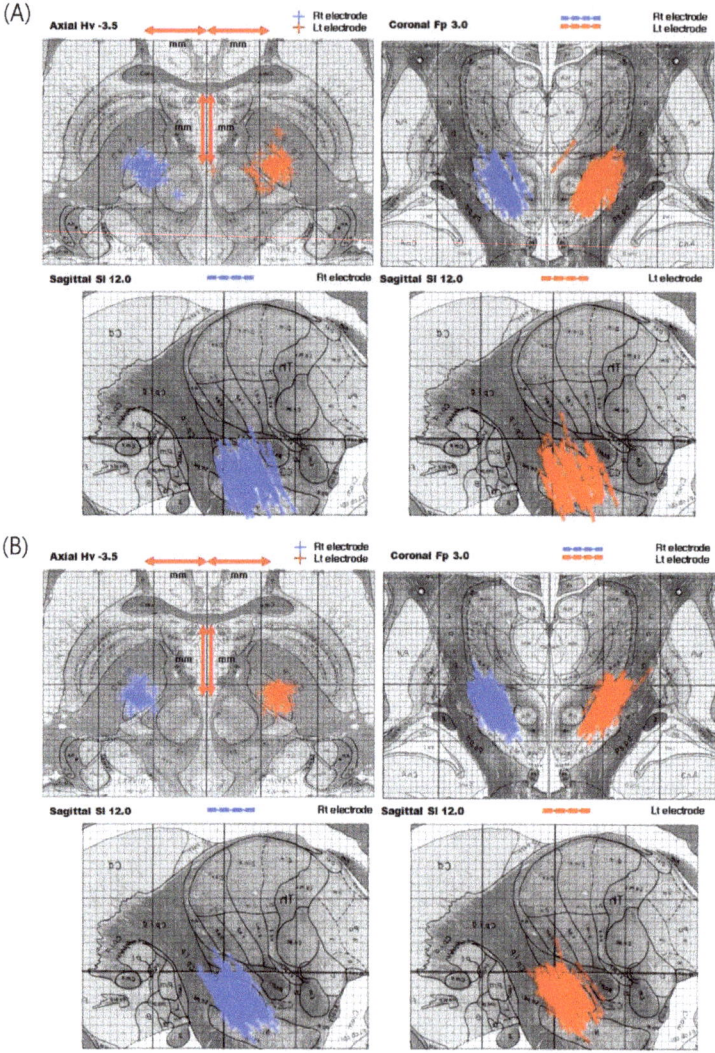

Figure 2. Plotting of the electrode location based on the plotted position of the electrode in the axial view which is 3.5 mm below the anterior commissure (AC)–posterior commissure (PC) line in the human brain atlas of Schaltenbrand and Wahren. (**A**) Local anesthesia (LA) cohort, (**B**) General anesthesia (GA) cohort. Compared to LA cohort, the GA cohort showed a higher tendency for the electrode to be located within the subthalamic nucleus (STN).

4. Future Direction

Studies published to date have shown that the rationale and technology of STN DBS surgery performed under GA are accurate, and they presented similar clinical results compared to STN DBS under LA cohort. A large-scale prospective randomized controlled trial is in progress to assess the degree of the improvement of non-motor symptoms in PD patients [120].

Care should be taken when interpreting and applying the conclusion, since the STN DBS surgery under GA data reported to date have been published in large centers with considerable experiences. In general, STN DBS surgery should be performed in the most convenient way for the surgeons and center to provide the best results to the patients. Traditionally, factors, such as claustrophobia, severe off-medication symptoms, or nonspecific fear of waking during surgery, made patients choose GA. However, based on the increasingly cumulative data showing similar or better results compared to LA, a surgeon may choose STN DBS surgery under GA.

Adaptive DBS is a promising technology because it can provide more selective stimulation trigger/parameter and reduce stimulation-induced dyskinesia by suppressing beta activity when it exceeds a certain threshold level [121,122]. There is still little literature on adaptive DBS implemented under general anesthesia, and further studies for application of adaptive DBS under general anesthesia should be conducted.

There are patients who cannot undergo STN DBS surgery due to various reasons or may not benefit from STN DBS surgery. Non-invasive lesion-based therapies, such as focused ultrasound and Gamma Knife radiosurgery (GKRS), have been proposed as alternatives to DBS because of their effectiveness and safety [123–126]. The further innovative refinement of noninvasive methods of Gamma Knife radiosurgery (GKRS) and focused ultrasound may allow advanced PD patients to receive surgical treatment more conveniently and efficiently in the near future.

5. Conclusions

The number of DBS surgeries continues to increase, as indications expand and the population is aging. Currently, STN DBS surgery is performed in various ways with or without MER under LA or GA in each center. Based on the reports of previously published studies and ours, it is likely that GA does not interfere with the MER signal from STN. In addition, STN DBS under GA without intraoperative stimulation shows similar or better clinical outcome without any additional complication compared to STN DBS under LA. Although there are various pros and cons of each method in each protocol in each protocol of STN DBS under LA and under GA, the stereotype that STN DBS surgery must be performed under LA to perform intraoperative macrostimulation and MER to obtain the best clinical outcome should be changed at the moment.

In conclusion, it is suggested that, if there is no significant difference in clinical treatment effects and complications between GA and LA, it would be reasonable to implement STN DBS under GA because it can minimize unnecessary inconvenience of the patients with PD. Long-term follow-up studies with the large number of the patients would be necessary to further validate the safety and efficacy of STN DBS under GA.

Author Contributions: Conceptualization, S.H.P. and B.J.; methodology, H.-J.K.; software, Y.H.L.; validation, W.-W.L., K.H.P. and K.P.; formal analysis, H.R.P.; investigation, E.J.S.; resources, J.M.L.; data curation, Y.H.L.; writing—original draft preparation, H.R.P. and S.H.P.; writing—review and editing, H.R.P., B.J. and S.H.P.; visualization, H.-J.K.; supervision, B.J.; project administration, S.H.P.; funding acquisition, H.R.P. and S.H.P. All authors have read and agreed to the published version of the manuscript.

Funding: This study was funded by the Korea Healthcare Technology R&D Project (grant HI11C21100200, HI18C0886), funded by the Ministry of Health & Welfare, Republic of Korea; the Industrial Strategic Technology Development Program (grant 10050154, Business Model Development for Personalized Medicine Based on Integrated Genome and Clinical Information) funded by the Ministry of Trade, Industry & Energy (MI, Korea); the Original Technology Research Program for Brain Science through the National Research Foundation of Korea (NRF) funded by the Ministry of Education, Science and Technology (grant 2015M3C7A1028926, 2017M3C7A1044367); the Original Technology Research Program for Brain Science through the NRF funded by the Ministry of Education, Science and Technology (2017M3C7A1047392); Basic Science Research Program through the NRF funded by the Ministry of Education (NRF-2017R1D1A1B03035556); and Soonchunhyang University Research Fund (2020).

Acknowledgments: Yona Kim contributed to this work by English proofreading.

Conflicts of Interest: The authors declare no conflict of interest.

References

1. Han, M.; Nagele, E.; DeMarshall, C.; Acharya, N.; Nagele, R. Diagnosis of Parkinson's disease based on disease-specific autoantibody profiles in human sera. *PLoS ONE* **2012**, *7*, e32383. [CrossRef] [PubMed]
2. Benabid, A.-L.; Pollak, P.; Louveau, A.; Henry, S.; De Rougemont, J. Combined (thalamotomy and stimulation) stereotactic surgery of the VIM thalamic nucleus for bilateral Parkinson disease. *Ster. Funct. Neurosurg.* **1987**, *50*, 344–346. [CrossRef] [PubMed]
3. Fasano, A.; Daniele, A.; Albanese, A. Treatment of motor and non-motor features of Parkinson's disease with deep brain stimulation. *Lancet Neurol.* **2012**, *11*, 429–442. [CrossRef]
4. Kleiner-Fisman, G.; Herzog, J.; Fisman, D.N.; Tamma, F.; Lyons, K.E.; Pahwa, R.; Lang, A.E.; Deuschl, G. Subthalamic nucleus deep brain stimulation: Summary and meta-analysis of outcomes. *Mov. Disord.* **2006**, *21*, S290–S304. [CrossRef]
5. Kim, H.-J.; Jeon, B.S.; Paek, S.H. Nonmotor symptoms and subthalamic deep brain stimulation in Parkinson's disease. *J. Mov. Disord.* **2015**, *8*, 83. [CrossRef] [PubMed]
6. Rezai, A.R.; Kopell, B.H.; Gross, R.E.; Vitek, J.L.; Sharan, A.D.; Limousin, P.; Benabid, A.L. Deep brain stimulation for Parkinson's disease: Surgical issues. *Mov. Disord.* **2006**, *21* (Suppl. 14), S197–S218. [CrossRef]
7. Lyons, M.K.; Ziemba, K.; Evidente, V. Multichannel microelectrode recording influences final electrode placement in pallidal deep brain stimulation for Parkinson's disease: Report of twenty consecutive cases. *Turk. Neurosurg.* **2011**, *21*, 555–558. [CrossRef]
8. Kinfe, T.M.; Vesper, J. The impact of multichannel microelectrode recording (MER) in deep brain stimulation of the basal ganglia. In *Stereotactic and Functional Neurosurgery*; Springer: Berlin/Heidelberg, Germany, 2013; pp. 27–33.
9. Chen, S.-Y.; Lee, C.-C.; Lin, S.-H.; Hsin, Y.-L.; Lee, T.-W.; Yen, P.-S.; Chou, Y.-C.; Lee, C.-W.; Hsieh, W.A.; Su, C.-F. Microelectrode recording can be a good adjunct in magnetic resonance image–directed subthalamic nucleus deep brain stimulation for parkinsonism. *Surg. Neurol.* **2006**, *65*, 253–260. [CrossRef]
10. Chang, W.S.; Kim, H.Y.; Kim, J.P.; Park, Y.S.; Chung, S.S.; Chang, J.W. Bilateral subthalamic deep brain stimulation using single track microelectrode recording. *Acta Neurochir.* **2011**, *153*, 1087–1095. [CrossRef]
11. Tsai, S.-T.; Hung, H.-Y.; Lee, C.-H.; Chen, S.-Y. Letter to the Editor: Deep brain stimulation and microelectrode recording. *J. Neurosurg.* **2014**, *120*, 580. [CrossRef]
12. Machado, A.; Rezai, A.R.; Kopell, B.H.; Gross, R.E.; Sharan, A.D.; Benabid, A.L. Deep brain stimulation for Parkinson's disease: Surgical technique and perioperative management. *Mov. Disord.* **2006**, *21* (Suppl. 14), S247–S258. [CrossRef] [PubMed]
13. Priori, A.; Egidi, M.; Pesenti, A.; Rohr, M. Do intraoperative microrecordings improve subthalamic nucleus targeting in stereotactic neurosurgery for Parkinson's disease? *J. Neurosurg. Sci.* **2003**, *47*, 56. [PubMed]
14. Benazzouz, A.; Breit, S.; Koudsie, A.; Pollak, P.; Krack, P.; Benabid, A.L. Intraoperative microrecordings of the subthalamic nucleus in Parkinson's disease. *Mov. Disord. Off. J. Mov. Disord. Soc.* **2002**, *17*, S145–S149. [CrossRef] [PubMed]
15. Su, X.-L.; Luo, X.-G.; Lv, H.; Wang, J.; Ren, Y.; He, Z.-Y. Factors predicting the instant effect of motor function after subthalamic nucleus deep brain stimulation in Parkinson's disease. *Transl. Neurodegener.* **2017**, *6*, 14. [CrossRef] [PubMed]
16. Ho, A.L.; Ali, R.; Connolly, I.D.; Henderson, J.M.; Dhall, R.; Stein, S.C.; Halpern, C.H. Awake versus asleep deep brain stimulation for Parkinson's disease: A critical comparison and meta-analysis. *J. Neurol. Neurosurg. Psychiatry* **2018**, *89*, 687–691. [CrossRef]
17. Saint-Cyr, J.A.; Hoque, T.; Pereira, L.C.; Dostrovsky, J.O.; Hutchison, W.D.; Mikulis, D.J.; Abosch, A.; Sime, E.; Lang, A.E.; Lozano, A.M. Localization of clinically effective stimulating electrodes in the human subthalamic nucleus on magnetic resonance imaging. *J. Neurosurg.* **2002**, *97*, 1152–1166. [CrossRef]

18. McClelland, S., 3rd; Ford, B.; Senatus, P.B.; Winfield, L.M.; Du, Y.E.; Pullman, S.L.; Yu, Q.; Frucht, S.J.; McKhann, G.M., 2nd; Goodman, R.R. Subthalamic stimulation for Parkinson disease: Determination of electrode location necessary for clinical efficacy. *Neurosurg. Focus* **2005**, *19*, E12. [CrossRef]
19. Zonenshayn, M.; Rezai, A.R.; Mogilner, A.Y.; Beric, A.; Sterio, D.; Kelly, P.J. Comparison of anatomic and neurophysiological methods for subthalamic nucleus targeting. *Neurosurgery* **2000**, *47*, 282–292, discussion 292–284. [CrossRef]
20. Lanotte, M.M.; Rizzone, M.; Bergamasco, B.; Faccani, G.; Melcarne, A.; Lopiano, L. Deep brain stimulation of the subthalamic nucleus: Anatomical, neurophysiological, and outcome correlations with the effects of stimulation. *J. Neurol. Neurosurg. Psychiatry* **2002**, *72*, 53–58. [CrossRef]
21. Bus, S.; Pal, G.; Ouyang, B.; van den Munckhof, P.; Bot, M.; Sani, S.; Verhagen Metman, L. Accuracy of Microelectrode Trajectory Adjustments during DBS Assessed by Intraoperative CT. *Stereotact. Funct. Neurosurg.* **2018**, *96*, 231–238. [CrossRef]
22. Starr, P.A.; Martin, A.J.; Ostrem, J.L.; Talke, P.; Levesque, N.; Larson, P.S. Subthalamic nucleus deep brain stimulator placement using high-field interventional magnetic resonance imaging and a skull-mounted aiming device: Technique and application accuracy. *J. Neurosurg.* **2010**, *112*, 479–490. [CrossRef] [PubMed]
23. Foltynie, T.; Zrinzo, L.; Martinez-Torres, I.; Tripoliti, E.; Petersen, E.; Holl, E.; Aviles-Olmos, I.; Jahanshahi, M.; Hariz, M.; Limousin, P. MRI-guided STN DBS in Parkinson's disease without microelectrode recording: Efficacy and safety. *J. Neurol. Neurosurg. Psychiatry* **2011**, *82*, 358–363. [CrossRef] [PubMed]
24. Nakajima, T.; Zrinzo, L.; Foltynie, T.; Olmos, I.A.; Taylor, C.; Hariz, M.I.; Limousin, P. MRI-guided subthalamic nucleus deep brain stimulation without microelectrode recording: Can we dispense with surgery under local anaesthesia? *Stereotact. Funct. Neurosurg.* **2011**, *89*, 318–325. [CrossRef] [PubMed]
25. Ostrem, J.L.; Galifianakis, N.B.; Markun, L.C.; Grace, J.K.; Martin, A.J.; Starr, P.A.; Larson, P.S. Clinical outcomes of PD patients having bilateral STN DBS using high-field interventional MR-imaging for lead placement. *Clin. Neurol. Neurosurg.* **2013**, *115*, 708–712. [CrossRef] [PubMed]
26. Saleh, S.; Swanson, K.I.; Lake, W.B.; Sillay, K.A. Awake neurophysiologically guided versus asleep MRI-guided STN DBS for Parkinson disease: A comparison of outcomes using levodopa equivalents. *Stereotact. Funct. Neurosurg.* **2015**, *93*, 419–426. [CrossRef]
27. Ostrem, J.L.; Ziman, N.; Galifianakis, N.B.; Starr, P.A.; San Luciano, M.; Katz, M.; Racine, C.A.; Martin, A.J.; Markun, L.C.; Larson, P.S. Clinical outcomes using ClearPoint interventional MRI for deep brain stimulation lead placement in Parkinson's disease. *J. Neurosurg.* **2016**, *124*, 908–916. [CrossRef]
28. Sidiropoulos, C.; Rammo, R.; Merker, B.; Mahajan, A.; LeWitt, P.; Kaminski, P.; Womble, M.; Zec, A.; Taylor, D.; Wall, J. Intraoperative MRI for deep brain stimulation lead placement in Parkinson's disease: 1 year motor and neuropsychological outcomes. *J. Neurol.* **2016**, *263*, 1226–1231. [CrossRef]
29. Chircop, C.; Dingli, N.; Aquilina, A.; Zrinzo, L.; Aquilina, J. MRI-verified "asleep" deep brain stimulation in Malta through cross border collaboration: Clinical outcome of the first five years. *Br J. Neurosurg.* **2018**, *32*, 365–371. [CrossRef]
30. Matias, C.M.; Frizon, L.A.; Nagel, S.J.; Lobel, D.A.; Machado, A.G. Deep brain stimulation outcomes in patients implanted under general anesthesia with frame-based stereotaxy and intraoperative MRI. *J. Neurosurg.* **2018**, *129*, 1572–1578. [CrossRef]
31. Mirzadeh, Z.; Chapple, K.; Lambert, M.; Evidente, V.G.; Mahant, P.; Ospina, M.C.; Samanta, J.; Moguel-Cobos, G.; Salins, N.; Lieberman, A.; et al. Parkinson's disease outcomes after intraoperative CT-guided "asleep" deep brain stimulation in the globus pallidus internus. *J. Neurosurg.* **2016**, *124*, 902–907. [CrossRef]
32. Hertel, F.; Züchner, M.; Weimar, I.; Gemmar, P.; Noll, B.; Bettag, M.; Decker, C. Implantation of electrodes for deep brain stimulation of the subthalamic nucleus in advanced parkinson's disease with the aid of intraoperative microrecording under general anesthesia. *Neurosurgery* **2006**, *59*, E1138. [CrossRef] [PubMed]
33. Lefaucheur, J.-P.; Gurruchaga, J.-M.; Pollin, B.; Von Raison, F.; Mohsen, N.; Shin, M.; Ménard-Lefaucheur, I.; Oshino, S.; Kishima, H.; Fénelon, G. Outcome of bilateral subthalamic nucleus stimulation in the treatment of Parkinson's disease: Correlation with intra-operative multi-unit recordings but not with the type of anaesthesia. *Eur. Neurol.* **2008**, *60*, 186–199. [CrossRef] [PubMed]
34. Lin, S.H.; Chen, T.Y.; Lin, S.Z.; Shyr, M.H.; Chou, Y.C.; Hsieh, W.A.; Tsai, S.T.; Chen, S.Y. Subthalamic deep brain stimulation after anesthetic inhalation in Parkinson disease: A preliminary study. *J. Neurosurg.* **2008**, *109*, 238–244. [CrossRef] [PubMed]

35. Fluchere, F.; Witjas, T.; Eusebio, A.; Bruder, N.; Giorgi, R.; Leveque, M.; Peragut, J.C.; Azulay, J.P.; Regis, J. Controlled general anaesthesia for subthalamic nucleus stimulation in Parkinson's disease. *J. Neurol. Neurosurg. Psychiatry* **2014**, *85*, 1167–1173. [CrossRef] [PubMed]
36. Patel, N.K.; Heywood, P.; O'Sullivan, K.; Love, S.; Gill, S.S. MRI-directed subthalamic nucleus surgery for Parkinson's disease. *Stereotact. Funct. Neurosurg.* **2002**, *78*, 132–145. [CrossRef] [PubMed]
37. Burchiel, K.J.; McCartney, S.; Lee, A.; Raslan, A.M. Accuracy of deep brain stimulation electrode placement using intraoperative computed tomography without microelectrode recording. *J. Neurosurg.* **2013**, *119*, 301–306. [CrossRef]
38. Mirzadeh, Z.; Chapple, K.; Lambert, M.; Dhall, R.; Ponce, F.A. Validation of CT-MRI fusion for intraoperative assessment of stereotactic accuracy in DBS surgery. *Mov. Disord.* **2014**, *29*, 1788–1795. [CrossRef]
39. Zrinzo, L.; Foltynie, T.; Limousin, P.; Hariz, M. Image-guided and image-verified deep brain stimulation. *Mov. Disord.* **2013**, *28*, 254. [CrossRef]
40. Ferroli, P.; Franzini, A.; Marras, C.; Maccagnano, E.; D'Incerti, L.; Broggi, G. A simple method to assess accuracy of deep brain stimulation electrode placement: Pre-operative stereotactic CT+ postoperative MR image fusion. *Stereotact. Funct. Neurosurg.* **2004**, *82*, 14–19. [CrossRef]
41. Fiegele, T.; Feuchtner, G.; Sohm, F.; Bauer, R.; Anton, J.V.; Gotwald, T.; Twerdy, K.; Eisner, W. Accuracy of stereotactic electrode placement in deep brain stimulation by intraoperative computed tomography. *Park. Relat. Disord.* **2008**, *14*, 595–599. [CrossRef]
42. Chen, T.; Mirzadeh, Z.; Chapple, K.M.; Lambert, M.; Shill, H.A.; Moguel-Cobos, G.; Troster, A.I.; Dhall, R.; Ponce, F.A. Clinical outcomes following awake and asleep deep brain stimulation for Parkinson disease. *J. Neurosurg.* **2018**, *130*, 109–120. [CrossRef]
43. Ko, A.L.; Magown, P.; Ozpinar, A.; Hamzaoglu, V.; Burchiel, K.J. Asleep Deep Brain Stimulation Reduces Incidence of Intracranial Air during Electrode Implantation. *Stereotact. Funct. Neurosurg.* **2018**, *96*, 83–90. [CrossRef] [PubMed]
44. Cui, Z.; Pan, L.; Song, H.; Xu, X.; Xu, B.; Yu, X.; Ling, Z. Intraoperative MRI for optimizing electrode placement for deep brain stimulation of the subthalamic nucleus in Parkinson disease. *J. Neurosurg.* **2016**, *124*, 62–69. [CrossRef] [PubMed]
45. Chen, T.; Mirzadeh, Z.; Ponce, F.A. "Asleep" Deep Brain Stimulation Surgery: A Critical Review of the Literature. *World Neurosurg.* **2017**, *105*, 191–198. [CrossRef] [PubMed]
46. Sheshadri, V.; Rowland, N.C.; Mehta, J.; Englesakis, M.; Manninen, P.; Venkatraghavan, L. Comparison of General and Local Anesthesia for Deep Brain Stimulator Insertion: A Systematic Review. *Can. J. Neurol. Sci.* **2017**, *44*, 697–704. [CrossRef]
47. Bot, M.; van den Munckhof, P.; Bakay, R.; Stebbins, G.; Metman, L.V. Accuracy of intraoperative computed tomography during deep brain stimulation procedures: Comparison with postoperative magnetic resonance imaging. *Stereotact. Funct. Neurosurg.* **2017**, *95*, 183–188. [CrossRef]
48. Kremer, N.I.; Oterdoom, D.L.M.; van Laar, P.J.; Piña-Fuentes, D.; van Laar, T.; Drost, G.; van Hulzen, A.L.J.; van Dijk, J.M.C. Accuracy of Intraoperative Computed Tomography in Deep Brain Stimulation-A Prospective Noninferiority Study. *Neuromodul. Technol. Neural Interface* **2019**, *22*, 472–477. [CrossRef]
49. Harries, A.M.; Kausar, J.; Roberts, S.A.; Mocroft, A.P.; Hodson, J.A.; Pall, H.S.; Mitchell, R.D. Deep brain stimulation of the subthalamic nucleus for advanced Parkinson disease using general anesthesia: Long-term results. *J. Neurosurg.* **2012**, *116*, 107–113. [CrossRef]
50. Kwon, W.K.; Kim, J.H.; Lee, J.H.; Lim, B.G.; Lee, I.O.; Koh, S.B.; Kwon, T.H. Microelectrode recording (MER) findings during sleep-awake anesthesia using dexmedetomidine in deep brain stimulation surgery for Parkinson's disease. *Clin. Neurol. Neurosurg.* **2016**, *143*, 27–33. [CrossRef] [PubMed]
51. Warnke, P. Deep brain stimulation: Awake or asleep: It comes with a price either way. *J. Neurol. Neurosurg. Psychiatry* **2018**, *89*, 672. [CrossRef] [PubMed]
52. Tsai, S.-T.; Kuo, C.-C.; Chen, T.-Y.; Chen, S.-Y. Neurophysiological comparisons of subthalamic deep-brain stimulation for Parkinson's disease between patients receiving general and local anesthesia. *Tzu Chi Med. J.* **2016**, *28*, 63–67. [CrossRef] [PubMed]
53. LaHue, S.C.; Ostrem, J.L.; Galifianakis, N.B.; San Luciano, M.; Ziman, N.; Wang, S.; Racine, C.A.; Starr, P.A.; Larson, P.S.; Katz, M. Parkinson's disease patient preference and experience with various methods of DBS lead placement. *Park. Relat. Disord.* **2017**, *41*, 25–30. [CrossRef] [PubMed]

54. Yamada, K.; Goto, S.; Kuratsu, J.; Matsuzaki, K.; Tamura, T.; Nagahiro, S.; Murase, N.; Shimazu, H.; Kaji, R. Stereotactic surgery for subthalamic nucleus stimulation under general anesthesia: A retrospective evaluation of Japanese patients with Parkinson's disease. *Park. Relat. Disord.* **2007**, *13*, 101–107. [CrossRef] [PubMed]
55. Chen, S.Y.; Tsai, S.T.; Lin, S.H.; Chen, T.Y.; Hung, H.Y.; Lee, C.W.; Wang, W.H.; Chen, S.P.; Lin, S.Z. Subthalamic deep brain stimulation in Parkinson's disease under different anesthetic modalities: A comparative cohort study. *Stereotact. Funct. Neurosurg.* **2011**, *89*, 372–380. [CrossRef] [PubMed]
56. Asha, M.J.; Fisher, B.; Kausar, J.; Garratt, H.; Krovvidi, H.; Shirley, C.; White, A.; Chelvarajah, R.; Ughratdar, I.; Hodson, J.A. Subthalamic deep brain stimulation under general anesthesia and neurophysiological guidance while on dopaminergic medication: Comparative cohort study. *Acta Neurochir.* **2018**, *160*, 823–829. [CrossRef] [PubMed]
57. Lettieri, C.; Rinaldo, S.; Devigili, G.; Pauletto, G.; Verriello, L.; Budai, R.; Fadiga, L.; Oliynyk, A.; Mondani, M.; D'Auria, S.; et al. Deep brain stimulation: Subthalamic nucleus electrophysiological activity in awake and anesthetized patients. *Clin. Neurophysiol. Off. J. Int. Fed. Clin. Neurophysiol.* **2012**, *123*, 2406–2413. [CrossRef] [PubMed]
58. Maltête, D.; Navarro, S.; Welter, M.-L.; Roche, S.; Bonnet, A.-M.; Houeto, J.-L.; Mesnage, V.; Pidoux, B.; Dormont, D.; Cornu, P. Subthalamic stimulation in Parkinson disease: With or without anesthesia? *Arch. Neurol.* **2004**, *61*, 390–392. [CrossRef]
59. Brodsky, M.A.; Anderson, S.; Murchison, C.; Seier, M.; Wilhelm, J.; Vederman, A.; Burchiel, K.J. Clinical outcomes of asleep vs awake deep brain stimulation for Parkinson disease. *Neurology* **2017**, *89*, 1944–1950. [CrossRef]
60. Sharma, M.; Deogaonkar, M. Accuracy and safety of targeting using intraoperative "O-arm" during placement of deep brain stimulation electrodes without electrophysiological recordings. *J. Clin. Neurosci. Off. J. Neurosurg. Soc. Australas* **2016**, *27*, 80–86. [CrossRef]
61. Carlson, J.D.; McLeod, K.E.; McLeod, P.S.; Mark, J.B. Stereotactic Accuracy and Surgical Utility of the O-Arm in Deep Brain Stimulation Surgery. *Oper. Neurosurg. (Hagerstown)* **2017**, *13*, 96–107. [CrossRef]
62. Sillay, K.A.; Rusy, D.; Buyan-Dent, L.; Ninman, N.L.; Vigen, K.K. Wide-bore 1.5 T MRI-guided deep brain stimulation surgery: Initial experience and technique comparison. *Clin. Neurol. Neurosurg.* **2014**, *127*, 79–85. [CrossRef] [PubMed]
63. Aviles-Olmos, I.; Kefalopoulou, Z.; Tripoliti, E.; Candelario, J.; Akram, H.; Martinez-Torres, I.; Jahanshahi, M.; Foltynie, T.; Hariz, M.; Zrinzo, L. Long-term outcome of subthalamic nucleus deep brain stimulation for Parkinson's disease using an MRI-guided and MRI-verified approach. *J. Neurol. Neurosurg. Psychiatry* **2014**, *85*, 1419–1425. [CrossRef] [PubMed]
64. Chabardes, S.; Isnard, S.; Castrioto, A.; Oddoux, M.; Fraix, V.; Carlucci, L.; Payen, J.F.; Krainik, A.; Krack, P.; Larson, P. Surgical implantation of STN-DBS leads using intraoperative MRI guidance: Technique, accuracy, and clinical benefit at 1-year follow-up. *Acta Neurochir.* **2015**, *157*, 729–737. [CrossRef] [PubMed]
65. Spiegelmann, R.; Nissim, O.; Daniels, D.; Ocherashvilli, A.; Mardor, Y. Stereotactic targeting of the ventrointermediate nucleus of the thalamus by direct visualization with high-field MRI. *Stereotact. Funct. Neurosurg.* **2006**, *84*, 19–23. [CrossRef] [PubMed]
66. Lee, P.S.; Richardson, R.M. Interventional MRI-Guided Deep Brain Stimulation Lead Implantation. *Neurosurg. Clin. N. Am.* **2017**, *28*, 535–544. [CrossRef]
67. Min, H.K.; Ross, E.K.; Lee, K.H.; Dennis, K.; Han, S.R.; Jeong, J.H.; Marsh, M.P.; Striemer, B.; Felmlee, J.P.; Lujan, J.L.; et al. Subthalamic nucleus deep brain stimulation induces motor network BOLD activation: Use of a high precision MRI guided stereotactic system for nonhuman primates. *Brain Stimul.* **2014**, *7*, 603–607. [CrossRef]
68. Kochanski, R.B.; Sani, S. Awake versus Asleep Deep Brain Stimulation Surgery: Technical Considerations and Critical Review of the Literature. *Brain Sci.* **2018**, *8*, 17. [CrossRef]
69. Kamiryo, T.; Laws, E.R., Jr. Stereotactic frame-based error in magnetic-resonance-guided stereotactic procedures: A method for measurement of error and standardization of technique. *Stereotact. Funct. Neurosurg.* **1996**, *67*, 198–209. [CrossRef]
70. Ko, A.L.; Ibrahim, A.; Magown, P.; Macallum, R.; Burchiel, K.J. Factors affecting stereotactic accuracy in image-guided deep brain stimulator electrode placement. *Stereotact. Funct. Neurosurg.* **2017**, *95*, 315–324. [CrossRef]

71. Chen, T.; Mirzadeh, Z.; Chapple, K.; Lambert, M.; Dhall, R.; Ponce, F.A. "Asleep" deep brain stimulation for essential tremor. *J. Neurosurg.* **2016**, *124*, 1842–1849. [CrossRef]
72. Holloway, K.; Docef, A. A quantitative assessment of the accuracy and reliability of O-arm images for deep brain stimulation surgery. *Neurosurgery* **2013**, *72*, 47–57. [CrossRef] [PubMed]
73. Geevarghese, R.; O'Gorman Tuura, R.; Lumsden, D.E.; Samuel, M.; Ashkan, K. Registration Accuracy of CT/MRI Fusion for Localisation of Deep Brain Stimulation Electrode Position: An Imaging Study and Systematic Review. *Stereotact. Funct. Neurosurg.* **2016**, *94*, 159–163. [CrossRef] [PubMed]
74. Ivan, M.E.; Yarlagadda, J.; Saxena, A.P.; Martin, A.J.; Starr, P.A.; Sootsman, W.K.; Larson, P.S. Brain shift during bur hole-based procedures using interventional MRI. *J. Neurosurg.* **2014**, *121*, 149–160. [CrossRef] [PubMed]
75. Deuschl, G.; Schade-Brittinger, C.; Krack, P.; Volkmann, J.; Schäfer, H.; Bötzel, K.; Daniels, C.; Deutschländer, A.; Dillmann, U.; Eisner, W. A randomized trial of deep-brain stimulation for Parkinson's disease. *N. Engl. J. Med.* **2006**, *355*, 896–908. [CrossRef]
76. Erickson, K.M.; Cole, D.J. Anesthetic considerations for awake craniotomy for epilepsy. *Anesthesiol. Clin.* **2007**, *25*, 535–555, ix. [CrossRef]
77. Grant, R.; Gruenbaum, S.E.; Gerrard, J. Anaesthesia for deep brain stimulation: A review. *Curr. Opin. Anaesthesiol.* **2015**, *28*, 505. [CrossRef]
78. Khan, M.F.; Mewes, K.; Gross, R.E.; Skrinjar, O. Assessment of brain shift related to deep brain stimulation surgery. *Stereotact. Funct. Neurosurg.* **2008**, *86*, 44–53. [CrossRef]
79. Pallavaram, S.; Dawant, B.M.; Remple, M.S.; Neimat, J.S.; Kao, C.; Konrad, P.E.; D'Haese, P.F. Effect of brain shift on the creation of functional atlases for deep brain stimulation surgery. *Int. J. Comput. Assist. Radiol. Surg.* **2010**, *5*, 221–228. [CrossRef]
80. Elias, W.J.; Durieux, M.E.; Huss, D.; Frysinger, R.C. Dexmedetomidine and arousal affect subthalamic neurons. *Mov. Disord.* **2008**, *23*, 1317–1320. [CrossRef]
81. Pollak, P.; Krack, P.; Fraix, V.; Mendes, A.; Moro, E.; Chabardes, S.; Benabid, A.L. Intraoperative micro- and macrostimulation of the subthalamic nucleus in Parkinson's disease. *Mov. Disord.* **2002**, *17* (Suppl. 3), S155–S161. [CrossRef]
82. Gorgulho, A.; De Salles, A.A.; Frighetto, L.; Behnke, E. Incidence of hemorrhage associated with electrophysiological studies performed using macroelectrodes and microelectrodes in functional neurosurgery. *J. Neurosurg.* **2005**, *102*, 888–896. [CrossRef] [PubMed]
83. Binder, D.K.; Rau, G.M.; Starr, P.A. Risk factors for hemorrhage during microelectrode-guided deep brain stimulator implantation for movement disorders. *Neurosurgery* **2005**, *56*, 722–732. [CrossRef] [PubMed]
84. Vesper, J.; Haak, S.; Ostertag, C.; Nikkhah, G. Subthalamic nucleus deep brain stimulation in elderly patients–analysis of outcome and complications. *BMC Neurol.* **2007**, *7*, 7. [CrossRef] [PubMed]
85. Guridi, J.; Rodriguez-Oroz, M.C.; Lozano, A.M.; Moro, E.; Albanese, A.; Nuttin, B.; Gybels, J.; Ramos, E.; Obeso, J.A. Targeting the basal ganglia for deep brain stimulation in Parkinson's disease. *Neurology* **2000**, *55*, S21–S28.
86. Houeto, J.-L.; Welter, M.-L.; Bejjani, P.-B.; du Montcel, S.T.; Bonnet, A.-M.; Mesnage, V.; Navarro, S.; Pidoux, B.; Dormont, D.; Cornu, P. Subthalamic stimulation in Parkinson disease: Intraoperative predictive factors. *Arch. Neurol.* **2003**, *60*, 690–694. [CrossRef]
87. Blasberg, F.; Wojtecki, L.; Elben, S.; Slotty, P.J.; Vesper, J.; Schnitzler, A.; Groiss, S.J. Comparison of Awake vs. Asleep Surgery for Subthalamic Deep Brain Stimulation in Parkinson's Disease. *Neuromodulation* **2018**, *21*, 541–547. [CrossRef]
88. Castrioto, A.; Marmor, O.; Deffains, M.; Willner, D.; Linetsky, E.; Bergman, H.; Israel, Z.; Eitan, R.; Arkadir, D. Anesthesia reduces discharge rates in the human pallidum without changing the discharge rate ratio between pallidal segments. *Eur. J. Neurosci.* **2016**, *44*, 2909–2913. [CrossRef]
89. Moll, C.K.; Payer, S.; Gulberti, A.; Sharrott, A.; Zittel, S.; Boelmans, K.; Köppen, J.; Gerloff, C.; Westphal, M.; Engel, A.K. STN stimulation in general anaesthesia: Evidence beyond 'evidence-based medicine'. In *Stereotactic and Functional Neurosurgery*; Springer: Berlin/Heidelberg, Germany, 2013; pp. 19–25.
90. Sanghera, M.K.; Grossman, R.G.; Kalhorn, C.G.; Hamilton, W.J.; Ondo, W.G.; Jankovic, J. Basal ganglia neuronal discharge in primary and secondary dystonia in patients undergoing pallidotomy. *Neurosurgery* **2003**, *52*, 1358–1373. [CrossRef]

91. Tsai, S.T.; Chuang, W.Y.; Kuo, C.C.; Chao, P.C.; Chen, T.Y.; Hung, H.Y.; Chen, S.Y. Dorsolateral subthalamic neuronal activity enhanced by median nerve stimulation characterizes Parkinson's disease during deep brain stimulation with general anesthesia. *J. Neurosurg.* **2015**, *123*, 1394–1400. [CrossRef]
92. Kim, W.; Song, I.H.; Lim, Y.H.; Kim, M.-R.; Kim, Y.E.; Hwang, J.H.; Kim, I.K.; Song, S.W.; Kim, J.W.; Lee, W.-W. Influence of propofol and fentanyl on deep brain stimulation of the subthalamic nucleus. *J. Korean Med. Sci.* **2014**, *29*, 1278–1286. [CrossRef]
93. Lee, W.-W.; Ehm, G.; Yang, H.-J.; Song, I.H.; Lim, Y.H.; Kim, M.-R.; Kim, Y.E.; Hwang, J.H.; Park, H.R.; Lee, J.M. Bilateral deep brain stimulation of the subthalamic nucleus under sedation with propofol and fentanyl. *PLoS ONE* **2016**, *11*, e0152619. [CrossRef] [PubMed]
94. Galvan, A.; Wichmann, T. GABAergic circuits in the basal ganglia and movement disorders. *Prog. Brain Res.* **2007**, *160*, 287–312. [PubMed]
95. Raz, A.; Eimerl, D.; Zaidel, A.; Bergman, H.; Israel, Z. Propofol decreases neuronal population spiking activity in the subthalamic nucleus of Parkinsonian patients. *Anesth. Analg.* **2010**, *111*, 1285–1289. [CrossRef] [PubMed]
96. Lin, S.H.; Lai, H.Y.; Lo, Y.C.; Chou, C.; Chou, Y.T.; Yang, S.H.; Sun, I.; Chen, B.W.; Wang, C.F.; Liu, G.T.; et al. Decreased Power but Preserved Bursting Features of Subthalamic Neuronal Signals in Advanced Parkinson's Patients under Controlled Desflurane Inhalation Anesthesia. *Front. Neurosci.* **2017**, *11*, 701. [CrossRef] [PubMed]
97. Kouvaras, E.; Asprodini, E.K.; Asouchidou, I.; Vasilaki, A.; Kilindris, T.; Michaloudis, D.; Koukoutianou, I.; Papatheodoropoulos, C.; Kostopoulos, G. Fentanyl treatment reduces GABAergic inhibition in the CA1 area of the hippocampus 24 h after acute exposure to the drug. *Neuropharmacology* **2008**, *55*, 1172–1182. [CrossRef]
98. Hutchison, W.D.; Lang, A.E.; Dostrovsky, J.O.; Lozano, A.M. Pallidal neuronal activity: Implications for models of dystonia. *Ann. Neurol.* **2003**, *53*, 480–488. [CrossRef]
99. Khatib, R.; Ebrahim, Z.; Rezai, A.; Cata, J.P.; Boulis, N.M.; John Doyle, D.; Schurigyn, T.; Farag, E. Perioperative events during deep brain stimulation: The experience at cleveland clinic. *J. Neurosurg. Anesthesiol.* **2008**, *20*, 36–40. [CrossRef]
100. Duque, P.; Mateo, O.; Ruiz, F.; de Viloria, J.G.; Contreras, A.; Grandas, F. Intraoperative microrecording under general anaesthesia with bispectral analysis monitoring in a case of deep brain stimulation surgery for Parkinson's disease. *Eur. J. Neurol.* **2008**, *15*, e76–e77. [CrossRef]
101. Lee, J.Y.; Deogaonkar, M.; Rezai, A. Deep brain stimulation of globus pallidus internus for dystonia. *Park. Relat. Disord.* **2007**, *13*, 261–265. [CrossRef]
102. Morace, R.; De Angelis, M.; Aglialoro, E.; Maucione, G.; Cavallo, L.; Solari, D.; Modugno, N.; Santilli, M.; Esposito, V.; Aloj, F. Sedation with α2 Agonist Dexmedetomidine During Unilateral Subthalamic Nucleus Deep Brain Stimulation: A Preliminary Report. *World Neurosurg.* **2016**, *89*, 320–328. [CrossRef]
103. Rozet, I. Anesthesia for functional neurosurgery: The role of dexmedetomidine. *Curr. Opin. Anaesthesiol.* **2008**, *21*, 537–543. [CrossRef] [PubMed]
104. Sassi, M.; Zekaj, E.; Grotta, A.; Pollini, A.; Pellanda, A.; Borroni, M.; Pacchetti, C.; Menghetti, C.; Porta, M.; Servello, D. Safety in the use of dexmedetomidine (precedex) for deep brain stimulation surgery: Our experience in 23 randomized patients. *Neuromodulation* **2013**, *16*, 401–406. [CrossRef] [PubMed]
105. Hans, P.; Bonhomme, V.; Born, J.D.; Maertens de Noordhoudt, A.; Brichant, J.F.; Dewandre, P.Y. Target-controlled infusion of propofol and remifentanil combined with bispectral index monitoring for awake craniotomy. *Anaesthesia* **2000**, *55*, 255–259. [CrossRef] [PubMed]
106. Johansen, J.W.; Sebel, P.S. Development and clinical application of electroencephalographic bispectrum monitoring. *Anesthesiology* **2000**, *93*, 1336–1344. [CrossRef] [PubMed]
107. Sutcliffe, A.; Mitchell, R.; Gan, Y.; Mocroft, A.; Nightingale, P. General anaesthesia for deep brain stimulator electrode insertion in Parkinson's disease. *Acta Neurochir.* **2011**, *153*, 621–627. [CrossRef]
108. Tsai, S.-T.; Chen, T.-Y.; Lin, S.-H.; Chen, S.-Y. Five-year clinical outcomes of local versus general anesthesia deep brain stimulation for Parkinson's disease. *Parkinson's Dis.* **2019**, *2019*, 5676345. [CrossRef]
109. Martin, A.J.; Larson, P.S.; Ziman, N.; Levesque, N.; Volz, M.; Ostrem, J.L.; Starr, P.A. Deep brain stimulator implantation in a diagnostic MRI suite: Infection history over a 10-year period. *J. Neurosurg.* **2017**, *126*, 108–113. [CrossRef]

110. Chen, T.; Mirzadeh, Z.; Chapple, K.; Lambert, M.; Ponce, F.A. Complication rates, lengths of stay, and readmission rates in "awake" and "asleep" deep brain simulation. *J. Neurosurg.* **2017**, *127*, 360–369. [CrossRef]
111. Jacob, R.L.; Geddes, J.; McCartney, S.; Burchiel, K.J. Cost analysis of awake versus asleep deep brain stimulation: A single academic health center experience. *J. Neurosurg.* **2016**, *124*, 1517–1523. [CrossRef]
112. Lefranc, M.; Zouitina, Y.; Tir, M.; Merle, P.; Ouendo, M.; Constans, J.M.; Godefroy, O.; Peltier, J.; Krystkowiak, P. Asleep Robot-Assisted Surgery for the Implantation of Subthalamic Electrodes Provides the Same Clinical Improvement and Therapeutic Window as Awake Surgery. *World Neurosurg.* **2017**, *106*, 602–608. [CrossRef]
113. Liu, Z.; He, S.; Li, L. General Anesthesia versus Local Anesthesia for Deep Brain Stimulation in Parkinson's Disease: A Meta-Analysis. *Stereotact. Funct. Neurosurg.* **2019**, *97*, 381–390. [CrossRef] [PubMed]
114. Paek, S.H.; Han, J.H.; Lee, J.Y.; Kim, C.; Jeon, B.S.; Kim, D.G. Electrode position determined by fused images of preoperative and postoperative magnetic resonance imaging and surgical outcome after subthalamic nucleus deep brain stimulation. *Neurosurgery* **2008**, *63*, 925–936, discussion 936–927. [CrossRef] [PubMed]
115. Paek, S.H.; Yun, J.Y.; Song, S.W.; Kim, I.K.; Hwang, J.H.; Kim, J.W.; Kim, H.J.; Kim, H.J.; Kim, Y.E.; Lim, Y.H.; et al. The clinical impact of precise electrode positioning in STN DBS on three-year outcomes. *J. Neurol. Sci.* **2013**, *327*, 25–31. [CrossRef] [PubMed]
116. Ryu, S.I.; Romanelli, P.; Heit, G. Asymptomatic transient MRI signal changes after unilateral deep brain stimulation electrode implantation for movement disorder. *Stereotact. Funct. Neurosurg.* **2004**, *82*, 65–69. [CrossRef] [PubMed]
117. Englot, D.J.; Glastonbury, C.M.; Larson, P.S. Abnormal T2-weighted MRI signal surrounding leads in a subset of deep brain stimulation patients. *Stereotact. Funct. Neurosurg.* **2011**, *89*, 311–317. [CrossRef] [PubMed]
118. Fenoy, A.J.; Villarreal, S.J.; Schiess, M.C. Acute and subacute presentations of cerebral edema following deep brain stimulation lead implantation. *Stereotact. Funct. Neurosurg.* **2017**, *95*, 86–92. [CrossRef]
119. Deogaonkar, M.; Nazzaro, J.M.; Machado, A.; Rezai, A. Transient, symptomatic, post-operative, non-infectious hypodensity around the deep brain stimulation (DBS) electrode. *J. Clin. Neurosci.* **2011**, *18*, 910–915. [CrossRef]
120. Holewijn, R.A.; Verbaan, D.; de Bie, R.M.A.; Schuurman, P.R. General Anesthesia versus Local Anesthesia in StereotaXY (GALAXY) for Parkinson's disease: Study protocol for a randomized controlled trial. *Trials* **2017**, *18*, 417. [CrossRef]
121. Little, S.; Pogosyan, A.; Neal, S.; Zavala, B.; Zrinzo, L.; Hariz, M.; Foltynie, T.; Limousin, P.; Ashkan, K.; FitzGerald, J. Adaptive deep brain stimulation in advanced Parkinson disease. *Ann. Neurol.* **2013**, *74*, 449–457. [CrossRef]
122. Little, S.; Beudel, M.; Zrinzo, L.; Foltynie, T.; Limousin, P.; Hariz, M.; Neal, S.; Cheeran, B.; Cagnan, H.; Gratwicke, J. Bilateral adaptive deep brain stimulation is effective in Parkinson's disease. *J. Neurol. Neurosurg. Psychiatry* **2016**, *87*, 717–721. [CrossRef]
123. Higuchi, Y.; Matsuda, S.; Serizawa, T. Gamma knife radiosurgery in movement disorders: Indications and limitations. *Mov. Disord.* **2017**, *32*, 28–35. [CrossRef] [PubMed]
124. Friedman, J.H.; Epstein, M.; Sanes, J.N.; Lieberman, P.; Cullen, K.; Lindquist, C.; Daamen, M. Gamma knife pallidotomy in advanced Parkinson's disease. *Ann. Neurol.* **1996**, *39*, 535–538. [CrossRef] [PubMed]
125. Magara, A.; Bühler, R.; Moser, D.; Kowalski, M.; Pourtehrani, P.; Jeanmonod, D. First experience with MR-guided focused ultrasound in the treatment of Parkinson's disease. *J. Ther. Ultrasound* **2014**, *2*, 11. [CrossRef] [PubMed]
126. Martínez-Fernández, R.; Rodríguez-Rojas, R.; Del Álamo, M.; Hernández-Fernández, F.; Pineda-Pardo, J.A.; Dileone, M.; Alonso-Frech, F.; Foffani, G.; Obeso, I.; Gasca-Salas, C. Focused ultrasound subthalamotomy in patients with asymmetric Parkinson's disease: A pilot study. *Lancet Neurol.* **2018**, *17*, 54–63. [CrossRef]

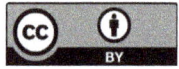

© 2020 by the authors. Licensee MDPI, Basel, Switzerland. This article is an open access article distributed under the terms and conditions of the Creative Commons Attribution (CC BY) license (http://creativecommons.org/licenses/by/4.0/).

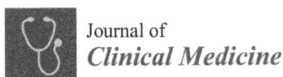

Article

Influence of Anesthesia and Clinical Variables on the Firing Rate, Coefficient of Variation and Multi-Unit Activity of the Subthalamic Nucleus in Patients with Parkinson's Disease

Michael J. Bos [1,2,*,†], Ana Maria Alzate Sanchez [2,†], Raffaella Bancone [2], Yasin Temel [2,3], Bianca T.A. de Greef [2,4], Anthony R. Absalom [5], Erik D. Gommer [2,6], Vivianne H.J.M. van Kranen-Mastenbroek [2,6], Wolfgang F. Buhre [1,2], Mark J. Roberts [7] and Marcus L.F. Janssen [2,6]

1. Department of Anesthesiology and Pain Medicine, Maastricht University Medical Center, P. Debyelaan 25, 6229 HX Maastricht, The Netherlands; wolfgang.buhre@mumc.nl
2. School for Mental Health and Neuroscience, Faculty of Health, Medicine and Life Sciences, Maastricht University, Universiteitssingel 40, 6229 ER Maastricht, The Netherlands; a.alzatesanchez@alumni.maastrichtuniversity.nl (A.M.A.S.); raffaellabancone@gmail.com (R.B.); y.temel@mumc.nl (Y.T.); bianca.greef@mumc.nl (B.T.A.d.G.); e.gommer@mumc.nl (E.D.G.); v.kranen.mastenbroek@mumc.nl (V.H.J.M.v.K.-M.); m.janssen@maastrichtuniversity.nl (M.L.F.J.)
3. Department of Neurosurgery, Maastricht University Medical Center, P. Debyelaan 25, 6229 HX Maastricht, The Netherlands
4. Department of Neurology, Maastricht University Medical Center, P. Debyelaan 25, 6229 HX, Maastricht, The Netherlands
5. Department of Anesthesiology, Groningen University, University Medical Center Groningen, Hanzeplein 1, 9713 GZ Groningen, The Netherlands; a.r.absalom@umcg.nl
6. Department of Clinical Neurophysiology, Maastricht University Medical Center, P. Debyelaan 25, 6229 HX Maastricht, The Netherlands
7. Faculty of Psychology and Neuroscience, Maastricht University, Universiteitssingel 40, 6229 ER Maastricht, The Netherlands; mark.roberts@maastrichtuniversity.nl
* Correspondence: Michael.bos@mumc.nl
† Authors contributed equally.

Received: 24 March 2020; Accepted: 17 April 2020; Published: 24 April 2020

Abstract: Background: Microelectrode recordings (MER) are used to optimize lead placement during subthalamic nucleus deep brain stimulation (STN-DBS). To obtain reliable MER, surgery is usually performed while patients are awake. Procedural sedation and analgesia (PSA) is often desirable to improve patient comfort, anxiolysis and pain relief. The effect of these agents on MER are largely unknown. The objective of this study was to determine the effects of commonly used PSA agents, dexmedetomidine, clonidine and remifentanil and patient characteristics on MER during DBS surgery. Methods: Data from 78 patients with Parkinson's disease (PD) who underwent STN-DBS surgery were retrospectively reviewed. The procedures were performed under local anesthesia or under PSA with dexmedetomidine, clonidine or remifentanil. In total, 4082 sites with multi-unit activity (MUA) and 588 with single units were acquired. Single unit firing rates and coefficient of variation (CV), and MUA total power were compared between patient groups. Results: We observed a significant reduction in MUA, an increase of the CV and a trend for reduced firing rate by dexmedetomidine. The effect of dexmedetomidine was dose-dependent for all measures. Remifentanil had no effect on the firing rate but was associated with a significant increase in CV and a decrease in MUA. Clonidine showed no significant effect on firing rate, CV or MUA. In addition to anesthetic effects, MUA and CV were also influenced by patient-dependent variables. Conclusion: Our results showed that PSA influenced neuronal properties in the STN and the dexmedetomidine (DEX) effect was dose-dependent. In addition, patient-dependent characteristics also influenced MER.

Keywords: deep brain stimulation; microelectrode recordings; subthalamic nucleus; procedural sedation and analgesia; Parkinson's disease; clonidine; dexmedetomidine; remifentanil

---

1. Introduction

Deep brain stimulation (DBS) of the subthalamic nucleus (STN) is a well-established procedure for the treatment of refractory Parkinson's disease (PD) [1]. The clinical outcome of the surgery largely depends on correct positioning of the stimulating electrode in the sensorimotor region of the STN [2,3]. Microelectrode recordings (MER) of single-cell and multi-unit neuronal activity are commonly used to verify the borders of the STN [4]. To obtain reliable MER, DBS surgery is traditionally performed under local anesthesia alone, as the sedative and anesthetic agents may interfere with neural activity. However, patients may experience pain, anxiety or other forms of discomfort. To improve patient comfort and tolerance of the DBS implantation procedure, procedural sedation and/or analgesia (PSA) may be applied [5].

Propofol is commonly used for sedation during DBS implantation. It exerts its clinical effect through an agonist effect on the gamma-aminobutyric acid type A ($GABA_A$) receptor [6]. Several studies have shown that GABAergic agents alter STN activity in a dose-dependent manner [7–9]. In the past decade experience has been gained with non-GABA-mediated agents, including the α_2-agonists clonidine (CLONI) and dexmedetomidine (DEX), which possess sedative and mild analgesic effects, and the ultrashort acting opioid, remifentanil (REMI) which provides potent analgesia and mild sedation. Since the pharmacokinetic effects of these drugs are not mediated by $GABA_A$ receptors, their influence on STN neuronal activity is postulated to be less pronounced than of GABAergic agents. However, the available literature on non-GABA-mediated PSA effects on STN neuronal activity is sparse and consists largely of small uncontrolled retrospective case series with poor control over heterogeneity in patient cohorts [10–16].

The primary aim of this study was to determine the effect of the non-GABAergic PSA agents DEX, CLONI and REMI on MER in patients with PD during DBS electrode implantation surgery. In addition to PSA-related effects on MER, we analyzed patient characteristics such as age, disease severity and disease duration to control for heterogeneity in the sample.

2. Materials and Methods

2.1. Subjects

After gaining the approval of the local ethical committee (METC Maastricht University Medical Center, the Netherlands, protocol number 184214) we conducted a retrospective analysis of data from all PD patients who underwent DBS surgery in Maastricht UMC+ between January 2009 and December 2018. We acquired patient demographics and anesthetic data and retrieved the raw MER data for offline processing and analysis.

2.2. Anesthetic Management

All patients underwent a multidisciplinary preoperative assessment of eligibility for DBS surgery. In the operating room, standard monitoring was applied including a five-lead electrocardiogram, pulse oximetry, inspiratory and expiratory O_2 and CO_2 monitoring and invasive blood pressure monitoring. DBS surgery was performed under local anesthesia alone or in combination with PSA administered at the discretion of the responsible anesthesiologist. The goal of PSA was to maintain mild to moderate sedation, with the patient responsive to verbal command (so-called conscious sedation). The skin puncture sites of the stereotactic frame pins, and the surgical incision sites, were infiltrated with a 50:50 mixture of lidocaine 1% and levobupivacaine 0.5% with epinephrine (1:100.000). During the procedure some patients received no sedative drugs, whereas some received one or more of DEX, CLONI or REMI by continuous intravenous infusion for PSA. Some patients received DEX only in the first phase of the surgery until around 20 min before the start of MER (Table 1). After DBS electrode implantation, all patients underwent general anesthesia for tunneling of the extension cables and placement of the pulse generator. Postoperatively, patients were transferred to the post-anesthesia care unit for hemodynamic- and neuro-monitoring.

Table 1. Demographic and clinical data of all patients.

Group		Patients M/F	Hemispheres (n)	Electrodes (n)	SU/MUA (n)	Age (y)	UPDRS III	Dose Range	
Awake	No PSA	15/6	42	149	165/1257	59.4 ± 8.3	38.2 ± 16.5		
	PSA discon	4/3	14	42	51/339	59.3 ± 7.6	42.0 ± 8.5		
Sedation	DEX	7/4	22	70	86/565	60.9 ± 5.9	33.4 ± 12.4	0.07–0.6 µg kg^{-1} h^{-1}	
	REMI	8/6	28	99	93/636	58.1 ± 8.0	37.9 ± 14.3	0.02–0.25 µg kg^{-1} min^{-1}	
	CLONI	6/2	16	56	41/339	64.8 ± 8.3	35.8 ± 11.9	20–50 µg h^{-1} or 30–150 µg IV in bolus	
	DEX + REMI	4/1	10	35	46/267	65.8 ± 6.5	34.3 ± 7.8	DEX 0.3–0.5 µg kg^{-1} h^{-1}	REMI 0.02–0.05 µg kg^{-1} min^{-1}
	CLONI + REMI	6/6	24	84	106/679	59.5 ± 7.3	36.4 ± 9.1	CLONI 20 µg h^{-1} or 45–150 µg IV in bolus	REMI 0.01–0.09 µg kg^{-1} min^{-1}
Total		50/28	156	535	588/4082	60.5 ± 7.7	37.0 ± 12.8		

Values are expressed in mean ± SD. UPDRS III scores are preoperative scores in OFF-state. DEX: dexmedetomidine; CLONI: clonidine; REMI: remifentanil; MUA: multi-unit activity; PSA: procedural sedation and analgesia; SU: single unit; UPDRS III: Unified Parkinson Disease Rating Scale part III; n: number; y: year.

2.3. Surgical Procedure

After placement of a Leksell stereotactic frame (Elekta, Stockholm, Sweden), a computed tomography (CT) scan of the head was performed. The CT-image was co-registered with a magnetic resonance imaging (MRI) that had been performed before surgery. Following target identification and trajectory planning, a burr hole was drilled, micro-electrodes (model 230766, Medizintechnik GmbH, Emmendingen, Germany) were implanted and recordings were performed. Visual and auditory confirmation of the target was performed by a neurophysiologist. Then, macrostimulation and neurological testing were carried out. The presence of good quality electrophysiological recordings and few or no side effects indicated the optimal contact point at which a quadripolar electrode (model 3387 or 3389; Medtronic, Minneapolis, USA) was placed. A postoperative CT scan was performed within 24 h in order to exclude intracerebral hemorrhages and to evaluate the final position of the electrodes.

2.4. MER Acquisition

Up to 5 microelectrodes were used to record neuronal activity along the planned trajectory in order to identify the target. Data were recorded from 10 mm above to 5 to 7 mm below the target in steps of 0.5–1 mm for approximately 30 s at each recording location (mean 35.94 s, SD 15.93). Data from a typical electrode track is shown in Figure 1A.

The target for all patients was the STN. The electrodes classically passed through the thalamus, zona incerta, STN and sometimes reached into the dorsal border of the substantia nigra reticulata. The electrode signal was sampled at 20 or 25 kHz, bandpass filtered online, (V3.15; Inomed Medizintechnik GmbH, Emmendingen, Germany) and saved for offline analysis. The first 41 patients were recorded with a high-pass filter 160 Hz, thereafter the high-pass filter was at 0 Hz, low-pass filter was at 5000 Hz.

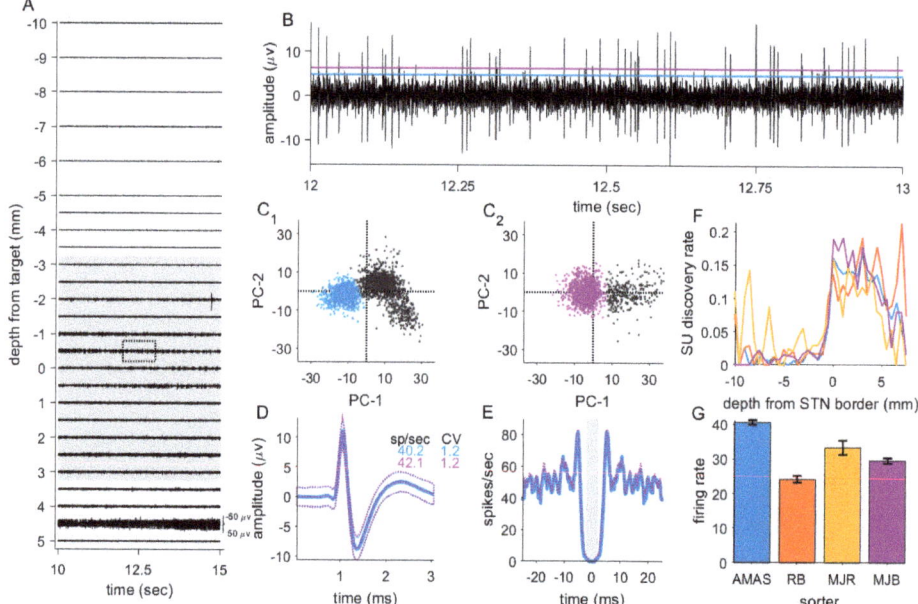

Figure 1. Overview of the sorting process. (**A**) Example recording trajectory of one electrode with 5 s of data shown at each site. Grey shading indicates sites identified as within the subthalamic nucleus (STN). (**B**) Expanded view of data from one recording site (region highlighted by a dashed box in A) with the spike detection threshold set by A.M.A.S. (blue) and M.J.B. (purple); (**C**) clusters of the spike waveforms identified from the example recording by A.M.A.S. and M.J.B.; (**D**) spike waveform (mean: thick lines, thin lines: standard deviation) of the spike sorted from the example recording by A.M.A.S. and M.J.B.; (**E**) Autocorrelation of the spike times from the example recording by A.M.A.S. and M.J.B.; (**F**) The proportion of sites with identified single units (SU)s (discovery rate) was quite similar, indicating that all sorters applied comparable criteria. (**G**) Nevertheless, the mean firing rate of STN neurons differed somewhat between sorters.

2.5. Data Processing and Analysis

Custom-written MATLAB scripts (V2017B; MathWorks) were used to conduct the data-analysis. For each recording, the raw data were high-pass filtered at 300 Hz prior to visual and auditory inspection. To identify single unit (SU) activity, periods of interest were manually selected to exclude periods of high noise or unstable SU activity. Spike times were identified by signal crossings of a manually set threshold (Figure 1B). Spikes representing SUs were selected using principal component analysis and K means clustering (Figure 1C). Manual selection was used for sorting SU clusters. SU clusters were confirmed as SUs by inspecting their autocorrelation, with a minimum gap of 2 ms between spikes representing the refractory period. For added robustness, this analysis was independently performed by 4 authors (A.M.A.S., M.J.B., R.B. and M.J.R.) (Figure 1C–G). For the main analysis data sorted by A.M.A.S. was used, who inspected all recording sites in our sample. Firing rate (spikes per second) of the SUs were calculated by dividing the number of spikes by the recording time. The coefficient of variation (CV) was defined by dividing the standard deviation of the inter-spike interval by the mean.

To identify multi-unit activity (MUA) we calculated the power-spectral density of the signal within the bandwidth of 100 and 500 Hz. Periods of high noise were automatically identified and rejected by calculating the root-mean squared (RMS) of the high-pass filtered data in segments of 50 ms. Periods in which the RMS exceeded the median RMS + 3 standard deviations were excluded from further analysis [17]. Following this procedure, the surviving raw (unfiltered) data were cut into non-overlapping snips of 250 ms and the power-spectral density was calculated using a multitaper method with discrete prolate spheroidal sequences using the Fieldtrip MATLAB toolbox [18]. To account for non-biological differences between recording tracts (electrode and tissue impedance etc.) power at each frequency was expressed as a ratio with respect to power at the first 5 recording sites. Finally, MUA total power, hereafter referred to simply as MUA, was calculated as the sum of all baseline corrected power above 300 Hz.

2.6. Statistical Analysis

Statistical analyses was performed using custom-written MATLAB scripts (V2017B; MathWorks) to test the effect of PSA agents and other variables on electrophysiological measures. For all tests, the threshold for statistical significance was set to $\alpha = 0.05$. Patients were divided into 7 groups according to their sedative administration (no PSA (control group)), PSA discontinued (discontinued before MER), DEX, REMI, CLONI, DEX and REMI, CLONI and REMI (Table 1)).

As a first step of the statistical analysis, one-way ANOVAs were conducted for each electrophysiological measure to test for differences between groups. This was followed by multiple two-sample *t*-tests comparing data from each PSA group with data from the no PSA group. *P*-values were corrected for multiple comparison using the Benjamini & Hochberg method for control of the false discovery rate (FDR) [19].

For further insight, linear regression analysis was conducted using the applied PSA drugs, and clinical and demographic variables as predictors to test their effect on firing rate, CV and MUA. Additional linear regression analysis with a random effect grouped by patient ID were conducted, considering the clustered nature of the data.

Finally, we tested the effect of the PSA dose. We focused on DEX since the dose of CLONI was not consistent, which made impossible to run a dose-dependent analysis, while the effect of REMI was small. We conducted a correlation analysis including data from patients who received either DEX alone, or a combination of DEX and REMI. A standard linear model (no random effects) was constructed.

3. Results

3.1. Demographics

From January 2009 to December 2018 a total of 93 PD patients underwent STN-DBS insertion. Data from 13 patients were excluded from analysis because of incomplete data. Two patients underwent surgery under general anesthesia and were also excluded from further analysis. Anesthetic and electrophysiological data from the remaining 78 patients were analyzed, thus yielding electrophysiological date from 156 cerebral hemispheres (Table 1).

Data were first grouped into clusters depending on whether data were acquired when patients were awake or sedated. The awake cluster included data from two patient groups: the first group received no sedatives and the second group of patients received DEX or a combination of DEX and REMI which was discontinued approximately 20 min before MER. The data in the sedation cluster was sub-divided according to the PSA applied during surgery: DEX, CLONI, REMI, or a combination of DEX and REMI or REMI and CLONI (Table 1).

To control for systematic differences between groups, we tested whether demographic characteristics (age, disease duration, Unified Parkinson Disease Rating Scale (UPDRS), side of onset, sex and weight) were equivalent across groups. One-way ANOVA showed no difference for any of these variables (respectively $F(6,71) = 1.14$, $p = 0.35$; $F(6,71) = 0.59$, $p = 0.74$; $F(6,71) = 0.40$, $p = 0.88$; $F(6,71) = 0.39$, $p = 0.88$; $F(6,71) = 0.46$, $p = 0.83$, $F(6,71) = 0.39$, $p = 0.88$ no correction for multiple comparisons were applied since we were here more concerned with minimizing type 2 errors).

3.2. Discontinuation of Sedative Agents

In 7 patients, PSA agents (DEX $n = 4$, DEX and REMI $n = 3$) were given during the first part of the operation and were discontinued approximately 20 min before the start of MER. While these patients appeared clinically to be awake during surgery, it is possible that these compounds might still have affected the electrophysiological properties of the STN even after their discontinuation [14]. Therefore, we tested whether the group who received no PSA drugs and the group of patients in whom PSA was discontinued should be considered as distinct groups for further analysis. We conducted a t-test for comparison of the electrophysiological measures (firing rate (sp/sec), CV and MUA) between these groups. In SU activity there was a trend towards decreased firing rate ($t(214) = 1.63$, $p = 0.11$), but no difference in the CV ($t(214) = -0.18$, $p = 0.86$). MUA was significantly reduced in the discontinued drug group ($t(1571) = 5.67$, $p < 0.0001$). Given these findings (Figure 2) we considered the patients in whom PSA agents were discontinued as a separate group from patients who received no PSA for further analysis.

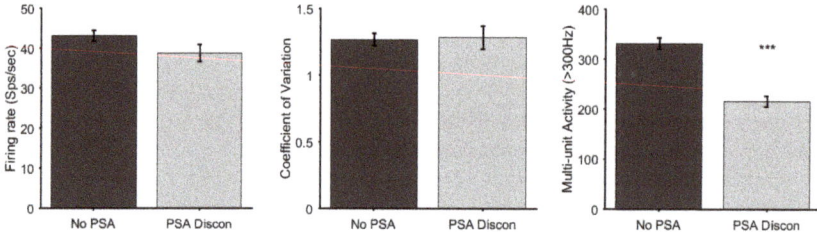

Figure 2. Bar plot and t-test for within awake group analysis for firing rate, defined in spikes per seconds, coefficient of variation and multi-unit activity, defined as activity above 300HZ. Mean and standard error are shown in each bar. *** $p < 0.001$. PSA: procedural sedation and analgesia.

3.3. Effect of PSA Agents on Firing Rate, Coefficient of Variation and Multi-Unit Activity

A one-way ANOVA was conducted between the seven groups for each electrophysiological measure. Significant, or trending differences between groups for all measures were observed (Firing rate, F(6,581) =2.08, $p < 0.054$; CV, F(6,581) = 3.69, $p < 0.001$; MUA, F(6,4088) = 15.93, $p < 0.0001$). To further test for differences between groups, a post-hoc two-sample t-tests was conducted to compare each PSA drug against the control group ($n = 165$) with respect to firing rate, CV and MUA.

No significant differences in the firing rate between groups after FDR correction for multiple comparisons were found, although DEX and REMI, and REMI in combination with CLONI showed a trend towards significance ($t(209) = 2.64$, $p = 0.0531$; $t(269) = 2.28$, $p = 0.0695$).

For CV, there were significant differences between the no drug group and the groups DEX ($t(249) = -3.84$, $p = 0.00092$), REMI ($t(256) = -2.65$, $p = 0.013$), DEX and REMI group ($t(209) = -3.05$, $p = 0.0078$), and REMI and CLONI ($t(269) = -2.62$, $p = 0.013$).

All PSA drug groups except REMI showed a significant decrease in MUA ($n = 1255$, PSA discontinued, $t(1594) = 4.95$, $p < 0.0001$; DEX, $t(1820) = 6.73$, $p < 0.0001$; CLONI, $t(1594) = 4.45$, $p < 0.0001$; DEX and REMI, $t(1522) = 3.94$, $p < 0.0001$; and REMI and CLONI, $t(1934) = 3.69$, $p < 0.0001$), REMI ($t(1891) = 1.31$, $p = 0.19$). All p values were corrected for multiple comparison using FDR (Figure 3).

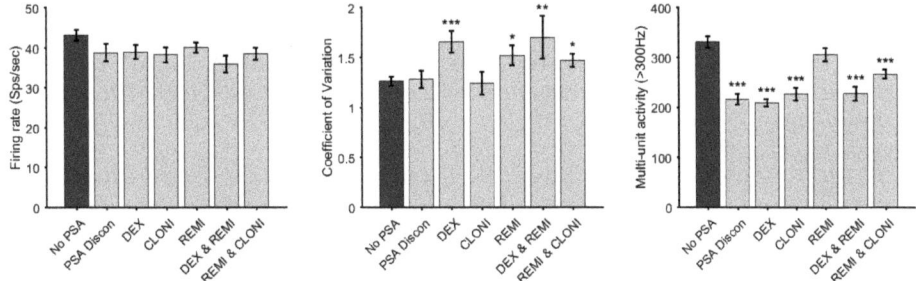

Figure 3. Bar plot (error bars show standard error) and t-test for the No PSA group against each PSA group for firing rate, coefficient of variation and multi-unit activity. * $p < 0.05$, ** $p < 0.01$, *** $p < 0.001$. CLONI: clonidine; DEX: dexmedetomidine; REMI: remifentanil; PSA: procedural sedation and analgesia.

To account for variance in the patient groups, we conducted a linear regression analysis to test the effect of the PSA agents with clinical and demographic variables included as factors. For DEX, CLONI, REMI, sex, recording location with respect to onset side of the disease, and left or right hemisphere were defined as categorical variables. We further included age at surgery (years), weight (Kg), UPDRS III pre-operative off medication, disease duration at surgery (months) and depth of the recording site within the STN (mm from the dorsal border) as continuous variables in the model (Table 2).

Table 2. Standard linear regression model for firing rate, CV and MUA.

Variable		Firing Rate		Coefficient of Variation		Multi-Unit Activity	
		Estimate	p-Value	Estimate	p-Value	Estimate	p-Value
DEX	Yes	−3.121	0.068	0.313	0.001	−88.814	<0.001
REMI	Yes	−2.105	0.141	0.163	0.040	2.607	0.806
CLONI	Yes	−2.156	0.203	−0.004	0.963	−50.923	0.675
PSA (DISCONTINUED)	Yes	−3.836	0.120	−0.011	0.933	−115.240	<0.001
SEX	Male	0.379	0.808	−0.031	0.720	−2.112	0.855
ONSET SIDE	Ipsilateral (*)	−1.840	0.152	0.100	0.161	−16.353	0.090
HEMISPHERE	Right	1.854	0.150	−0.087	0.222	24.785	0.010
AGE	Years	−0.091	0.314	0.001	0.788	−43.996	<0.001
WEIGHT	Kg	−0.004	0.931	−0.003	0.337	0.452	0.181
UPDRS III		0.068	0.196	0.002	0.428	−0.026	0.946
DISEASE DURATION	Months	−0.002	0.914	−0.002	0.020	−0.018	0.882
STN DEPTH	mm	0.560	0.130	−0.008	0.681	25.024	<0.001
Model data		R-squared: 0.035 Adjusted R-Squared 0.0149 p-value = 0.0553		R-squared: 0.0511 Adjusted R-Squared 0.0313 p-value = 0.00241		R-squared: 0.0586 Adjusted R-Squared 0.0558 p-value = 9.1e^{-46}	

In the analysis, we included demographic and clinical variables as sex, onset side (recording site ipsi- or contralateral to the onset side of the disease), hemisphere (right or left), age, weight, UPDRS III pre-operative off medication and disease duration. Estimate indicate the slope of the line, when negative indicates decrease and positive indicates increase. * ipsilateral to body side with onset of disease. CLONI: clonidine; DEX: dexmedetomidine; REMI: remifentanil; PSA: procedural sedation and analgesia; UPDRS III: Unified Parkinson's Disease Rating Scale part III.

There were no significant effects of the PSA agents in the firing rate, but we could observe some trends. Notably, DEX was weakly associated with a reduced firing rate. For CV, DEX showed a significant effect and REMI showed a small effect. DEX and PSA discontinued showed significant effects in the MUA, while CLONI and REMI did not. The slope (estimates) indicated the direction of the effect. In this sense, the effect of the PSA agents in CV indicates an increase, while the slope for MUA indicates a decrease. These findings supported our previous analysis, except CLONI, where effects identified in the t-test were not significant in this analysis.

In addition to effects of PSA agents, we found that electrophysiological measures were affected by several clinical and demographic variables. Disease duration showed a negative effect on CV, thus CV decreased as disease advanced. Age showed a significant impact on MUA, thus MUA decreased with increased age. Hemisphere (left or right) was also significantly associated with MUA, thus right hemisphere showed higher power than the left hemisphere. Finally, STN depth had a significant impact on MUA (Table 2).

Taking into consideration that we were working with multiple observations within each patient, we also conducted a linear regression model with a random effect grouped by patient for all three electrophysiological measures. This more conservative analysis brings a reduction in the statistical power, nevertheless for CV, the effect of DEX, REMI and disease duration remained significant. For MUA, the effect of DEX, PSA discontinued, hemisphere and age also remained significant. The non-significant effect on firing rate also remained (supplementary material Table S1).

3.4. Interrater Reliability

SUs were identified and sorted by hand which is an inevitably subjective process (Figure 1). To test whether the effects we report were robust, every recording was inspected by at least two individuals (every site was inspected A.M.A.S. and one of M.J.B., M.J.R. or R.B.). We repeated the linear regression analysis for SU data (spikes/seconds and CV) using data for units identified by M.J.B., M.J.R. or R.B., including the sorter ID as an additional categorical variable. All main effects we report on were replicated in this analysis (supplementary material Table S2).

3.5. Dose-Dependent Effect of DEX

Our analysis showed that DEX had a significant impact on electrophysiological measures. To test whether these effects were dose-dependent, we conducted further analysis focused only on patients who received DEX during surgery. We first performed a simple correlation analysis between each measure and DEX dose (Figure 4). The correlations were significant, but the correlation coefficient was low for all measures. For illustration, we extrapolated the regression line to include 0 dose and plotted the data for the 0 dose patients (not included PSA discontinued group). For both firing rate and CV the regression line passed close to the mean of the 0 dose data, while this was not the case for MUA. This may indicate a non-linear effect of DEX on MUA whereby even a small dose leads to strong suppression. This interpretation would be in line with our finding that discontinuation of DEX, 20 min before recordings MUA also had a large impact. One interesting point is that the analysis of firing rate was significant, showing a decrease in firing rate with increased dose. This might mean that the trend observed in the *t*-test and linear regression analysis is a true effect.

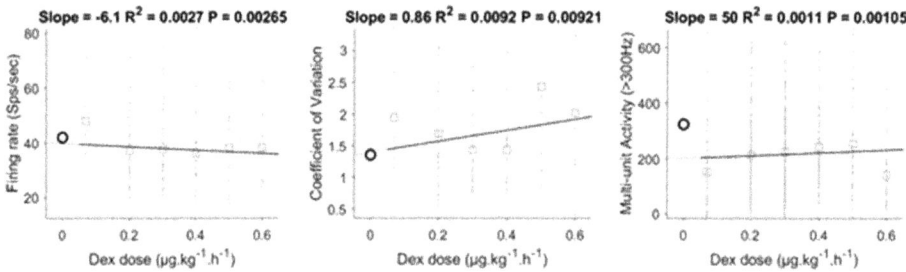

Figure 4. Correlation analysis on the dose of DEX for the electrophysiological measures. Correlations were significant. Data of the no PSA drug group is shown in black for comparison but was excluded from the regression analysis. DEX: dexmedetomidine.

4. Discussion

In this retrospective analysis, we studied the influence of the non-GABAergic drugs DEX, CLONI and REMI on the firing rate and CV of single neuron activity, as well as the power of MUA in the STN of PD patients undergoing DBS surgery. The results of the present study demonstrated that, even when PSA was discontinued around 20 min prior to MER, this still had significant effect on MUA. A trend was observed for a reduced firing rate by DEX, which was significant on the correlation analysis. Both DEX and REMI showed an increase in CV, but only DEX showed a decrease in MUA. The effect of DEX was dose-dependent. CLONI showed no effect on all measures. Lastly, several patient-dependent variables, such as age, disease duration and left or right hemisphere influenced MUA and CV.

4.1. Effect of Procedural Sedation and Analgesia on Micro-Electrode Recordings

The use of PSA agents and their effects on neuronal activity has been debated since the initiation of DBS surgery. Traditionally, the anesthetic management approach comprised local anesthesia with monitored care to facilitate MER. However, recent work has shown that 40% of patients suffer from pain, severe OFF-symptoms and intolerable exhaustion during the hours of awake surgery [5]. To improve patient acceptance, sedation is thus commonly administered. Propofol, a GABAergic agent, has been most frequently used when sedation is required. As stated before, several clinical reports showed a dose-dependent effect of propofol on STN neuronal activity in patients with PD [7–9,20]. Propofol reduces neuronal activity by enhancing inhibitory neurotransmission and reducing excitatory neurotransmission [21]. Although some studies showed good quality MER with low-dose propofol, potent GABAergic agents such as propofol should not be the first choice for PSA during DBS surgery [22–24].

Alternatively, α_2-agonists (non-GABAergic) are useful in this regard. Currently, two different α_2-agonists are commonly used in clinical practice: CLONI and DEX. While both drugs have anxiolytic, sedative and analgesic properties, DEX is a more selective α_2-receptor agonist than CLONI. Since central α_1-receptor activation counteracts sedative α_2 effects, DEX has a more profound sedative effect [25]. The sedative effects of α_2-agonists are mediated through activation of pre- and postsynaptic α_2-receptors in the locus coeruleus which has noradrenergic afferent connections with the STN [26,27]. This route provides a plausible mechanism for the effects observed in the current study, since it has been shown that noradrenergic modulation with α_1 and α_2-agonists change firing rate and firing patterns of STN neurons, in line with our findings [28,29].

4.1.1. Dexmedetomidine

In this study we analyzed quantitative effects of DEX on MER following two different PSA protocols. In the first protocol PSA agents (DEX alone or DEX and REMI) were discontinued approximately 20 min before the start of MER. It can be speculated that the effects on MER in the discontinued group are solely DEX effects, since REMI has a very short context-sensitive half-time of 3–4 min. In these patients, MUA was significantly suppressed while, SU activity showed a trend towards a lower firing rate but no change in CV. Interestingly, an earlier study by Mathews et al., in which a similar PSA protocol was used (discontinuation of PSA agents before the MER), reported no difference in firing rate, but showed a significant decrease in CV [14]. Their protocol was not identical to ours. Patients received either REMI in bolus (the control group in that study), or DEX and REMI in bolus prior to MER. Moreover, the dose of DEX was higher in their study (0.1–1.0 µg kg^{-1} h^{-1} versus 0.2–0.5 µg kg^{-1} h^{-1}). In another case series by Kwon et al., patients received a loading dose of DEX 0.9 µg kg^{-1} followed by a maintenance dose of 0.5 µg kg^{-1} h^{-1} combined with REMI at 0.05 µg kg^{-1} min^{-1} and propofol was administered in small boluses. Using this protocol, the depth of sedation was maintained at a level of slight sedation (Bispectral index (BIS) of 80). All PSA agents were discontinued 20 min before MER. In that study, firing rates of STN neurons were significantly reduced compared to the control group who received no sedatives [15]. The suppression of firing rates in this protocol (that included higher DEX dose in addition to the high loading does) is in line with our finding of a dose-dependent suppression, although it is challenging to compare previous studies in which DEX was discontinued before MER with our findings, due to different dose regimens. Taken together, the previous literature and our data suggest that DEX still has an effect on MER after 20 min of discontinuation.

In our study, a second group of patients received continuous DEX infusions, alone or in combination with REMI during MER. Firing rates were not significantly altered, but there was a trend to lowering. Both CV and MUA were significantly affected whereby CV was increased and MUA decreased. Correlation analysis showed that these effects were dose-dependent, including lowering of the firing rate. A small case series reported a suppression of neuronal activity in patients who received DEX sedation throughout the full procedure (range 0.1–0.4 $\mu g\ kg^{-1}\ h^{-1}$) in comparison to patients in which DEX was discontinued before recordings [12]. In another study, patients received a bolus DEX of 0.5–1.0 $\mu g\ kg^{-1}$ followed by a maintenance infusion of 0.1–1.0 $\mu g\ kg^{-1}\ h^{-1}$. They reported a slight increase in firing rate and a significant decrease in burst index (decreased number of spikes within a burst) compared to patients who received no sedation [13]. Thus, these findings appear contradictory to our findings as well as with previous literature. A possible explanation for the differences with our findings is the dose they used, which included a bolus followed by a relatively high maintenance dose.

To summarize our results, dexmedetomidine caused a trend toward decreased firing rates, significantly suppressed MUA and increased CV. These effects were present even at low dose and even after discontinuation of DEX. However, direct comparison of our findings with previous studies is challenging, because of the variability of the sedation protocols, patients groups and methodology.

4.1.2. Clonidine

CLONI is a α_2-receptor agonist with a pharmacodynamic profile almost identical to DEX but is less selective for the α_2-receptor than DEX. As a consequence, effects on the locus coeruleus are less profound and therefore CLONI would be expected to have less impact on STN neural firing compared to DEX. To our knowledge, no studies have yet reported effects of CLONI on MER during DBS surgery.

In our study, patients received CLONI alone or in combination with REMI. Compared to the no PSA group, these patients showed no significant differences in neuronal firing rates, CV or MUA, although firing rates and MUA showed a trend towards a decrease. Moreover, in our linear regression analysis the effect estimate associated with CLONI was consistently lower than the estimate associated with DEX. Thus, in line with our expectation, CLONI appeared to show a similar but less profound effect on STN neurons compared to DEX. It should be noted however, that direct comparison between the two agents is complex because of the difference in pharmacokinetic profiles. In our study the comparison was further limited due to the heterogeneity in CLONI doses and the lower number of patients in the CLONI group.

4.1.3. Remifentanil

The last PSA agent we investigated was remifentanil. Remifentanil is an ultrashort-acting μ-receptor opioid agonist with a rapid time to peak activity after a bolus dose and a short context-sensitive half-time of less than 4 min without regard to infusion duration [30]. In rats, opioids have been reported to exert an inhibitory modulation of GABAergic and glutamatergic synaptic transmission in the STN via presynaptic μ- and δ-receptors [31,32]. Only a limited number of studies have addressed effects of opioids during STN-DBS surgery [9,22,23,33]. In these studies, neurophysiological data were obtained while patients received propofol in combination with opioids. Therefore, the opioid effects on neuronal activity could not be well characterized. To our knowledge only one other study has assessed the effect of REMI on STN neurons in PD patients [24]. In that study, single cell activity of 4 neurons were analyzed before and after a bolus of 0.5 $\mu g\ kg^{-1}$. REMI did not significantly alter short interval discharge activity, a measure related to firing rate. Our results also showed no significant effect of REMI on firing rates or MUA. The use of REMI was only associated with a significant increase in CV compared to the control group.

4.2. Effect of Clinical and Demographic Variables on Microelectrode Recordings

In addition to the effects of the PSA agents, clinical and demographic variables might affect neuronal firing properties of the STN. Therefore, we tested the effect of these variables on electrophysiological recordings.

One interesting finding was that the CV increased in patients with a longer disease duration. An increase in burst activity is generally observed in animal models of PD [34,35]. One potential explanation of this phenomenon is that neuronal firing becomes more strongly locked to a more powerful beta rhythm, seen with advanced disease, thereby reducing variability in the interspike-interval. The underlying mechanism of our finding therefore remains elusive. Finally, while CV was related to disease duration, no relation with the UPDRS III score, side of onset or age of the patients was observed.

The hemisphere of the recordings significantly influenced MUA with the right STN having higher power than the left. Currently no study to our knowledge has reported lateralization of MUA in the STN during rest. Interestingly, several studies in humans and animals have shown that the left and right cortex are related to different functions. In line with functional lateralization in the cortex, emotions seems to be processed in the right STN [36–39]. We therefore speculate that the difference we observed may be related to functional lateralization of the STN; a hypothesis that needs further validation.

Finally, the age of the patient significantly influenced MUA. Within the STN, older patients showed lower power compared to younger patients. An effect of aging on neuronal power spectrum in the cortex has been reported previously [40–42]. In contrast to our findings, these studies all reported an increase in high frequency power with age, which they discuss in terms of the neuronal noise hypothesis of aging [43]. A number of interesting hypothesis may account for the reversal of this pattern that we observed in STN. First, our population was generally older than the older adults in these papers, to the extent that our younger patients would be considered to belong to their 'older' groups. One interpretation of these data could be that the relationship between age and neural population power is non-linear such that adults in late middle age show the highest power. Second, there may be task effects, since our data were recorded with the patient not performing a cognitive task, while previous reports have all been in the context of active cognitive tasks. Third, our data may show a genuine difference in the effect of aging in the STN compared to the cortex. Finally, the possibility exists that the change in power we observed reflects age-related changes in shape and location of the STN [44]. According to this hypothesis, recording sites at the same stereotaxic coordinates may represent different functional domains, with different neuronal properties, within the STN in different age groups. Future work may elucidate these possibilities.

Multi-Unit Activity

MUA is an important measure to identify the entrance of the STN. Both through visual and auditory inspection and by automatic identification algorithms, an increase in neuronal activity, compared to the overlying white matter zone, is one of the most widely used signs of the dorsal border of the STN [45]. Our results show that sedatives, either continuous or discontinued, as well as a number of patient specific characteristics, influence MUA. To our knowledge, no previous studies have investigated the effect of PSA agents on MUA, despite its usefulness as a clinical marker. More research is necessary to define whether these effects are large enough to be clinically relevant.

4.3. Limitations

Our study had some limitations. First, it was a retrospective study, involving patients for whom there was no standardized PSA protocol and uncontrolled variability in PSA drug choices and doses. We found that demographic and clinical characteristics did not differ systematically between the groups, therefore these factors could be accounted for with a regression analysis thanks to our large overall sample size. Since no standardized PSA protocol was used we were limited when testing for dose-dependent effects. Second, while we compared our findings to previous reports, the available literature is sparse and characterized by heterogeneity in PSA protocols, patient characteristics and MER data analysis. Our findings suggest that some differences among previous reports may be accounted for by dose-dependent effects (e.g. on firing rates). Prospective studies with standardized PSA protocols are required to confirm these findings. Also, we did not assess spectral changes in the local field potential. Investigating the effect of PSA on the presence of pathologic oscillations remains unanswered. Another limitation is that this study did not assess the effects of the various agents on intraoperative clinical measures such as tremor. A follow-up study is needed to assess the effects of the various PSA protocols on STN depth and size. Moreover, it is important for clinical practice to address in future studies whether the use of PSA influences clinical outcome of STN DBS.

5. Conclusions

When administering sedation during DBS electrode implantation, the aim is always to achieve an optimal balance between patient comfort and good quality MER, to allow optimal placement of the probe. Our results showed that PSA influenced neuronal properties in the STN and that the DEX effect was dose-dependent. Moreover, patient dependent characteristics influenced MER. Whether these effects are large enough to be clinically relevant was not addressed in this study.

Supplementary Materials: The following are available online at http://www.mdpi.com/2077-0383/9/4/1229/s1, Table S1: random effects modeling with patient as a random variable, Table S2: random effects modeling with sorter as a random variable.

Author Contributions: Conceptualization, M.J.R. and M.L.F.J.; Formal analysis, M.J.R., A.M.A.S., R.B., M.J.R. and M.L.F.J.; Investigation, M.J.B., A.M.A.S., M.J.R. and M.L.F.J; Methodology, A.M.A.S., B.T.A.d.G., M.J.R. and M.L.F.J.; Software, M.J.R.; Supervision, Y.T. and M.L.F.J.; Writing – original draft, M.J.B., A.M.A.S. and M.J.R.; Writing – review & editing, M.J.B., R.B., Y.T., B.T.A.d.G., A.R.A., E.D.G., V.H.J.M.v.K.-M., W.F.B., M.J.R. and M.L.F.J. All authors have read and agreed to the published version of the manuscript.

Funding: This study was supported by a grant from de Stichting Weijerhorst.

Conflicts of Interest: The authors declare no conflict of interest.

References

1. Fasano, A.; Daniele, A.; Albanese, A. Treatment of motor and non-motor features of Parkinson's disease with deep brain stimulation. *Lancet Neurol.* **2012**, *11*, 429–442. [CrossRef]
2. Welter, M.-L.; Schüpbach, M.; Czernecki, V.; Karachi, C.; Fernandez-Vidal, S.; Golmard, J.-L.; Serra, G.; Navarro, S.; Welaratne, A.; Hartmann, A.; et al. Optimal target localization for subthalamic stimulation in patients with Parkinson disease. *Neurology* **2014**, *82*, 1352–1361. [CrossRef] [PubMed]
3. McNeely, M.E.; Hershey, T.; Campbell, M.C.; Tabbal, S.D.; Karimi, M.; Hartlein, J.M.; Lugar, H.M.; Revilla, F.J.; Perlmutter, J.S.; Earhart, G.M. Effects of deep brain stimulation of dorsal versus ventral subthalamic nucleus regions on gait and balance in Parkinson's disease. *J. Neurol. Neurosurg. Psychiatry* **2011**, *82*, 1250–1255. [CrossRef] [PubMed]
4. Campbell, B.; Machado, A.G.; Baker, K.B. Electrophysiologic mapping for deep brain stimulation for movement disorders. *Handb. Clin. Neurol.* **2019**, *160*, 345–355. [CrossRef] [PubMed]
5. Mulroy, E.; Robertson, N.; Macdonald, L.; Bok, A.; Simpson, M. Patients' Perioperative Experience of Awake Deep-Brain Stimulation for Parkinson Disease. *World Neurosurg.* **2017**, *105*, 526–528. [CrossRef] [PubMed]
6. Sahinovic, M.M.; Struys, M.; Absalom, A. Clinical Pharmacokinetics and Pharmacodynamics of Propofol. *Clin. Pharmacokinet.* **2018**, *57*, 1539–1558. [CrossRef]
7. Raz, A.; Eimerl, D.; Zaidel, A.; Bergman, H.; Israel, Z. Propofol Decreases Neuronal Population Spiking Activity in the Subthalamic Nucleus of Parkinsonian Patients. *Anesthesia Analg.* **2010**, *111*, 1285–1289. [CrossRef]
8. Martinez-Simon, A.; Alegre, M.; Honorato-Cia, C.; Nuñez-Cordoba, J.M.; Cacho-Asenjo, E.; Trocóniz, I.F.; Carmona-Abellan, M.; Valencia, M.; Guridi, J. Effect of Dexmedetomidine and Propofol on Basal Ganglia Activity in Parkinson Disease. *Anesthesiology* **2017**, *126*, 1033–1042. [CrossRef]

9. Moll, C.K.E.; Payer, S.; Gulberti, A.; Sharrott, A.; Zittel, S.; Boelmans, K.; Köppen, J.; Gerloff, C.; Westphal, M.; Engel, A.K.; et al. STN Stimulation in General Anaesthesia: Evidence Beyond 'Evidence-Based Medicine'. *Stereotact. Funct. Neurosurg.* **2013**, *117*, 19–25. [CrossRef]
10. Rozet, I.; Muangman, S.; Vavilala, M.S.; Lee, L.A.; Souter, M.J.; Domino, K.J.; Slimp, J.C.; Goodkin, R.; Lam, A.M. Clinical Experience with Dexmedetomidine for Implantation of Deep Brain Stimulators in Parkinson's Disease. *Anesthesia Analg.* **2006**, *103*, 1224–1228. [CrossRef]
11. Morace, R.; De Angelis, M.; Aglialoro, E.; Maucione, G.; Cavallo, L.; Solari, D.; Modugno, N.; Santilli, M.; Esposito, V.; Aloj, F. Sedation with α2 Agonist Dexmedetomidine During Unilateral Subthalamic Nucleus Deep Brain Stimulation: A Preliminary Report. *World Neurosurg.* **2016**, *89*, 320–328. [CrossRef] [PubMed]
12. Elias, W.J.; Durieux, M.; Huss, D.; Frysinger, R.C. Dexmedetomidine and arousal affect subthalamic neurons. *Mov. Disord.* **2008**, *23*, 1317–1320. [CrossRef] [PubMed]
13. Krishna, V.; Elias, G.J.; Sammartino, F.; Basha, D.; King, N.K.K.; Fasano, A.; Munhoz, R.; Kalia, S.K.; Hodaie, M.; Venkatraghavan, L.; et al. The effect of dexmedetomidine on the firing properties of STN neurons in Parkinson's disease. *Eur. J. Neurosci.* **2015**, *42*, 2070–2077. [CrossRef] [PubMed]
14. Mathews, L.; Camalier, C.R.; Kla, K.M.; Mitchell, M.D.; Konrad, P.E.; Neimat, J.S.; Smithson, K.G. The Effects of Dexmedetomidine on Microelectrode Recordings of the Subthalamic Nucleus during Deep Brain Stimulation Surgery: A Retrospective Analysis. *Ster. Funct. Neurosurg.* **2017**, *95*, 40–48. [CrossRef]
15. Kwon, W.-K.; Kim, J.H.; Lee, J.-H.; Lim, B.-G.; Lee, I.-O.; Koh, S.B.; Kwon, T.H. Microelectrode recording (MER) findings during sleep–awake anesthesia using dexmedetomidine in deep brain stimulation surgery for Parkinson's disease. *Clin. Neurol. Neurosurg.* **2016**, *143*, 27–33. [CrossRef]
16. Bos, M.J.; Buhre, W.; Temel, Y.; Joosten, E.A.; Absalom, A.R.; Janssen, M.L. Effect of Anesthesia on Microelectrode Recordings during Deep Brain Stimulation Surgery. *J. Neurosurg. Anesthesiol.* **2020**. [CrossRef]
17. Tepper, Á.; Henrich, M.C.; Schiaffino, L.; Rosado-Muñoz, A.; Gutiérrez, A.; Martínez, J.G. Selection of the Optimal Algorithm for Real-Time Estimation of Beta Band Power during DBS Surgeries in Patients with Parkinson's Disease. *Comput. Intell. Neurosci.* **2017**, *2017*, 1–9. [CrossRef]
18. Oostenveld, R.; Fries, P.; Maris, E.; Schoffelen, J.-M. FieldTrip: Open Source Software for Advanced Analysis of MEG, EEG, and Invasive Electrophysiological Data. *Comput. Intell. Neurosci.* **2010**, *2011*, 1–9. [CrossRef]
19. Benjamini, Y.; Hochberg, Y. Controlling the False Discovery Rate: A Practical and Powerful Approach to Multiple Testing. *J. R. Stat. Soc. Ser. B (Stat. Methodol.)* **1995**, *57*, 289–300. [CrossRef]
20. Hertel, F.; Züchner, M.; Weimar, I.; Gemmar, P.; Noll, B.; Bettag, M.; Decker, C. Implantation of electrodes for deep brain stimulation of the subthalamic nucleus in advanced Parkinson's disease with the aid of intraoperative microrecording under general anesthesia. *Neurosurgery* **2006**, *59*, 1138. [CrossRef]
21. Brohan, J.; Goudra, B.G. The Role of GABA Receptor Agonists in Anesthesia and Sedation. *CNS Drugs* **2017**, *31*, 845–856. [CrossRef] [PubMed]
22. Lee, W.W.; Ehm, G.; Yang, H.J.; Song, I.H.; Lim, Y.H.; Kim, M.R.; Kim, Y.E.; Hwang, J.H.; Park, H.R.; Lee, J.M.; et al. Bilateral Deep Brain Stimulation of the Subthalamic Nucleus under Sedation with Propofol and Fentanyl. *PLoS ONE* **2016**, *11*, e0152619. [CrossRef] [PubMed]
23. Duque, P.; Mateo, O.; Ruiz, F.; De Viloria, J.G.; Contreras, A.; Grandas, F. Intraoperative microrecording under general anaesthesia with bispectral analysis monitoring in a case of deep brain stimulation surgery for Parkinsons disease. *Eur. J. Neurol.* **2008**, *15*, 76–77. [CrossRef] [PubMed]
24. Maciver, M.B.; Bronte-Stewart, H.M.; Henderson, J.M.; Jaffe, R.A.; Brock-Utne, J.G.; Henderson, J.M. Human Subthalamic Neuron Spiking Exhibits Subtle Responses to Sedatives. *Anesthesiology* **2011**, *115*, 254–264. [CrossRef]
25. Bhana, N.; Goa, K.L.; McClellan, K.J. Dexmedetomidine. *Drugs* **2000**, *59*, 263–268. [CrossRef]
26. Weerink, M.; Struys, M.; Hannivoort, L.N.; Barends, C.R.M.; Absalom, A.R.; Colin, P. Clinical Pharmacokinetics and Pharmacodynamics of Dexmedetomidine. *Clin. Pharmacokinet.* **2017**, *56*, 893–913. [CrossRef]
27. Jamadarkhana, S.; Gopal, S. Clonidine in Adults as a Sedative Agent in the Intensive Care Unit. *J. Anaesthesiol. Clin. Pharmacol.* **2010**, *26*, 439–445.
28. Delaville, C.; Zapata, J.; Cardoit, L.; Benazzouz, A. Activation of subthalamic alpha 2 noradrenergic receptors induces motor deficits as a consequence of neuronal burst firing. *Neurobiol. Dis.* **2012**, *47*, 322–330. [CrossRef]

29. Belujon, P.; Bezard, E.; Taupignon, A.; Bioulac, B.; Benazzouz, A. Noradrenergic Modulation of Subthalamic Nucleus Activity: Behavioral and Electrophysiological Evidence in Intact and 6-Hydroxydopamine-Lesioned Rats. *J. Neurosci.* **2007**, *27*, 9595–9606. [CrossRef]
30. Michelsen, L.G.; Hug, C.C., Jr. The pharmacokinetics of remifentanil. *J. Clin. Anesthesia* **1996**, *8*, 679–682. [CrossRef]
31. Stanford, I.M.; Cooper, A.J. Presynaptic mu and delta opioid receptor modulation of GABAA IPSCs in the rat globus pallidus in vitro. *J. Neurosci.* **1999**, *19*, 4796–4803. [CrossRef] [PubMed]
32. Shen, K.Z.; Johnson, S.W. Presynaptic modulation of synaptic transmission by opioid receptor in rat subthalamic nucleusin vitro. *J. Physiol.* **2002**, *541*, 219–230. [CrossRef] [PubMed]
33. Kim, W.; Song, I.H.; Lim, Y.H.; Kim, M.R.; Kim, Y.E.; Hwang, J.H.; Kim, I.K.; Song, S.W.; Kim, J.W.; Lee, W.W.; et al. Influence of Propofol and Fentanyl on Deep Brain Stimulation of the Subthalamic Nucleus. *J. Korean Med. Sci.* **2014**, *29*, 1278–1286. [CrossRef] [PubMed]
34. Janssen, M.L.; Zwartjes, D.G.; Tan, S.K.; Vlamings, R.; Jahanshahi, A.; Heida, T.; Hoogland, G.; Steinbusch, H.W.; Visser-Vandewalle, V.; Temel, Y. Mild dopaminergic lesions are accompanied by robust changes in subthalamic nucleus activity. *Neurosci. Lett.* **2012**, *508*, 101–105. [CrossRef]
35. Bergman, H.; Wichmann, T.; Karmon, B.; DeLong, M.R. The primate subthalamic nucleus. II. Neuronal activity in the MPTP model of parkinsonism. *J. Neurophysiol.* **1994**, *72*, 507–520. [CrossRef]
36. Bočková, M.; Chladek, J.; Jurak, P.; Halamek, J.; Balaz, M.; Rektor, I. Involvement of the subthalamic nucleus and globus pallidus internus in attention. *J. Neural Transm.* **2010**, *118*, 1235–1245. [CrossRef]
37. Baunez, C.; Robbins, T.W. Bilateral lesions of the subthalamic nucleus induce multiple deficits in an attentional task in rats. *Eur. J. Neurosci.* **1997**, *9*, 2086–2099. [CrossRef]
38. Asanowicz, D.; Marzecová, A.; Jaśkowski, P.; Wolski, P. Hemispheric asymmetry in the efficiency of attentional networks. *Brain Cogn.* **2012**, *79*, 117–128. [CrossRef]
39. Eitan, R.; Shamir, R.R.; Linetsky, E.; Rosenbluh, O.; Moshel, S.; Ben-Hur, T.; Bergman, H.; Israel, Z. Asymmetric right/left encoding of emotions in the human subthalamic nucleus. *Front. Syst. Neurosci.* **2013**, *7*, 69. [CrossRef]
40. Voytek, B.; Kramer, M.A.; Case, J.; Lepage, K.Q.; Tempesta, Z.R.; Knight, R.T.; Gazzaley, A. Age-related changes in 1/f neural electrophysiological noise. *J. Neurosci.* **2015**, *35*, 13257–13265. [CrossRef]
41. Dave, S.; Brothers, T.A.; Swaab, T.Y. 1/f neural noise and electrophysiological indices of contextual prediction in aging. *Brain Res.* **2018**, *1691*, 34–43. [CrossRef]
42. Leenders, M.P.; Lozano-Soldevilla, D.; Roberts, M.; Jensen, O.; De Weerd, P. Diminished Alpha Lateralization During Working Memory but Not During Attentional Cueing in Older Adults. *Cereb. Cortex* **2016**, *28*, 21–32. [CrossRef] [PubMed]
43. Hong, S.L.; Rebec, G.V. A new perspective on behavioral inconsistency and neural noise in aging: Compensatory speeding of neural communication. *Front. Aging Neurosci.* **2012**, *4*, 27. [CrossRef]
44. Dunnen, W.F.D.; Staal, M.J. Anatomical alterations of the subthalamic nucleus in relation to age: A postmortem study. *Mov. Disord.* **2005**, *20*, 893–898. [CrossRef] [PubMed]
45. Valsky, D.; Marmor-Levin, O.; Deffains, M.; Eitan, R.; Blackwell, K.T.; Bergman, H.; Israel, Z. Stop! border ahead: Automatic detection of subthalamic exit during deep brain stimulation surgery. *Mov. Disord.* **2017**, *32*, 70–79. [CrossRef] [PubMed]

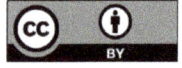

© 2020 by the authors. Licensee MDPI, Basel, Switzerland. This article is an open access article distributed under the terms and conditions of the Creative Commons Attribution (CC BY) license (http://creativecommons.org/licenses/by/4.0/).

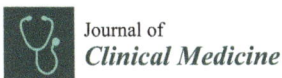

Perspective

Methodological Considerations for Neuroimaging in Deep Brain Stimulation of the Subthalamic Nucleus in Parkinson's Disease Patients

Bethany R. Isaacs [1,2,*], Max C. Keuken [3], Anneke Alkemade [1], Yasin Temel [2], Pierre-Louis Bazin [1,4] and Birte U. Forstmann [1]

1. Integrative Model-based Cognitive Neuroscience Research Unit, University of Amsterdam, 1018 WS Amsterdam, The Netherlands; jmalkemade@gmail.com (A.A.); pilou.bazin@uva.nl (P.-L.B.); buforstmann@gmail.com (B.U.F.)
2. Department of Experimental Neurosurgery, Maastricht University Medical Center, 6202 AZ Maastricht, The Netherlands; y.temel@mumc.nl
3. Municipality of Amsterdam, Services & Data, Cluster Social, 1000 AE Amsterdam, The Netherlands; mckeuken@gmail.com
4. Max Planck Institute for Human Cognitive and Brain Sciences, D-04103 Leipzig, Germany
* Correspondence: broseisaacs@gmail.com

Received: 24 August 2020; Accepted: 25 September 2020; Published: 27 September 2020

Abstract: Deep brain stimulation (DBS) of the subthalamic nucleus is a neurosurgical intervention for Parkinson's disease patients who no longer appropriately respond to drug treatments. A small fraction of patients will fail to respond to DBS, develop psychiatric and cognitive side-effects, or incur surgery-related complications such as infections and hemorrhagic events. In these cases, DBS may require recalibration, reimplantation, or removal. These negative responses to treatment can partly be attributed to suboptimal pre-operative planning procedures via direct targeting through low-field and low-resolution magnetic resonance imaging (MRI). One solution for increasing the success and efficacy of DBS is to optimize preoperative planning procedures via sophisticated neuroimaging techniques such as high-resolution MRI and higher field strengths to improve visualization of DBS targets and vasculature. We discuss targeting approaches, MRI acquisition, parameters, and post-acquisition analyses. Additionally, we highlight a number of approaches including the use of ultra-high field (UHF) MRI to overcome limitations of standard settings. There is a trade-off between spatial resolution, motion artifacts, and acquisition time, which could potentially be dissolved through the use of UHF-MRI. Image registration, correction, and post-processing techniques may require combined expertise of traditional radiologists, clinicians, and fundamental researchers. The optimization of pre-operative planning with MRI can therefore be best achieved through direct collaboration between researchers and clinicians.

Keywords: Parkinson's disease; magnetic resonance imaging; deep brain stimulation; ultra-high field

1. Introduction

Longevity is increasing and consequently triggering a surge in age-related, multimorbid neurodegenerative diseases [1,2]. One of these diseases is Parkinson's disease (PD). PD is the second most common neurodegenerative disorder worldwide and typically occurs after 50 years of age [3]. This is a multi-systems disease primarily characterized by symptoms that affect movement control, such as bradykinesia, tremor, rigidity, postural instability, and gait difficulties [3].

Drug treatments for PD are symptomatic in nature and function to replace the dopamine deficiency within the brain that occurs due to loss of nigrostriatal dopamine neurons [4–6]. While dopaminergic medications relieve the motor-related symptoms of PD, they do not address non-motor symptoms, further complications, or disease progression [6]. Moreover, drug therapy in PD is associated with side effects that include but are not limited to nausea and vomiting, sleep disorders, hallucinations, and delusions. Furthermore, as the disease progresses, initially beneficial drug treatments become less effective in about 40% of patients. At this stage, the therapeutic window begins to narrow and the medication may wear off faster, resulting in the re-emergence or worsening of motor fluctuations [7,8]. Chronic drug treatment and disease progression are also associated with levodopa-induced dyskinesias, which refer to involuntary, uncontrolled movements that occur when medications are most effective [7–9]. Increasing the dosages in response to reduced durability of levodopa or dopamine agonists is not always feasible. Alternative treatments such as device-aided therapies may then be considered.

The next step for a subset of patients is neurosurgery intervention by means of deep brain stimulation (DBS) of the subthalamic nucleus (STN) [10–13]. The STN is a small, glutamatergic, biconvex structure with a high iron content that is located within the subcortex [14,15]. DBS involves the implantation of electrodes that emit persistent high frequency stimulation in this nucleus [11–13]. The STN is a viable target for DBS as it modulates output of both the indirect and hyper-direct cortico-basal pathways, whose functions are assumed to suppress undesirable motor behavior and inappropriate movements, respectively [16,17]. In PD, dopaminergic degradation of the substantia nigra (SN) is thought to result in inhibition of direct pathways, as well as disinhibition of indirect and hyper-direct pathways. Collectively, this leads to the functional disinhibition of output to motor-related areas of the cortex, which is thought to produce impaired movement and reduced movement control [16]. However the exact mechanisms underlying DBS are still poorly understood, although the general consensus is that DBS results in a functional normalization of pathologically overactive circuits [17–19].

While DBS may ameliorate between 60 to 90% of the motor-related symptoms of PD, it can produce neuropsychiatric side effects and emotional or associative disturbances, with side effects ranging from hypomania; apathy; hallucinations; and, as well as general changes in moral competency, personality and reckless behavior [20–23]. A fraction of patients will fail to exhibit a long-term clinical benefit in the reduction of parkinsonian symptoms [24,25]. Revisions or removals of the DBS system occur in between 15 and 34% of operated patients, 17% of which are attributed solely to electrode misplacement [26,27]. Additional risks can arise from the surgery itself, with implantation posing a 15% risk of "minor and reversible problems", and a 2–3% risk of fatal or hemorrhagic events, infection, lead fracture, and dislocation [28]. Between 2013 and 2017, there were 711 bilateral DBS placement surgeries in The Netherlands, a subset of which were suffering from PD. Of those 711 surgeries, 169 patients required the DBS system to be either replaced or removed entirely [29]. These side effects and adverse outcomes can partially be attributed to suboptimal placement of the DBS lead, which is dependent on the accuracy of the preoperative planning procedures [30,31].

2. Using MRI to Target the STN in PD for DBS

As noted, the success of DBS treatment is partly determined by the accuracy of targeting the STN. Further, targeting is dependent on stereotaxic precision, neuroimaging methods, and electrophysiological mappings [32]. Identification of the STN can be achieved in two ways: indirectly or directly. Indirect targeting refers to identification of the DBS target via application of reformatted anatomical atlases, formulae coordinates, and distances from anatomical landmarks. These standard targets can be applied to a patient's individual magnetic resonance imaging (MRI), or can be used as a coordinate for navigation with a stereotaxic reference system (see next paragraph). Additionally, intra-operative microelectrode recordings, macrostimulation, and intraoperative behavioral feedback are commonly used for verification with indirect targeting [32,33]. Direct targeting refers to visualization of the STN on patient-specific MRI images [34,35].

For indirect targeting, the most common landmarks are the mid-way point between the anterior and posterior commissure (AC and PC, respectively), which are visualized and marked on a T1-weighted

(T1w) MRI, computer tomography (CT), or ventriculography [33,36]. The native brain is commonly realigned to the AC-PC with a Euclidean transform [37,38]. This transform provides an augmented matrix with a 3D homogenous coordinate system, allowing for application of formulae coordinates and distances. The standardized STN coordinates are defined as 12 mm lateral, 4 mm posterior, and 5 mm inferior to the mid commissural point [39]. Some centers may utilize their own reference points, such as the top of the red nucleus [40–42].

Direct targeting with patient-specific MRI is generally preferred as the STN is known to shift with both age and disease, as well as vary in size, shape, and location across individuals [43–47]. Clinical MRI typically visualizes the STN using T2-weighted (T2w) images, which present the nucleus as a hypointense region relative to surrounding tissue. The optimal part of the STN is considered to be the ventral dorsolateral portion, also termed the somatosensory region, and is assumed to have direct connections with pre-motor cortical areas [48]. As with indirect targeting, direct targeting also incorporates AC-PC alignment, which provides the common reference system required for frame-based stereotaxic surgeries. Additionally, AC-PC alignment allows for comparisons between planned target location, actual target location, and postoperative verification. Therefore, clinical identification of the STN is usually achieved with a combination of both direct and indirect targeting methods.

The presence of extreme side effects and lack of clinical effect that can occur with DBS may arise from either direct or indirect targeting. One method for increasing the success and efficacy of DBS is to optimize preoperative planning procedures via neuroimaging techniques. For instance, advanced MRI can be used to increase visualization and understanding of anatomy, connectivity, and functioning of the STN. This information can then be used to inform on optimal electrode placement on a patient-specific basis.

The goal of this paper is to explain the current procedures for structural target identification of the STN for DBS in PD using MRI. We identify limitations that may contribute to suboptimal identification of the STN and provide alternatives for optimizing MRI in order to visualize the STN. The organization of topics is as follows: field strength; current procedures for intra and post-operative verification with microelectrode recordings; SAR limitations; shimming and magnetic field corrections; sequence types and contrasts; voxel sizes; motion correction; registration and image fusion; quantitative maps; complications unrelated to pre-operative planning; and conclusions. The suggestions are presented with the underlying expectation that more accurate visualization can translate into targeting and implantation with increased precision.

3. Field Strength

Pre-operative MRIs are obtained to both visualize the DBS target and to assess for potential comorbidity and identify venous architecture to ensure a safe entry route for surgery. The quality of MRI is dependent on a large number of factors. One of these factors is the signal-to-noise ratio (SNR), which is strongly influenced by field strength (Tesla or T for short) (see Figure 1) [24,49,50]. SNR can be defined as the difference in signal intensity, effectively determining the amount of signal that represents the true anatomy compared to noise and random variation [51,52]. Low-field MRIs such as 1.5 or 3 T are routinely used for DBS targeting. However, recently, an ultra-high field (UHF) 7 T MRI system has been approved for medical neuroimaging [53]. Compared to 7 T, 1.5 and 3 T MRI tend to suffer from both inherently lower SNR and low contrast-to-noise (CNR). CNR reflects the difference in SNR between different tissue types, which is therefore essential for specificity [54,55]. Moreover, the STN is an inherently difficult structure to visualize as it is a small structure located within a very deep and dense portion of the basal ganglia and is surrounded by structures containing similar chemical compositions. This is exemplified by vast inconsistencies in observed volumetric measures, size, and location estimates of subcortical nuclei reported at low field strengths [44–46].

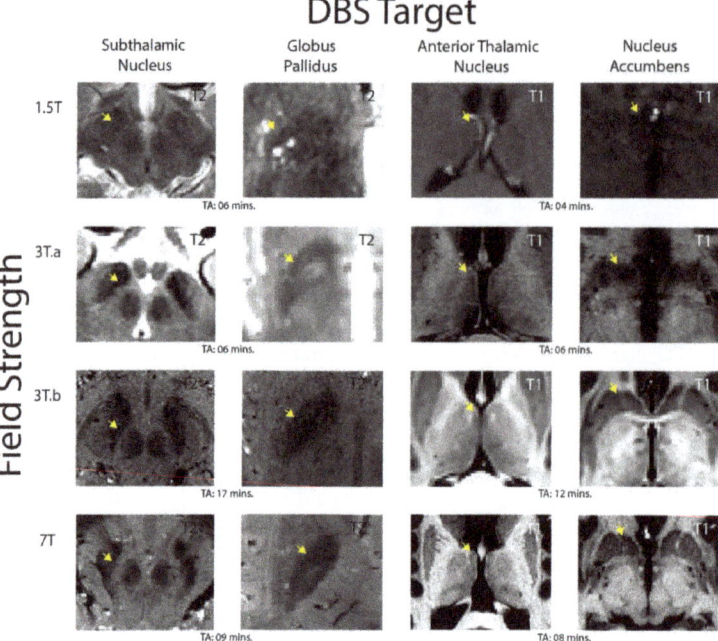

Figure 1. Visualizing deep brain stimulation (DBS) targets with different magnetic resonance imaging (MRI) field strengths (adapted from [24] illustrating DBS targets across field strengths, requiring different contrasts. We obtained 1.5 T images from a 52-year-old male Parkinson's disease patient at the Maastricht University Medical Center (MUMC). Clinical 3 T and 7 T images were obtained from a from 57-year-old male Parkinson's disease patient at the Maastricht University Medical Center (MUMC), and the optimized 3 T images were obtained from a healthy male age-matched subject at the Spinoza Center for Neuroimaging, Amsterdam. All images are shown in the axial plane and are present in their native space with no post-processing to replicate the visualization of each nucleus as performed on neurosurgical planning software. The T1 contrasts show the anterior thalamic nucleus and nucleus accumbens at all field strengths. The subthalamic nucleus and globus pallidus (GP) are shown with a T2 contrast at 1.5 T and clinical 3 T scan. Note that in the 7 T contrast, the medial medullary lamina is visible, allowing us to distinguish between the internal and external segment of the GP. For optimized 3 T and 7 T, the STN and GP are shown with a T2* contrast. The acquisition times (TA) for each scan are included to highlight the fact that optimized 3 T can provide high-quality images similar to those at 7 T but take nearly twice as long to obtain. While the STN and GP are visible in both 3 T images, the contrast and sharpness of borders increases at 7 T.

The quality of the magnetic field is also determined by magnetic field gradients. MRI gradients are characterized by the change in the magnetic field as a function of distance. The MRI gradient arises from gradient coils, which are a set of electromagnetic components within the scanner that are used to control the magnetic field [56,57]. Weaker gradients arising from lower magnetic fields cause g-factor penalties, whereby an inhomogeneous B1 field causes artificial signal differences and noise amplification in tissues further from the coil in the subcortex at 3 T compared with 7 T MRI [58,59]. SNR is therefore lower in subcortical structures relative to the cortex due to the larger distance between the center of the brain and receiver coil elements. These differences are amplified at low field compared to UHF [60–62].

However, SNR scales supra-linearly with the static magnetic field, with up to a sixfold increase at 7 T compared to 3 T MRI [54,55]. This means that UHF-MRI can provide better quality images at a higher spatial resolution, increased contrast, and shorter acquisition times [51,63,64]. Reduced acquisition is essential, as clinical radiologists are often under strict time pressures that are intrinsically linked to value-based healthcare systems and cost-effectiveness rather than scientific value [65]. Numerous empirical studies and reviews have noted the advantages of utilizing UHF-MRI in clinical settings, performing direct comparisons between low- and high-field strengths for visualizing finer details of smaller nuclei, which are common targets for DBS [34,52,66–70].

Developments in array coil designs and parallel imaging techniques have resulted in the possibility to measure specific portions of tissue simultaneously. The simultaneous measurement increases SNR by a factor of 3 to 10 when compared to standard volume coils used at clinical field strengths, which are unable to selectively excite separate portions of tissue [60,63]. This is discussed in more detail later in the paper.

Importantly, there are caveats with regards to the implementation of UHF-MRI. Firstly, the Siemens 7 T MAGNETOM Terra is the only UHF-MR system to have obtained Food and Drug Administration (FDA) 510(k) clearance for clinical neuroradiology, and other applications of 7 T MRI are therefore considered experimental. Expense and accessibility is among the most important and most time-limiting factors in implementing UHF-MRI into clinical settings; less than one hundred 7 T systems exist worldwide, making up about 0.2% of all MRI systems [24,71]. Moreover, increased specific absorption rates (SAR), field inhomogeneities, local signal intensity variations, and signal dropout are factors that can reduce the benefits of 7 T MRI when not properly accounted for [72]. These can be countered with optimized shimming and pre-processing techniques such as bias field correction. However, these techniques require expertise that is not typically available within clinical settings [73–75].

4. Current Procedures for Intra- and Post-Operative Verification with Microelectrode Recordings

Current standard practices within The Netherlands includes both pre-operative planning with neuroimaging methods and intra-operative verification with microelectrode recordings (MER). In this case, once the target has been decided, the DBS system will be implanted in two steps. First, the surgeon will create a burr hole in the skull on both hemispheres. If microelectrode recordings (MER) are used, the MER leads will be inserted into predefined coordinates. In 0.5 to 2 mm intervals from around 10 mm above the target coordinate, MER will start recording activity through macrostimulation. Multiple MERs may be placed into the STN at around 2 mm apart within the anterior, posterior, central, medial, and lateral portions. The MER lead that outputs consistent oscillations of beta bursts that are indicative of STN activity will be selected for test stimulation and subsequent implantation. If the patient is awake, additional intraoperative behavioral testing may be performed to assess the therapeutic effect of specific stimulation programs. Once the target has been verified via intra-operative neuroimaging (CT or ultra-low field MRI), the leads will be permanently implanted and then connected to a cortical grid and a stimulator will be inserted under the chest [76–79].

Not all centers use pre-operative CT or MRI and instead rely on standard coordinates with MER verification (and vice versa). There are reports that suggest MER significantly improves DBS outcomes [80], and that MER fails to show any significant benefit compared to direct targeting [81]. Moreover, there remains a mismatch of around 20% in the planned target coordinate based on MRI, compared to the actual optimal location identified with MER when using 1.5 and 3 T [82,83]. Further, the use of intra-operative ultra-low field MRI for identification of the test leads during surgery has shown to be as effective as MER in improving post-operative motor symptoms [84]. Moreover, while not a strictly scientific issue, the application of MER more than doubles the cost of a bilateral STN surgery [85]. See [86] for an extensive overview on comparisons between MER and MRI for STN identification in PD.

Lastly, post-operative management requires the identification of optimal stimulation parameters. These parameters can vary per patient, and some patients may require DBS in combination with medication. Microlesioning effects and acute foreign body reactions can impact the homeostasis of

STN function and lead to a misinterpretation of DBS efficacy. Therefore the patient should ideally be assessed several times at different stages after the surgery [87]. Baseline motor function is initially obtained after total withdrawal of dopaminergic medication [88]. Axial motor symptoms such as bradykinesia, rigidity, stability, gait, posture, and dysarthria are assessed with rating scales such as the Unified Parkinson's Disease Rating Scale Part 3 (UPDRS, III) or Movement Disorders Society (MDS)-UPDRS [79,89]. As the DBS lead consists of multiple contact points, each point is tested separately through monopolar stimulation, beginning with a standard frequency of 130 Hz and pulse width of 60 μs [90]. Amplitudes are varied in a step-wise manner and the lowest amplitude that results in the highest suppression of clinical symptoms with the absence of sustained adverse effects will be chosen as the optimal stimulation parameters [27]. More in-depth literature on practices for post-operative verification, stimulation programming, and care can be found in [91–93] and the references therein.

5. SAR Limitations

SAR refers to the amount of energy deposited into the body due to the radio frequency (RF) pulses applied with MRI sequences. RF pulses are emitted via electrical currents through coils, being used to generate the B1 field [74]. RF deposition can result in tissue heating, and to ensure that the absorbed energy does not induce local thermal damage, there are SAR limitations based on the region of interest, with the amount of SAR depending on tissue type [94,95]. However, field inhomogeneities increase with field strength, as the RF wavelength scales according to the size of the object being imaged, which then reduces its ability to penetrate the brain with a uniform power [96,97]. In the case of UHF-MRI, stronger gradients are required to magnetize tissues in the middle of the brain and to create a homogenous field, which results in higher SAR. Therefore, the safety limits are reached sooner at UHF than with lower field. Moreover, SAR can vary person to person due to individual differences in anatomy. This means that scan acquisition can require real-time parameter adaptation. Maintaining a low SAR can be achieved by increasing the repetition time (TR), reducing the flip angle (FA), or by reducing the number of acquired slices. Unfortunately, introducing these parameter changes to MR sequences can negatively affect the quality of the scan [98,99]. This invites an ethical debate as to whether future FDA-approved sequences and image pre-processing methods at UHF would allow for such real-time deviations in a clinical protocol where SAR limitations are reached and sequence amendments are required.

Further, there are more absolute and relative contraindications at UHF including pacemakers, surgical implants and prosthesis, and foreign bodies, even if they are not metallic or comprised of diamagnetic materials due to potential local heating and subsequent torque and increased SAR. Moreover, in our experience, many DBS candidates may not be scanned due to site-specific criteria. For instance, while a non-metallic or non-paramagnetic dental bridge is not listed as a contraindication, the guidelines for the 7 T site at some locations required such patients to be excluded. Even more contraindications exist at 7 T, including circulatory and clotting disorders, which makes UHF-MRI less compatible with a larger portion of the elderly population, including the majority of PD DBS patients [100]. Therefore, optimizing 3 T remains a viable option where UHF-MRI cannot be applied. However, while 3 T may theoretically be optimized to allow for increased visualization of subcortical nuclei, it is essential to remember that acquisition times will be much longer than that of an analogous 7 T sequence [24,101–103]; this concept will be discussed throughout the paper.

6. Shimming and Magnetic Field Corrections

Shimming refers to the process of homogenizing either the main magnetic field (B0) or the radiofrequency field (B1). Inhomogeneity of the B0 field occurs when materials with different magnetic properties and susceptibility enter the bore, resulting in image distortion and signal loss. For example, the interface between brain tissue and air arising from the sinuses can cause artifacts within the frontal and temporal areas. These brain–air interface-induced artifacts can result in large shifts in the observed anatomical locations of nearby brain structures and cortical surfaces [104]. While post-processing techniques exist to correct some of these erroneous signals, they cannot control for complete signal loss and dropout. Therefore, the field needs to be shimmed prior to the acquisition of the main MRI scan.

Shimming the B0 field can occur passively by strategically placing ferromagnetic sheets within the bore itself to form the distribution of the magnetic field toward a more uniform state [105] or by using patient-related inserts such as an intra-oral pyrolytic carbon plate [106]. This process is useful for removing field imperfections related to hardware, although is not generally utilized in clinical practice as it is laborious, inflexible, and temperature-dependent. More commonly, the field can be actively shimmed, which uses currents within the MRI system to generate corrective magnetic fields in areas showing inhomogeneous signals [105].

Active shimming is limited by the ability to model and reproduce the distortions that occur within the field. Shimming is generally based on the principles of spherical harmonics (SH), which use orthonormal equations to index changes in signal waveforms representative of field inhomogeneity. The mapping and the correction of the inhomogeneity is achieved by superimposing the magnetic field with an opposing corrective field equal to and a reversal of the polarity within a spatial distribution deemed erroneous by the SH coefficients [107,108].

The order of SH is dependent on the number of dedicated current-driven coils. Traditional clinical and low-field MR systems will employ lower-order shimming methods mainly due to cost and space restraints [57]. Low-order shims primarily utilize linear terms including addition, scaling, and rotation of the SH coefficients to model the magnetic field. Linear SH coefficients function to resemble and compensate large-scale, shallow magnetic field components that can be corrected with a current offset applied with a standard gradient coil. This is typically achieved automatically with the use of a pre-scan B0 map. More local changes can be compensated for with dynamic shimming. However, this is most commonly used for multi-slice MR, which is prone to additional eddy current distortions and requires dedicated amplifier hardware. Further, the optimal shim method will depend on the desired contrast [109]. Ideally, each sequence should require an additional shim.

As field inhomogeneities increase with field strength, higher order harmonics are therefore required for UHF. Higher order SH allows for correcting more complex-shaped inhomogeneities by incorporating an additional non-linear quadratic field variation that allows for modelling the bending of curves in space. This requires supplementary dedicated shim coils, which can counter-intuitively induce additional distortions in the middle of the brain. Despite efforts to harmonize parameters, shimming is often site- and field-dependent, and manual iterative shimming is not always possible due to time constraints and/or limited expertise.

Additional B1 mapping is essential for accurate quantitative measures of signal intensities within the correct geometric space. Inhomogeneous B1 fields can result in distorted flip angles (FAs). FAs index the amount of net magnetization rotation experienced during the application of an RF pulse. If FAs are incorrectly calculated, geometric distortions occur, which reduces the accuracy in T1 and T2 values. B1 mapping allows for the correction of FA values prior to acquiring a structural scan. Primary B1+ mapping methods can be incorporated into sequence acquisition. This is most commonly achieved with the double angle method (DAM), which estimates local FAs from the ratio of two images obtained with different FA values. An additional 3D multi-shot method can be incorporated, which uses non-selective excitation to minimize inhomogeneous spin excitation across slices. Alternatively, spoiled gradient echo (GRE) sequences with variable FAs (VFA) and actual FA imaging (AFI) are commonly employed, which sample multiple T1 values to simulate signal differences across tissues [110–113].

Pre-processing of gradient non linearities (GNL) and intensity non-uniformity with retrospective image-based interpolation is also possible. Corrections for GNL are rarely accomplished in clinical settings but are commonplace for research-based applications. The magnitude of GNL increases with distance from the isocenter and can cause the visualization of structures to shift by up to 5 mm, which is detrimental for preoperative planning [114]. Correcting for GNL can be achieved by incorporating a low-pass filter to remove smooth spatially varying functions. Other GNL correction schemes include surface fitting and feature matching that rely on intensity-based methods. Intensity-based methods assume that different tissue intensities do not vary significantly unless they are subject to an erroneous bias field, where variations within one area can be corrected from the field of another spatial location within the image. Alternatively, histogram-based methods use a priori knowledge and manual input of known intensity and gradient probability distributions to correct images. B1 corrections can be achieved offline via image pre-processing steps with the FMRIB Software Library (FSL), Statistical Parametric Mapping (SPM), or Advanced Normalization Tools (ANTs) [115–118]. However, these methods must be considered experimental and their use in image correction for MRI in pre-operative planning is not currently FDA-approved.

7. Sequence Types and Contrasts

7.1. T1

As discussed, accurate DBS implantation requires careful trajectory planning and identification of vasculature to limit the risk of hemorrhagic complications. Visualization of larger venous architecture is most commonly achieved with an anatomical T1w scan with added gadolinium [119,120]. In its most basic form, T1w can be viewed as an anatomical scan that approximates the appearance of macroscopic tissues. T1w will visualize white matter as hyperintense; fluid, e.g., cerebral spinal fluid (CSF) as hypointense; and grey matter at intermediate intensity. A T1w contrast is achieved with a short echo time (TE) and repetition time (TR) and is a function of the longitudinal relaxation time, referring to the time it takes excited protons to return to their equilibrium subsequent to the application of an RF pulse. T1 is more sensitive to fat and fluid and therefore provides excellent differentiation between grey and white matter. Additional intravenous contrast agents will cause the recovery of the longitudinal magnetization of blood to quicken and therefore increase further contrast between veins and white matter [121–123]. For visualization of venous architecture, some centers may use any or a combination of T1w structural imaging, or they may use post-processing techniques such as susceptibility weighted imaging (SWI) and venography, which can be created from GRE-based sequences with flow compensation, or time-of-flight angiography. These types of sequences apply multiple RF pulses with short TRs to over-saturate static tissues and therefore suppress their signal, causing moving components such as blood to appear more hyperintense [124–126]. T1w MRI can also be used to rule out co-morbidities such as oedema, tumors, or other brain pathologies. See Figure 2 for an example of different contrasts.

7.2. T2

T2w images visualize grey matter as intermediate intensity and white matter as hypointense, although deep grey matter structures can appear even darker depending on the ferromagnetism of their tissue composition. As mentioned, visualization of STN is traditionally achieved with T2w sequences [127–129]. T2w MRI represents transverse relaxation, referring to the amount of time it takes excited protons to lose phase coherence. This dephasing is a tissue-specific process and takes longer for areas with high paramagnetic metal deposition such as iron. As the STN is iron-rich, the contrast is increased, and the nucleus appears hypointense compared to white matter tracts and surrounding grey matter structures. Typically, T2w contrasts within the clinic will come from fast-spin echo sequences that have both a long TE and TR, which are relatively immune to magnetic susceptibility artifacts. However, there is no general consensus as to the optimal sequence required for prime STN imaging. Theoretically, various sequences can achieve the same weighting but vary significantly in terms of their ability to accurately visualize the STN [130]. Moreover, the type of sequence will depend on the field strength, and contrasts are not always analogous across, for instance, 3 and 7 T [131]. Similarly, different MRI vendors will supply similar contrasts via sequences and sequence parameters with different names, making it difficult to draw comparisons between them [50,132,133].

7.3. T2 and Susceptibility-Based Contrasts*

Traditional clinical T2w sequences suffer from low signal and contrast. An alternative contrast that can be used to image the STN directly comes from 3D gradient echo (GRE) sequences, which can be used to create T2* images. Typically, GRE sequences will include a low FA, long TEs, and long TRs. Moreover, gradients are applied to initiate dephasing, as opposed to an RF pulse in traditional spin echo sequences [109,134]. These gradients do not refocus field inhomogeneities such as RF pulses do. Therefore the T2* contrast arising from GRE reflects magnetic field inhomogeneities caused by the dephasing of neighboring areas that occurs at different rates, and further interact with the signal of adjacent voxels [135]. As GRE sequences assess macroscopic intervoxel and microscopic intravoxel magnetic susceptibilities, it is important to adapt sequence parameters according to the tissue of interest [136]. The tissue characteristics of the STN undergo PD-specific changes, such as dopaminergic denervation and excessive iron deposit, which require adjusted parameters such as TE for optimal contrast [137,138]. Similarly, iron increases with normal aging requires different adaptations to TEs [139]. GRE sequences also incorporate multiple echoes to account for differences in magnetic susceptibility across tissues. Further, susceptibility effects are stronger for smaller voxel sizes as the dephasing is reduced [135]. This makes T2* imaging more appropriate for higher field strength MR, as smaller voxel sizes can be achieved with faster acquisition times [130,140]. These T2* images can be further processed to create quantitative maps that will be discussed in later sections.

Alternatively, susceptibility weighted images (SWI) can be created from T2*-based sequences by independently processing magnitude and phase images. Magnitude images reflect the overall MR signal, and their corresponding phase image contains information about field inhomogeneity, differences in local precession frequencies, and motion [141]. Phase images were largely discarded before the implementation of SWI as they require complex unwrapping, referring to the extraction of their original numerical range, which is constrained in the outputted image to $[-\pi, +\pi]$ [142]. However, phase can be used to visualize information that would otherwise be barely visible in magnitude images. Small structures result in field variations with high spatial frequencies, which can be used to enhance contrast by applying a high pass filter. The resulting SWI image is the product of multiplying the phase mask with the magnitude image [142–144]. It remains somewhat controversial to what extent SWI signal increases from 1.5 T to 3 T MRI. Moreover there is little evidence for increased accuracy for SWI at 3 T compared to classic T2 imaging [145]. However, SWI is significantly more accurate compared to traditional contrasts at higher field strengths [146–148]. GRE-based sequences and T2* contrasts can provide more detail regarding the shape, surface, and location of the STN compared to standard T2w spin echo-based sequences. This could translate to more accurate DBS targeting if it were used for preoperative planning. Improvements can refer to a smaller deviation between planned and actual lead location, a reduction in reimplantation or removal requirements, increased clinical efficacy, or decrease in associated side effects. However, the use of T2* contrasts and UHF-MRI remains widely debated and requires further validation [37,70,144,148–150].

We attempted to use a T2*-based UHF-MRI with a GRE-ASPIRE sequence [151] on a 7 T Siemens MAGNETOM system (Siemens Healthcare, Erlangen, Germany) for STN DBS planning in PD patients. The 7 T T2* scan consisted of a partial volume covering the subcortex, obtained with multiple echoes (TE1–4 = 2.47, 6.75, 13.50, 20.75) and 0.5 mm isotropic voxel sizes in just under 8 min. This was overlaid with a 3 T T2w turbo field echo sequence obtained on a 3 Tesla Phillips Ingenia system, with a single TE of 80 ms and voxel sizes of $0.45 \times 0.45 \times 2$ mm, and an acquisition time of around 6 min. When merging the 3 T and 7 T data, the STN appeared elongated along the posterior direction on 7 T. The optimal target coordinate appeared more superior, posterior, and lateral on the 7 T image than the optimal coordinate on 3 T. Here, the 7 T coordinate was used as the posterior test site sampled with MER was used as a target for DBS surgery. Typical STN activity was not observed, although intraoperative behavioral testing revealed that patients would exhibit a beneficial clinical effect. Such a finding may be explained by the fact that the test electrode was instead stimulating white matter fibers exciting the STN, such as the fasciculus lenticularis or medial fiber bundles. It is, however, unclear as to whether this discrepancy in optimal STN coordinate is due to errors in registration across field strength, smoothing factors and interpolation automatically applied by the pre-operative planning system that reduced the resolution of the 7 T data, magnetic field inhomogeneity, or geometric distortions of the T2* image. The issues regarding image correction and manipulation are discussed in later sections. It is entirely plausible that the discrepancy in optimal target location across field strength was due to human error, and the operating surgeons perhaps were not used to interpreting the high-resolution susceptibility-based images. Therefore, factors other than contrast and sequence type can influence the usability and accuracy of susceptibility-based imaging for neurosurgical applications.

It is important to note that the sequences described in this specific instance are not standardized across centers, and scanner vendors, field strengths, contrasts, and sequence parameters, even within the same sequence type, will differ across DBS centers and research institutes. This makes a direct comparison across the quality and replicability of MRI scans very difficult, and unless systems are harmonized, interpretations should be site-specific. See [86,130] for a comprehensive review on sequences used for imaging the STN.

7.4. Multi-Contrast MRI

Multi-contrast sequences may offer a novel alternative for eliminating the requirement of registration and resampling of separate scans while simultaneously reducing scan acquisition time (Figure 2) [152]. A recently developed multiparametric imaging sequence is the Multi Echo (ME) MP2RAGE, which is largely unaffected by B1 inhomogeneities [153–160]. This allows for the acquisition of T2*-based contrasts from which subsequent SWI and quantitative susceptibility maps (QSM) can be created in the same space as the T1 images [158,160]. Other benefits of multiple contrasts is that they contain complimentary information that can be used to jointly denoise and improve the SNR of the acquired images [161–163].

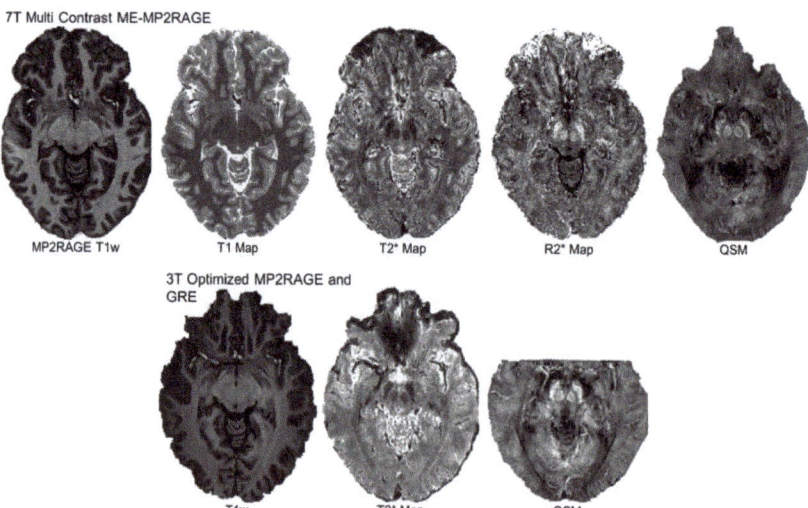

Figure 2. Multi-contrast imaging. The top row shows MP2RAGE T1-weighted, T1, T2*, and R2* maps and a quantitative susceptibility map (QSM) image obtained at 7 T within a single multi echo (ME) MP2RAGE sequence. Below are a 3 T T1-weighted map, a T2* map, and a QSM image, where each T1 and T2* were obtained with different sequences but were optimized to provide a contrast comparable to those obtainable at 7 T but without the inversions required for creating T1 maps. Both the 3 and 7 T images came from the same subject and are shown in the axial plane. The contrast and visibility of subcortical structures is indeed comparable across field strengths [164].

8. Voxel Sizes

Clinical T2w images often incorporate anisotropic voxel sizes with large slice thickness in the z direction. This allows for higher in-plane resolution along the axial plane, which is primarily used for targeting (Figure 3) [145,149]. Voxel sizes will typically range between 0.45 × 0.45 × 2 mm and 1 × 1 × 3 mm. Lower resolution allows for shorter acquisition times of around 5 min, simultaneously limiting the effect of artifacts due to subject movement. However, anisotropic voxels suffer from partial voluming effects (PVE), which refer to the blurring of signals across voxels, resulting in averaging different tissue types and reducing specificity [165]. PVE are especially problematic for small structures such as the STN. Volume estimates are commonly used as an index of scan quality, and have shown consistent deviations of more than 50% from ground truths when slice thicknesses were three times the size of the alternate planes [166]. Moreover, anisotropic voxels will decrease the accuracy of resampling to super resolutions, which is an automatically incorporated step of pre-operative planning systems [167].

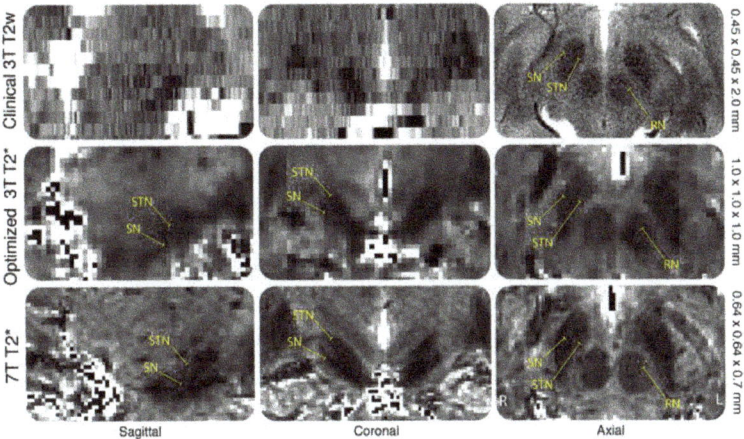

Figure 3. The effects of voxel geometry on the visualization of subcortical structures (adapted from [164]). Figure 3 shows clinical 3 T T2-weighted (T2w) with 0.45 × 0.45 × 2.0 mm voxel sizes, optimized 3 T T2* with 1.0 × 1.0 × 1.0 mm voxel sizes, and 7 T T2* maps with 0.64 × 0.64 × 0.7 mm voxel sizes. All images are acquired from a single subject and are shown at approximately the same anatomical level. The subthalamic nucleus (STN) and substantia nigra (SN) are shown at sagittal, coronal, and axial planes, with the red nucleus (RN) also highlighted in the axial plane. The anisotropic nature of the sagittal and coronal planes on the clinical 3 T do not allow for identification of any structure.

As spatial resolution is dependent on voxel size; smaller voxels should allow for more detailed and finer grained visualization of smaller structures. Voxel sizes can be reduced by increasing the acquisition matrix, reducing slice thickness, or decreasing the field of view. However, these factors can each negatively affect the SNR. The loss of SNR can be compensated by simply including more repetitions per sequence, which is an issue for PD populations as it necessitates an increase in acquisition time and requires the patient to be still. However this is often not possible for patients with movement disorders [166]. The loss of SNR caused by decreasing voxel sizes at lower fields can be counteracted through the use of UHF-MRI [130].

When targets in clinical MRI are verified with MER, the large slice thickness means that the spatial resolution is penalized along the z-axis. Therefore the depth of the electrode cannot be optimally planned and electrophysiological samplings are conducted to identify the ideal electrode placement [32,38,40]. This testing often requires that the patient is awake and endures behavioral assessments, which are stressful and physically demanding, prolong the time of the surgery, and can increase the risk of infection or hemorrhaging [168–170]. If smaller voxels can increase spatial resolution, three-dimensional anatomical accuracy, and tissue specificity, the requirement for intraoperative microelectrode recordings, multiple test electrode implantations, and awake behavioral testing could be eliminated, ultimately increasing patient comfort and reducing operation time.

However, voxels with a sub millimeter isotropic resolution used purely for identification of DBS targets, rather than for instance venous architecture, may not directly improve targeting accuracy. This is because the spatial resolution of stereotaxic coordinate systems is around 1.2 mm and chronically implanted conventional DBS electrodes are larger than 1 mm [171]. In addition, segmented DBS leads with directional steering may offer increased spatial resolution when recording local field potentials compared to traditional omnidirectional contacts [172,173]. Further, the development of microscale DBS contacts via multiresolution electrodes would allow for finer control of the stimulation volume and more precise targeting of smaller regions, matching the order and spatial resolution of submillimeter resolution MRI [174].

9. Motion Correction

Generally, clinical imaging for preoperative planning for DBS does not correct for motion, and the scans do not tend to incorporate acceleration methods such as parallel imaging. Accurate imaging requires the subject to remain still. If a patient scan exhibits severe motion artifacts, the scan is simply run again. MR images can be distorted by multiple sources of motion arising from breathing, cardiac movement, blood flow, pulsation of cerebrospinal fluid, and patient movement [104]. This can cause distortions in the image such as ghosting, signal loss, and blurring, as well as Gibb's and chemical shift artifacts [175]. Such artifacts can mask or simulate pathological effects [104]. Motion artifacts are particularly prevalent when imaging patients with movement disorders but can be controlled for in a number of ways such as timing medication to be most optimal during the time of scanning or administering additional sedatives during the scan. Moreover, the head and neck should be supported with pads to improve patient comfort, which will also limit movement.

The most logical method of limiting motion artifacts is to decrease the acquisition time. Sequence paraments can be manipulated to shorten the acquisition time by obtaining larger voxel sizes, a partial field of view (FOV), incorporating simultaneous multi slice 3D imaging and parallel imaging techniques, signal averaging, or obtaining multi contrast images. To correctly utilize these potential solutions, each factor should be considered relative to one another. For instance, partial FOVs can induce aliasing, fold over artifacts, and reduce the SNR, which can, to a certain extent, be countered by isolating the excitation to a localized region by using either multiple pulses, signal averaging, or fat suppression methods. Contrary to this, it may increase the effects of field inhomogeneity, but be combated with factors such as spatial pre-saturation. Such issues highlight the dynamic nature and interplay of sequence parameters and hardware, which can be largely overcome through the use of stronger field strengths such as 7 T.

Parallel imaging (PI) is a reconstruction technique rather than a sequence commonly employed to accelerate acquisition time [176]. Magnetic resonance (MR) images are not directly collected but are instead stored in a Cartesian grid, representing a spatial frequency domain known as k-space. K-space data is collected via superimposing spatially varying magnetic field gradients onto the main magnetic field [55,177]. Generalized auto-calibrating partially parallel acquisition (GRAPPA) methods speed up acquisition n time under-sampling each line of k-space in the phase-encoding direction. Additionally, partial FOVs are collected independently, corrected, and then reconstructed within the frequency domain [178–180]. Alternatively, sensitive encoding methods (SENSE or ASSET) can shorten scan times, and these methods occur in the image domain where data are obtained using multiple independent receiver channels where each coil is sensitive to a specific volume of tissue, which is then unfolded and recombined to form the MR image [177]. However, PI methods are associated with a number of artifacts including ghosting, speckling, wrap around, and g factor penalties and ought to be used with caution [181–183].

Motion correction can be conducted prospectively in real time by updating the image geometry during the scan, or retrospectively by post-acquisition registration techniques and manipulations during image reconstructions [184]. Additional hardware is required for prospective methods that are implemented within the scanner itself. In this case, fiducials can be attached to the patient's head, which assesses the extent of movement and adjusts the gradients accordingly. Alternatively, you can employ optical tracking or reflective markers, which are linked to a camera inside the bore. Motion correction is then achieved by either re-registration slice-by-slice during the scan, adjusting first order shims, and/or varying the gradient system online [185,186]. As discussed, motion artifacts do not have to come from patient movement but can arise on a much smaller scale at the proton level. Protons in blood, for example, exhibit a non-static magnetic field due to the variation of gradients in space. That is, they can miss rephasing pulses and therefore decay in signal before it can be read out by the scanner, especially for spin echo sequences that are used for obtaining T2w images [187]. This phenomenon is known as flow-related dephasing and results in artifactual phase shifts and signal distortion. In some instances, this can be useful, for example in angiography sequences, the negative effect is larger in sequences with longer TEs, such as those required for accurately imaging the STN. Adding in flow compensation or gradient moment nulling, which applies additional gradient pulses prior to the signal readout to compensate for signal decay, can compensate for this dephasing [188,189]. However, this is a computationally heavy process and is largely only suitable for partial FOVs. Alternatively, the sequence may be synchronized so that the acquisition occurs in time with the cardiac or respiratory cycle, which is known as cardiac gating and simultaneously requires pulse recordings or electrocardiograms [104].

10. Registration and Image Fusion

Using MRI to visualize deep brain structures such as the STN for DBS is a multi-stage process that involves the acquisition of multiple separate contrasts that require registration to a common, patient-specific native space. For pre-operative planning, at least two sets of image registrations are required: (i) anatomical T2 to T1 and (ii) pre-registered anatomical T1 and T2 to stereotaxic space defined by the CT or MRI including the coordinate frame. In this section, we focus on registration and fusion of MRI. For literature including alternative imaging modalities such as CT and ventriculography, see [190,191].

Image registration refers to the process of aligning a moving source image onto a fixed target through an estimated mapping between the pair of images. While the exact parameters incorporated within pre-operative planning systems are mostly proprietary, the general process will require a rigid registration, defined by six parameters: translation and rotations along the x-, y-, and z-axes. This refers to the spatial transformation of how a voxel can move from one space to another [192]. Transformations also require additional parameters such as interpolation and cost function. Interpolation refers to the process of re-gridding voxels from the source image to the target, an essential procedure as each pixel within the transformed image may not represent a whole integer within the target image. This is especially true when T2w images consist of anisotropic voxel sizes and the T1 images are isotropic. Therefore, the goal of interpolation is to piece back together the voxels that have been moved. Clinical neuroimaging traditionally employs the simplest intensity-based methods such as nearest neighbor interpolation, also known as point sampling, which assumes that similar values in different images are closer together and therefore constitute the same location [193,194]. Cost functions are used to assess the suitability of a given transform. This can be achieved with either similarity metrics such as mutual information, which compares, on the basis of pixel intensities, the differences between the transformed source and target image [195]. These registration steps are all conducted automatically within pre-operative planning systems, with the only manual alterations relating to viewing criteria such as brightness and intensity. This is suboptimal, as registrations often need tweaking and optimizing, and it becomes challenging to suggest exact methods for optimizing registrations with regards to pre-operative planning systems as it remains unclear as to what exact parameters are employed.

Linear within-subject registrations typically employ intensity-based similarity metrics, matching images on the basis of intensities or intensity distributions. Intensity methods can be optimized to incorporate local patches that account for textures and geometric information that are missed when assessing for global identical intensities. An example is boundary-based registration, which forms the basis of intra-subject registration of T2 to T1 images within the Human Connectome Project minimal processing pipeline [196,197]. Registrations could be optimized to include an additional affine transform that incorporates scaling or sheering [198]. Alternatively, deformable registrations via attribute matching and mutual saliency (DRAMMS) can be achieved. DRAMMS applies confidence weightings for matching voxels across contrast and will relax deformation in local regions where contrast-specific tissues are mutually exclusive to image type. DRAMMS has proven useful in accounting for pathology, subcortical structures, and cortical thinning, which are all factors to consider when imaging PD patients [199].

Further, no quality or standardized evaluation for registration accuracy currently exists in clinical neuroimaging beyond subjective visual assessment. This is problematic as it becomes unclear as to whether the initial rigid body transforms are an accurate spatial representation of individual anatomy, which, if erroneous, could result in targeting errors and DBS lead placement. The gold standard of accuracy is instead dependent on the stereotaxic frame, which is an extrinsic marker and does not include information directly related to the MR image.

Medical imaging often incorporates automated image fusion, which refers to the process of aligning, resampling, smoothing, and combining the information of multiple images into a more informative and descriptive output; for instance, by combining T1 and T2 into a single image. Fusion occurs after registration with the goal of interpolating and smoothing MRI images to make them more visually appealing, which can theoretically recover a signal within the data despite the noise [200]. However, smoothing and resampling voxel sizes will reduce anatomical variability and location accuracy as they can include signal from neighboring structures, leading to an erroneous increase in the size of the nucleus and PVEs [166,201]. Such smoothing methods may not be compatible with quantitative images such as T2* maps and QSM, as these images represent distinct signal intensities of specific voxels that are outside the predefined values of the planning system. In effect, this could be a simple viewing error, rather than a total incompatibility.

11. Quantitative Maps

Broadly speaking, MR contrasts are driven by how much T1 or T2 signal contributes to the image. These T1w or T2w images are qualitative in nature and fail to accurately assess tissue parameters such as recovery or relaxation time. However, certain sequences allow for parametric mapping (quantitative MRI or qMRI), where the intensities within each pixel are proportional to the T1 or T2. These values can be used to quantify intrinsic, biologically meaningful tissue information [202]. Additionally, qMRI allows for direct comparison across time, across subjects, and across scanners or sites, which is essential for the development of neuroscientific research and its application to the clinical situation [203]. Moreover, quantitative measures can aid identification and visualization of target structures with an objective approach and can minimize human error resulting from subjective interpretation. qMRI can only be made from specific sequences that comply with the principles of differential weightings, which incorporate an inversion or saturation recovery parameter with multiple inversion times or spoiled gradient echo sequences with variable flip angles [204]. However, in our experience, quantitative sequences at 3 T take at least twice as long as weighted MRI sequences used in clinical settings.

As mentioned, quantitative maps are used to index anatomical composition. For instance, the observed relaxation of T1 is extremely fast in myelinated white matter. The inverse of longitudinal relaxation rates, known as R1 [205], is thought to be linearly related to myelin concentrations [206,207]. T1 maps have been utilized clinically, for example, with quantifying perfusion; imaging hemorrhages and infarctions; evaluating contrast uptake; monitoring of tumors, gliosis, and multiple sclerosis lesions [205,208,209]. Quantitative T1 maps will usually require post-processing, most commonly achieved with the look-up table method, which functions to relate pixelwise T1 values within the native map with predefined and validated intensity values [159]. The automated creation of these T1 parametric maps can be built into the sequence at a cost of both time and capacity. Further post-processing is often required and relies on expertise that is again typically not available within a standard clinical setting [160,210].

For DBS of the STN, T2* maps can be used to improve visualization of the STN because iron content causes the T2* relaxation time to shorten, which for the STN at 7 T is around 15 ms [61,211]. A frequently used method to create T2* maps is done by fitting an exponential decay curve to the signal intensities per pixel from each of the multiple echoes obtained from a GRE sequence [212]. Moreover, the pixel intensities of reciprocal T2* maps (R2*) are proportional to iron load, with STN R2* values hovering around 67 s^{-1} (1/15 ms) at 7 T [155,213–216]. Alternatively, T2* images can be post-processed to create quantitative susceptibility maps (QSM), which quantify a tissue's magnetic susceptibility distribution on the basis of its perturbation of the magnetic field [213]. They are similar to SWI in that they are made from the separate magnitude and phase images of a GRE sequence, but they comprise multiple echoes and allow for quantitative measures rather than weightings. QSM requires initial phase unwrapping, background field extraction, and calculation of locally generated phase offsets, which refer to the fact that the phase of a single voxel can be expressed as either positive of negative, depending on its orientation relative to the magnetic field [214]. These phase-offsets are then deconvolved, typically with a dipole kernel, from which the underlying tissue susceptibility can be extracted per voxel, independently of surrounding voxels [215]. Moreover, QSMs are preferred over SWI, as SWI is limited by the non-local orientation-dependent effects of phase, which means that the same tissues can appear with different intensities on the basis of their location, whereas QSM solves this problem by convolving dipole fields [216,217]. Background removal methods based on principles of sophisticated harmonic artifact reduction for phase data (SHARP, also known as spherical mean value (SMV) filtering) and projection onto dipole fields (PDF) are commonly employed. SHARP is based on a theory similar to shimming, in that static magnetic fields and the corresponding phase maps are represented by harmonic functions. In regions of inhomogeneous susceptibility, the field will be non-harmonic, and background fields that are harmonic are eliminated from the phase data by subtraction [213,218]. The PDF method removes background fields by comparing the magnetic fields of dipoles inside a region of interest with those directly outside [219,220]. Alternatively, Laplacian boundary values can be used, which are based on a finite difference scheme [221]. However, quantifying an arbitrary distribution of susceptibility from the phase signal is challenging and poses an inverse problem whereby effects are first calculated from which parameters or causes are then determined, resulting in a noise amplification of the ensuing signal. The inversion problem can be solved with calculation of susceptibility through multiple orientation sampling (COSMOS). However, this method requires the acquisition of multiple head orientations, which is time-consuming and impractical for clinical use [222,223]. Morphology-enabled dipole inversion, or MEDI, will match the boundaries of each dipole with those observed in the T2*-weighted magnitude images [222]. Quantitative susceptibility and residual mapping (QUASAR) accounts for biophysical frequency contributions, which acknowledges that the notion that the local Larmor frequency is affected by the static field perturbations related to tissue susceptibility, as well as the magnetic field, chemical shifts, directional alignment of axons, and energy exchange between water and macromolecules [224]. Alternatively, some algorithms solve the entire equation within a single step by incorporating SHARP principles with simultaneous total generalized variation (TGV)-regularized dipole inversion [225,226]. Similarly phase removal using the Laplacian operator (HARPERELLA) simultaneously combines phase unwrapping and background removal [227]. These methods comprise tool boxes that are largely available in Matlab or Python (see [228] and the references therein).

The clinical potential of QSM lies in its sensitivity to variations in iron stored in ferritin and hemosiderin, lipids and calcium, levels of differential oxygenation-saturation present in venous blood, and identification of sub millimeter white matter microstructure [229–231]. Further, QSM has been shown to be superior to T2* in parcellations of the STN, which could translate into better visualization and targeting for DBS [223,228,232]. T2 relaxometry has been shown to predict motor outcome in some PD patients with STN DBS, where patients who have low T2 values may fail to show a clinical benefit [233]. It is possible that this can be explained by the fact that patients with low T2 relaxometry will have less contrast between the STN and the surrounding tissue, hindering the accurate visualization and targeting of the structure, which could be solved by employing QSM. However, QSM obtained during a scanning session is still experimental and under development. Further, there are many competing post-processing methods for creating QSM images, which makes translation challenging.

12. Complications Unrelated to Pre-Operative Planning

Lastly, we would like to mention that while this paper specifically refers to suboptimal placement of DBS leads due to the limitations of neuroimaging, negative outcomes of DBS application can arise independently of planning procedures and surgical expertise. For example, neurosurgery has been linked to brain deformation and shift, changes in cerebral spinal fluid volume, and intracranial pressure, which may induce spatial variability both during the surgery and cause a shift in the implanted lead location during recovery [27,234]. Similarly, DBS surgeries are associated with infection (mostly found in the chest and connector) [235]; reactive gliosis and gliotic scarring [236]; hemorrhage either during the surgery or delayed (in less than 5%) [237]; and, although rare, cerebral pneumocephalus [238]. In all these cases, the DBS system may require reimplantation, replacement, or removal.

13. Conclusions

In this paper, we have discussed some of the differences in current clinical MRI practices with optimized and UHF-MRI methods commonly employed in research environments. Clinical MRI hinges on weighted imaging with anisotropic voxel sizes and maintaining short acquisition, therefore being limited in signal and resolution. These current clinical practices are FDA-approved and are therefore deemed acceptable for neurosurgical purposes. However, the presence of side effects and non-responding patients nonetheless exist. Optimized 3 T and UHF-MRI tend to incorporate isotropic high-resolution imaging with quantitative and susceptibility-based contrasts for better visualization of deep brain structures, which, however, require more complex pre-processing and longer scan durations. The limitations incurred regarding reduced signal in clinical MRI and increased acquisition time with optimized 3 T can be largely overcome with the use of UHF-MRI. However, many of the image registration, correction, and post-processing techniques will typically require expertise that is outside the realm of traditional clinical settings. Importantly, the use of UHF-MRI and alternative contrasts such as QSM can only be implemented once pre-operative planning systems allow for their compatibility, which will require further FDA approval, not only for the MRI system but also for specific sequences. Additional approval for clinical use may be required for pre- and post-processing, such as the algorithms used for registration or calculation of quantitative maps.

We therefore propose that where UHF-MRI is not accessible, higher quality imaging can be obtained with optimized 3 T, although this will take longer than is perhaps clinically feasible for patients with severe movement disorders. Continued direct collaboration and combined efforts between fundamental neuroscience researchers and clinicians will be essential for the development of optimized 3 T and UHF-MRI in the pre-operative planning process for DBS of the STN in PD. Multi-site clinical trials can facilitate the optimization and validation of certain sequences. Sequences with identical parameters should be compared on identical MRI systems and different sites to ensure harmonization and reliability, as well as to validate the desired sequences. Rates of deviations between planned and actual target locations should be compared across vendors and systems as well as across sequences. Similarly, access agreements to work-in-progress protocols from MR vendors would facilitate the development and optimization of sequences, and would open access to underling algorithms and adjustable parameters within to pre-operative planning software vendors (e.g., Medtronic, St. Judes, Brainlab, Abott, Nextim, and Boston Scientific).

Of note, while this paper focused specifically on the STN as the most popular target for DBS in PD, alternative targets also exist (for example, see Figure 1). Some centers have long preferred the internal segment of the globus pallidus, and more recent research is being conducted on the suitability of alternate areas such as the ventral intermediate nucleus or the pedunculopontine nucleus for DBS targets. For a more in-depth review, please see [10,239,240] and the references therein.

Author Contributions: Conceptualization, B.R.I., M.C.K., A.A., Y.T., P.-L.B., and B.U.F.; validation, B.R.I., M.C.K., A.A., Y.T., P.-L.B., and B.U.F.; investigation, B.R.I., M.C.K., A.A., Y.T., P.-L.B., and B.U.F.; resources, Y.T. and B.U.F.; data curation, X.X.; writing—original draft preparation, B.R.I., M.C.K., and B.U.F.; writing—review and editing, B.R.I., M.C.K., A.A., Y.T., P.-L.B., and B.U.F.; visualization, B.R.I. and A.A.; supervision, B.U.F. and P.-L.B.; project administration, B.R.I. and M.C.K. All authors have read and agreed to the published version of the manuscript.

Funding: The work was supported by a Vici grant by the Dutch Organization for Scientific Research (NWO 016.Vici.185.052) (B.U.F.) and a starter grant from the European Research Council (ERC-Stg 313481) (B.U.F.).

Conflicts of Interest: The authors declare no conflict of interest.

References

1. Van Oostrom, S.H.; Gijsen, R.; Stirbu, I.; Korevaar, J.C.; Schellevis, F.G.; Picavet, H.S.J.; Hoeymans, N. Time trends in prevalence of chronic diseases and multimorbidity not only due to Aging: Data from general practices and health Surveys. *PLoS ONE* **2016**, *11*, e0160264. [CrossRef] [PubMed]
2. Rossi, A.; Berger, K.; Chen, H.; Leslie, D.L.; Mailman, R.B.; Huang, X. Projection of the prevalence of Parkinson's disease in the coming decades: Revisited. *Mov. Disord.* **2018**, *33*, 156–159. [CrossRef] [PubMed]
3. Sveinbjornsdottir, S. The clinical symptoms of Parkinson's disease. *J. Neurochem.* **2016**, *139*, 318–324. [CrossRef] [PubMed]
4. Evans, A.H.; Lees, A.J. Dopamine dysregulation syndrome in Parkinson's disease. *Curr. Opin. Neurol.* **2004**, *17*, 393–398. [CrossRef] [PubMed]
5. Olanow, C.W.; Obeso, J.A.; Stocchi, F. Continuous dopamine-receptor treatment of Parkinson's disease: Scientific rationale and clinical implications. *Lancet Neurol.* **2006**, *5*, 677–687. [CrossRef]
6. Lang, A.E.; Obeso, J.A. Challenges in Parkinson's disease: Restoration of the nigrostriatal dopamine system is not enough. *Lancet Neurol.* **2004**, *3*, 309–316. [CrossRef]
7. Ahlskog, J.E.; Muenter, M.D. Frequency of levodopa-related dyskinesias and motor fluctuations as estimated from the cumulative literature. *Mov. Disord.* **2001**, *16*, 448–458. [CrossRef]
8. Holloway, R.; Shoulson, I.; Kieburtz, K. Pramipexole vs. Levodopa as initial treatment for Parkinson disease: A randomized controlled trial. *J. Am. Med. Assoc.* **2000**, *284*, 1931–1938. [CrossRef]
9. Ahlskog, J.E. Medical Treatment of later-stage motor problems of Parkinson disease. *Mayo. Clin. Proc.* **1999**, *74*, 1239–1254. [CrossRef]
10. Odekerken, V.J.; Boel, J.A.; Schmand, B.A.; De Haan, R.J.; Figee, M.; Munckhof, P.V.D.; Schuurman, P.R.; De Bie, R.M.; For the NSTAPS study group; Bour, L. GPi vs. STN deep brain stimulation for Parkinson disease. *Neurology* **2016**, *86*, 755–761. [CrossRef]
11. Benabid, A.L.; Chabardes, S.; Mitrofanis, J.; Pollak, P. Deep brain stimulation of the subthalamic nucleus for the treatment of Parkinson's disease. *Lancet Neurol.* **2009**, *8*, 67–81. [CrossRef]
12. Limousin, P.; Krack, P.; Pollak, P.; Benazzouz, A.; Ardouin, C.; Hoffmann, D.; Benabid, A.L. Electrical stimulation of the subthalamic nucleus in advanced Parkinson's disease. *N. Engl. J. Med.* **2002**, *339*, 1105–1111. [CrossRef] [PubMed]
13. Limousin, P.; Pollak, P.; Benazzouz, A.; Hoffmann, D.; Le Bas, J.F.; Perret, J.; Benabid, A.L.; Broussolle, E. Effect on parkinsonian signs and symptoms of bilateral subthalamic nucleus stimulation. *Lancet* **1995**, *345*, 91–95. [CrossRef]
14. De Hollander, G.; Keuken, M.C.; Bazin, P.L.; Weiss, M.; Neumann, J.; Reimann, K.; Wähnert, M.; Turner, R.; Forstmann, B.U.; Schäfer, A. A gradual increase of iron toward the medial-inferior tip of the subthalamic nucleus. *Hum. Brain Mapp.* **2014**, *35*, 4440–4449. [CrossRef] [PubMed]

15. Alkemade, A.; De Hollander, G.; Miletic, S.; Keuken, M.C.; Balesar, R.; De Boer, O.; Swaab, D.F.; Forstmann, B.U. The functional microscopic neuroanatomy of the human subthalamic nucleus. *Brain Struct. Funct.* **2019**, *224*, 3213–3227. [CrossRef]
16. Chiken, S.; Nambu, A. Mechanism of deep brain stimulation. *Neuroscientist* **2016**, *22*, 313–322. [CrossRef]
17. Stefani, A.; Cerroni, R.; Mazzone, P.; Liguori, C.; Di Giovanni, G.; Pierantozzi, M.; Galati, S. Mechanisms of action underlying the efficacy of deep brain stimulation of the subthalamic nucleus in Parkinson's disease: Central role of disease severity. *Eur. J. Neurosci.* **2018**, *49*, 805–816. [CrossRef] [PubMed]
18. Petsko, G.A. The coming epidemic of neurologic disorders: What science is—And should be—Doing about it. *Daedalus* **2012**, *141*, 98–107. [CrossRef]
19. Bosco, D.A.; Lavoie, M.J.; Petsko, G.A.; Ringe, D. Proteostasis and movement disorders: Parkinson's disease and amyotrophic lateral sclerosis. *Cold Spring Harb. Perspect. Biol.* **2011**, *3*, a007500. [CrossRef]
20. Weaver, F.M.; Follett, K.; Stern, M.; Hur, K.; Harris, C.; Marks, W.J.; Rothlind, J.; Sagher, O.; Reda, D.; Moy, C.S.; et al. Bilateral deep brain stimulation vs. best medical therapy for patients with advanced parkinson disease. A randomized controlled Trial. *JAMA* **2009**, *301*, 63–73. [CrossRef]
21. Obeso, J.A.; Olanow, C.W.; Rodriguez-Oroz, M.C.; Krack, P.; Kumar, R.; Lang, A.E. Deep-brain stimulation of the subthalamic nucleus or the pars interna of the globus pallidus in Parkinson's disease. *N. Engl. J. Med.* **2001**, *345*, 956–963. [CrossRef] [PubMed]
22. Deuschl, G.; Schade-Brittinger, C.; Krack, P.; Volkmann, J.; Schafer, H.; Bötzel, K.; Daniels, C.; Deutschländer, A.; Dillmann, U.; Eisner, W.; et al. A randomized trial of deep-brain stimulation for Parkinson's disease. *N. Engl. J. Med.* **2006**, *355*, 896–908. [CrossRef]
23. Cyron, D. Mental side effects of deep brain stimulation (DBS) for movement disorders: The futility of denial. *Front. Integr. Neurosci.* **2016**, *10*, 17. [CrossRef] [PubMed]
24. Forstmann, B.U.; Isaacs, B.R.; Temel, Y. Ultra high field MRI-guided deep brain stimulation. *Trends Biotechnol.* **2017**, *35*, 904–907. [CrossRef] [PubMed]
25. Temel, Y.; Blokland, A.; Steinbusch, H.W.M.; Visser-Vandewalle, V. The functional role of the subthalamic nucleus in cognitive and limbic circuits. *Prog Neurobiol.* **2005**, *76*, 393–413. [CrossRef] [PubMed]
26. Rolston, J.D.; Englot, D.J.; Starr, P.A.; Larson, P.S. An unexpectedly high rate of revisions and removals in deep brain stimulation surgery: Analysis of multiple databases. *Park Relat Disord.* **2016**, *33*, 72–77. [CrossRef]
27. Hartmann, C.J.; Fliegen, S.; Groiss, S.J.; Wojtecki, L.; Schnitzler, A. An update on best practice of deep brain stimulation in Parkinson's disease. *Ther Adv Neurol Disord.* **2019**, *12*, 175628641983809. [CrossRef]
28. Fenoy, A.J.; Simpson, R.K. Risks of common complications in deep brain stimulation surgery: Management and avoidance—Clinical article. *J Neurosurg.* **2014**, *120*, 132–139. [CrossRef]
29. DIS Open Data. Available online: https://www.opendisdata.nl/ (accessed on 24 February 2020).
30. Kloc, M.; Kosutzka, Z.; Steno, J.; Valkovic, P. Prevalent placement error of deep brain stimulation electrode in movement disorders (technical considerations). *Bratislava Med. J.* **2017**, *118*, 647–653. [CrossRef]
31. Nagy, A.M.; Tolleson, C.M. Rescue procedures after suboptimal deep brain stimulation outcomes in common movement disorders. *Brain Sci.* **2016**, *6*, 46. [CrossRef]
32. Tonge, M.; Kocabicak, E.; Ackermans, L.; Kuijf, M.; Temel, Y. Final electrode position in subthalamic nucleus deep brain stimulation surgery: A comparison of indirect and direct targeting methods. *Turk Neurosurg.* **2016**, *26*, 900–903. [CrossRef] [PubMed]
33. Tu, P.H.; Liu, Z.H.; Chen, C.C.; Lin, W.Y.; Bowes, A.L.; Lu, C.S.; Lee, S.-T. Indirect targeting of subthalamic deep brain stimulation guided by stereotactic computed tomography and microelectrode recordings in patients with Parkinson's disease. *Front Hum Neurosci.* **2018**, *12*, 470. [CrossRef] [PubMed]
34. Cho, Z.H.; Min, H.K.; Oh, S.H.; Han, J.Y.; Park, C.W.; Chi, J.G.; Kim, Y.B.; Paek, S.H.; Lozano, A.M.; Lee, K.H. Direct visualization of deep brain stimulation targets in Parkinson disease with the use of 7-tesla magnetic resonance imaging. *J Neurosurg.* **2010**, *113*, 639–647. [CrossRef]
35. Machado, A.; Rezai, A.R.; Kopell, B.H.; Gross, R.E.; Sharan, A.D.; Benabid, A.-L. Deep brain stimulation for Parkinson's disease: Surgical technique and perioperative management. *Mov Disord.* **2006**, *21*, 247–258. [CrossRef] [PubMed]
36. Landi, A.; Grimaldi, M.; Antonini, A.; Parolin, M.; Marina, Z.A. MRI indirect stereotactic targeting for deep brain stimulation in Parkinson's disease. *J. Neurosurg. Sci.* **2003**, *47*, 26–32.
37. Duchin, Y.; Shamir, R.R.; Patriat, R.; Kim, J.; Vitek, J.L.; Sapiro, G.; Harel, N. Patient-specific anatomical model for deep brain stimulation based on 7 Tesla MRI. Toft M, ed. *PLoS ONE* **2018**, *13*, e0201469. [CrossRef]

38. Rabie, A.; Metman, L.V.; Slavin, K.V. Using "Functional" target coordinates of the subthalamic nucleus to assess the indirect and direct methods of the preoperative planning: Do the anatomical and functional targets coincide? *Brain Sci.* **2016**, *6*, 65. [CrossRef]
39. Starr, P.A. Placement of deep brain stimulators into the subthalamic nucleus or Globus pallidus internus: Technical approach. *Stereotact Funct Neurosurg.* **2002**, *79*, 118–145. [CrossRef]
40. Andrade-Souza, Y.M.; Schwalb, J.M.; Hamani, C.; Eltahawy, H.; Hoque, T.; Saint-Cyr, J.; Lozano, A.M. Comparison of three methods of targeting the subthalamic nucleus for chronic stimulation in Parkinson's disease. *Neurosurgery* **2005**, *56*, 360–368. [CrossRef]
41. Bejjani, B.P.; Dormont, D.; Pidoux, B.; Yelnik, J.; Damier, P.; Arnulf, I.; Bonnet, A.-M.; Marsault, C.; Agid, Y.; Philippon, J.; et al. Bilateral subthalamic stimulation for Parkinson's disease by using three-dimensional stereotactic magnetic resonance imaging and electrophysiological guidance. *J Neurosurg* **2000**, *92*, 615–625. [CrossRef]
42. Pallavaram, S.; D'Haese, P.F.; Lake, W.; Konrad, P.E.; Dawant, B.M.; Neimat, J.S. Fully automated targeting using nonrigid image registration matches accuracy and exceeds precision of best manual approaches to subthalamic deep brain stimulation targeting in parkinson disease. *Neurosurgery* **2015**, *76*, 756–763. [CrossRef] [PubMed]
43. Ashkan, K.; Blomstedt, P.; Zrinzo, L.; Tisch, S.; Yousry, T.; Limousin-Dowsey, P.; Hariz, M.I. Variability of the subthalamic nucleus: The case for direct MRI guided targeting. *Br. J. Neurosurg.* **2007**, *21*, 197–200. [CrossRef] [PubMed]
44. Isaacs, B.R.; Trutti, A.C.; Pelzer, E.; Tittgemeyer, M.; Temel, Y.; Forstmann, B.U.; Keuken, M.C. Cortico-basal white matter alterations occurring in Parkinson's disease. *PLoS ONE* **2019**, *14*, e0214343. [CrossRef] [PubMed]
45. Kaya, M.O.; Ozturk, S.; Ercan, I.; Gonen, M.; Kocabicak, E.; Erol, F.S. Statistical shape analysis of subthalamic nucleus in patients with Parkinson disease. *World Neurosurg.* **2019**, *126*, e835–e841. [CrossRef]
46. Keuken, M.C.; Bazin, P.L.; Crown, L.; Hootsmans, J.; Laufer, A.; Müller-Axt, C.; Sier, R.; Van Der Putten, E.; Schäfer, A.; Turner, R.; et al. Quantifying inter-individual anatomical variability in the subcortex using 7 T structural MRI. *NeuroImage* **2014**, *94*, 40–46. [CrossRef]
47. Xiao, Y.; Jannin, P.; D'Albis, T.; Guizard, N.; Haegelen, C.; Lalys, F.; Verin, M.; Collins, D.L. Investigation of morphometric variability of subthalamic nucleus, red nucleus, and substantia nigra in advanced Parkinson's disease patients using automatic segmentation and PCA-based analysis. *Hum. Brain Mapp.* **2014**, *35*, 4330–4344. [CrossRef]
48. Welter, M.L.; Schüpbach, M.; Czernecki, V.; Karachi, C.; Fernandez-Vidal, S.; Golmard, J.L.; Serra, G.; Navarro, S.; Welaratne, A.; Hartmann, A.; et al. Optimal target localization for subthalamic stimulation in patients with Parkinson disease. *Neurology* **2014**, *82*, 1352–1361. [CrossRef]
49. Rutt, B.K.; Lee, D.H. The impact of field strength on image quality in MRI. *J. Magn. Reson. Imaging* **1996**, *6*, 57–62. [CrossRef]
50. McRobbie, D.W.; Moore, E.A.; Graves, M.J. *Prince MR. MRI From Picture to Proton*; Cambridge University Press: Cambridge, UK, 2006.
51. Edelstein, W.A.; Glover, G.H.; Hardy, C.J.; Redington, R.W. The intrinsic signal-to-noise ratio in NMR imaging. *Magn. Reson. Med.* **1986**, *3*, 604–618. [CrossRef]
52. Springer, E.; Dymerska, B.; Cardoso, P.L.; Robinson, S.; Weisstanner, C.; Wiest, R.; Schmitt, B.; Trattnig, S. Comparison of Routine Brain Imaging at 3 T and 7 T. *Investig. Radiol.* **2016**, *51*, 469–482. [CrossRef]
53. U.S. Food and Drug Administration. *FDA Clears First 7T Magnetic Resonance Imaging Device*. FDA News Release. Available online: https://www.fda.gov/news-events/press-announcements/fda-clears-first-7t-magnetic-resonance-imaging-device (accessed on 3 February 2020).
54. Pohmann, R.; Speck, O.; Scheffler, K. Signal-to-noise ratio and MR tissue parameters in human brain imaging at 3, 7, and 9.4 tesla using current receive coil arrays. *Magn. Reson. Med.* **2015**, *75*, 801–809. [CrossRef] [PubMed]
55. De Zwart, J.A.; Ledden, P.J.; Kellman, P.; Van Gelderen, P.; Duyn, J.H. Design of a SENSE-optimized high-sensitivity MRI receive coil for brain imaging. *Magn. Reson. Med.* **2002**, *47*, 1218–1227. [CrossRef] [PubMed]
56. Turner, R. Gradient coil design: A review of methods. *Magn. Reson. Imaging* **1993**, *11*, 903–920. [CrossRef]
57. Winkler, S.A.; Schmitt, F.; Landes, H.; De Bever, J.; Wade, T.; Alejski, A.; Rutt, B.K. Gradient and shim technologies for Ultra High Field MRI. *NeuroImage* **2018**, *168*, 59–70. [CrossRef] [PubMed]

58. Hendriks, A.D.; Luijten, P.R.; Klomp, D.W.J.; Petridou, N. Potential acceleration performance of a 256-channel whole-brain receive array at 7 T. *Magn. Reson. Med.* **2019**, *81*, 1659–1670. [CrossRef]
59. Setsompop, K.; Gagoski, B.A.; Polimeni, J.R.; Witzel, T.; Wedeen, V.J.; Wald, L.L. Blipped-controlled aliasing in parallel imaging for simultaneous multislice echo planar imaging with reduced g -factor penalty. *Magn. Reson. Med.* **2011**, *67*, 1210–1224. [CrossRef]
60. Wiggins, G.C.; Polimeni, J.R.; Potthast, A.; Schmitt, M.; Alagappan, V.; Wald, L.L. 96-Channel receive-only head coil for 3 Tesla: Design optimization and evaluation. *Magn. Reson. Med.* **2009**, *62*, 754–762. [CrossRef]
61. De Hollander, G.; Keuken, M.C.; Van Der Zwaag, W.; Forstmann, B.U.; Trampel, R. Comparing functional MRI protocols for small, iron-rich basal ganglia nuclei such as the subthalamic nucleus at 7 T and 3 T. *Hum. Brain Mapp.* **2017**, *38*, 3226–3248. [CrossRef]
62. Forstmann, B.U.; De Hollander, G.; Van Maanen, L.; Alkemade, A.; Keuken, M.C. Towards a mechanistic understanding of the human subcortex. *Nat. Rev. Neurosci.* **2016**, *18*, 57–65. [CrossRef]
63. Duyn, J.H. The future of ultra-high field MRI and fMRI for study of the human brain. *NeuroImage* **2012**, *62*, 1241–1248. [CrossRef]
64. Van Der Zwaag, W.; Schäfer, A.; Marques, J.P.; Turner, R.; Trampel, R. Recent applications of UHF-MRI in the study of human brain function and structure: A review. *NMR Biomed.* **2015**, *29*, 1274–1288. [CrossRef] [PubMed]
65. Van Beek, E.J.R.; Kuhl, C.; Anzai, Y.; Desmond, P.; Ehman, R.L.; Gong, Q.; Gold, G.; Gulani, V.; Hall-Craggs, M.A.; Leiner, T.; et al. Value of MRI in medicine: More than just another test? *J. Magn. Reson. Imaging* **2018**, *49*, e14–e25. [CrossRef] [PubMed]
66. Beisteiner, R.; Robinson, S.; Wurnig, M.; Hilbert, M.; Merksa, K.; Rath, J.; Höllinger, I.; Klinger, N.; Marosi, C.; Trattnig, S.; et al. Clinical fMRI: Evidence for a 7T benefit over 3T. *NeuroImage* **2011**, *57*, 1015–1021. [CrossRef] [PubMed]
67. Cho, Z.H.; Kim, Y.B.; Han, J.Y.; Min, H.K.; Kim, K.N.; Choi, S.H.; Veklerov, E.; Shepp, L.A. New brain atlas—Mapping the human brain in vivo with 7.0 T MRI and comparison with postmortem histology: Will these images change modern medicine? *Int. J. Imaging Syst. Technol.* **2008**, *18*, 2–8. [CrossRef]
68. Duchin, Y.; Abosch, A.; Yacoub, E.; Sapiro, G.; Harel, N. Feasibility of using ultra-high field (7 T) MRI for clinical surgical targeting. *PLoS ONE* **2012**, *7*, e37328. [CrossRef]
69. Kraff, O.; Fischer, A.; Nagel, A.M.; Mönninghoff, C.; Ladd, M.E. MRI at 7 tesla and above: Demonstrated and potential capabilities. *J. Magn. Reson. Imaging* **2014**, *41*, 13–33. [CrossRef]
70. Plantinga, B.R.; Temel, Y.; Duchin, Y.; Uludag, K.; Patriat, R.; Roebroeck, A.; Kuijf, M.; Jahanshahi, A.; Romenij, B.T.H.; Vitek, J.; et al. Individualized parcellation of the subthalamic nucleus in patients with Parkinson's disease with 7T MRI. *NeuroImage* **2018**, *168*, 403–411. [CrossRef]
71. Straub, S.; Zaiss, M. Pros and cons of ultra-high-field MRI/MRS for human application. *Prog. Nucl. Magn. Reson. Spectrosc.* **2018**, *109*, 1–50. [CrossRef]
72. Truong, T.-K.; Chakeres, D.W.; Beversdorf, D.Q.; Scharre, D.; Schmalbrock, P. Effects of static and radiofrequency magnetic field inhomogeneity in ultra-high field magnetic resonance imaging. *Magn. Reson. Imaging* **2006**, *24*, 103–112. [CrossRef]
73. Stockmann, J.P.; Witzel, T.; Keil, B.; Polimeni, J.R.; Mareyam, A.; Lapierre, C.; Setsompop, K.; Wald, L.L. A 32-channel combined RF and B0 shim array for 3T brain imaging. *Magn. Reson. Med.* **2016**, *75*, 441–451. [CrossRef]
74. Mao, W.; Smith, M.B.; Collins, C. Exploring the limits of RF shimming for high-field MRI of the human head. *Magn. Reson. Med.* **2006**, *56*, 918–922. [CrossRef] [PubMed]
75. Available online: https://www.ismrm.org/20/program_files/DP13-02.htm (accessed on 3 February 2020).
76. Anderson, W.S.; Lenz, F.A. Surgery Insight: Deep brain stimulation for movement disorders. *Nat. Clin. Pr. Neurol.* **2006**, *2*, 310–320. [CrossRef] [PubMed]
77. Ashkan, K.; Wallace, B.; Bell, B.A.; Benabid, A.L. Deep brain stimulation of the subthalamic nucleus in Parkinson's disease 1993-2003: Where are we 10 years on? *Br. J. Neurosurg.* **2004**, *18*, 19–34. [CrossRef] [PubMed]
78. Gielen, F.L.H. Deep brain stimulation: Current practice and challenges for the future. In Proceedings of the First International IEEE EMBS Conference on Neural Engineering, Capri Island, Italy, 20–22 March 2003. [CrossRef]

79. Aviles-Olmos, I.; Kefalopoulou, Z.; Tripoliti, E.; Candelario, J.; Akram, H.; Martinez-Torres, I.; Jahanshahi, M.; Foltynie, T.; Hariz, M.; Zrinzo, L.; et al. Long-term outcome of subthalamic nucleus deep brain stimulation for Parkinson's disease using an MRI-guided and MRI-verified approach. *J. Neurol. Neurosurg. Psychiatry* **2014**, *85*, 1419–1425. [CrossRef]
80. Chen, S.Y.; Lee, C.C.; Lin, S.H.; Hsin, Y.L.; Lee, T.W.; Yen, P.S.; Chou, Y.C.; Lee, C.W.; Hsieh, W.A.; Su, C.F.; et al. Microelectrode recording can be a good adjunct in magnetic resonance image–directed subthalamic nucleus deep brain stimulation for parkinsonism. *Surg. Neurol.* **2006**, *65*, 253–260. [CrossRef]
81. Patel, N.K.; Heywood, P.; O'Sullivan, K.; Love, S.; Gill, S.S. MRI-directed subthalamic nucleus surgery for Parkinson's disease. *Ster. Funct. Neurosurg.* **2002**, *78*, 132–145. [CrossRef]
82. Lozano, C.S.; Ranjan, M.; Boutet, A.; Xu, D.S.; Kucharczyk, W.; Fasano, A.; Lozano, A.M. Imaging alone versus microelectrode recording–guided targeting of the STN in patients with Parkinson's disease. *J. Neurosurg.* **2019**, *130*, 1847–1852. [CrossRef]
83. Frequin, H.L.; Bot, M.; Dilai, J.; Scholten, M.N.; Postma, M.; Bour, L.J.; Contarino, M.F.; De Bie, R.M.; Schuurman, P.R.; Munckhof, P.V.D. Relative contribution of magnetic resonance imaging, microelectrode recordings, and awake test stimulation in final lead placement during deep brain stimulation surgery of the subthalamic nucleus in Parkinson's disease. *Ster. Funct. Neurosurg.* **2020**, *98*, 118–128. [CrossRef]
84. Ostrem, J.L.; Galifianakis, N.B.; Markun, L.C.; Grace, J.K.; Martin, A.J.; Starr, P.A.; Larson, P.S. Clinical outcomes of PD patients having bilateral STN DBS using high-field interventional MR-imaging for lead placement. *Clin. Neurol. Neurosurg.* **2013**, *115*, 708–712. [CrossRef]
85. McClelland, S. A cost analysis of intraoperative microelectrode recording during subthalamic stimulation for Parkinson's disease. *Mov. Disord.* **2011**, *26*, 1422–1427. [CrossRef]
86. Habets, J.; Isaacs, B.; Vinke, S.; Kubben, P. Controversies in deep brain stimulation surgery: Micro-electrode recordings. In *Evidence for Neurosurgery*; Springer: Cham, Switzerland, 2019; pp. 97–109. [CrossRef]
87. Tykocki, T.; Nauman, P.; Koziara, H.; Mandat, T. Microlesion effect as a predictor of the effectiveness of subthalamic deep brain stimulation for Parkinson's disease. *Ster. Funct. Neurosurg.* **2013**, *91*, 12–17. [CrossRef] [PubMed]
88. Slotty, P.; Wille, C.; Kinfe, T.M.; Vesper, J. Continuous perioperative apomorphine in deep brain stimulation surgery for Parkinson's disease. *Br. J. Neurosurg.* **2013**, *28*, 378–382. [CrossRef] [PubMed]
89. Kleiner-Fisman, G.; Herzog, J.; Kleiner-Fisman, G.; Tamma, F.; Lyons, K.E.; Pahwa, R.; Lang, A.E.; Deuschl, G. Subthalamic nucleus deep brain stimulation: Summary and meta-analysis of outcomes. *Mov. Disord.* **2006**, *21* (Suppl. S14), S290–S304. [CrossRef]
90. Moro, E.; Esselink, R.J.; Xie, J.; Hommel, M.; Benabid, A.L.; Pollak, P. The impact on Parkinson's disease of electrical parameter settings in STN stimulation. *Neurology* **2002**, *59*, 706–713. [CrossRef] [PubMed]
91. Esselink, R.A.J.; Kuijf, M.L. Organization of Care for Patients Treated by Deep Brain Stimulation. In *Fundamentals and Clinics of Deep Brain Stimulation*; Springer: Cham, Switzerland, 2020; pp. 161–168. [CrossRef]
92. Aubignat, M.; Lefranc, M.; Tir, M.; Krystkowiak, P. Deep brain stimulation programming in Parkinson's disease: Introduction of current issues and perspectives. *Rev. Neurol.* **2020**. [CrossRef]
93. De Oliveira Godeiro, C.; Moro, E.; Montgomery, E.B. Programming: General aspects. In *Fundamentals and Clinics of Deep Brain Stimulation*; Springer: Cham, Switzerland, 2020. [CrossRef]
94. Food and Drug Administration. Guidance for the Submission of Premarket Notifications for Magnetic Resonance Diagnostic Devices. Available online: https://www.fda.gov/regulatory-information/search-fda-guidance-documents/submission-premarket-notifications-magnetic-resonance-diagnostic-devices (accessed on 3 February 2020).
95. International Electrochemical Commission. *Medical Electrical Equipment: Part 2-33. Particular Requirements for the Safety of Magnetic Resonance Equipment for Medical Diagnosis*; IEC—International Electrotechnical Commission: Geneva, Switzerland, 2010.
96. Vaughan, J.; Garwood, M.; Collins, C.; Liu, W.; DelaBarre, L.; Adriany, G.; Andersen, P.; Merkle, H.; Goebel, R.; Smith, M.; et al. 7T vs. 4T: RF power, homogeneity, and signal-to-noise comparison in head images. *Magn. Reson. Med.* **2001**, *46*, 24–30. [CrossRef]
97. Balchandani, P.; Naidich, T.P. Ultra-high-field MR neuroimaging. *Am. J. Neuroradiol.* **2015**, *36*, 1204–1215. [CrossRef]

98. Bergen, B.V.D.; Berg, C.V.D.; Bartels, L.W.; Lagendijk, J.J.W. 7 T body MRI:B1shimming with simultaneous SAR reduction. *Phys. Med. Biol.* **2007**, *52*, 5429–5441. [CrossRef]
99. Allison, J.; Yanasak, N. What MRI sequences produce the highest specific absorption rate (SAR), and is there something we should be doing to reduce the SAR during standard examinations? *Am. J. Roentgenol.* **2015**, *205*, W140. [CrossRef]
100. Ghadimi, M.; Sapra, A. *Magnetic Resonance Imaging (MRI), Contraindications*; StatPearls Publishing: Treasure Island, FL, USA, 2019.
101. Horn, A.; Reich, M.; Vorwerk, J.; Li, N.; Wenzel, G.; Fang, Q.; Schmitz-Hübsch, T.; Nickl, R.; Kupsch, A.; Volkmann, J.; et al. Connectivity Predicts deep brain stimulation outcome in Parkinson disease. *Ann. Neurol.* **2017**, *82*, 67–78. [CrossRef]
102. Schmitz, B.L.; Aschoff, A.J.; Hoffmann, M.H.K.; Grön, G. Advantages and pitfalls in 3T MR brain imaging: A pictorial review. *Am. J. Neuroradiol.* **2006**, *26*, 2229–2237.
103. Marques, J.P.; Simonis, F.; Webb, A.G. Low-field MRI: An MR physics perspective. *J. Magn. Reson. Imaging* **2019**, *49*, 1528–1542. [CrossRef] [PubMed]
104. Bekiesińska-Figatowska, M. Artifacts in magnetic resonance imaging. *Pol. J. Radiol.* **2015**, *80*, 93–106. [CrossRef]
105. Wachowicz, K. Evaluation of active and passive shimming in magnetic resonance imaging. *Res. Rep. Nucl. Med.* **2014**, *4*, 1. [CrossRef]
106. Wilson, J.L.; Jenkinson, M.; Jezzard, P. Optimization of static field homogeneity in human brain using diamagnetic passive shims. *Magn. Reson. Med.* **2002**, *48*, 906–914. [CrossRef]
107. Golay, M.J.E. Field homogenizing coils for nuclear spin resonance instrumentation. *Rev. Sci. Instruments* **1958**, *29*, 313–315. [CrossRef]
108. Roméo, F.; Hoult, D.I. Magnet field profiling: Analysis and correcting coil design. *Magn. Reson. Med.* **1984**, *1*, 44–65. [CrossRef]
109. Bitar, R.; Leung, G.; Perng, R.; Tadros, S.; Moody, A.R.; Sarrazin, J.; McGregor, C.; Christakis, M.; Symons, S.; Nelson, A.; et al. MR Pulse sequences: What every radiologist wants to know but is afraid to ask. *Radiographics* **2006**, *26*, 513–537. [CrossRef]
110. Cheng, H.L.M.; Wright, G.A. Rapid high-resolutionT1 mapping by variable flip angles: Accurate and precise measurements in the presence of radiofrequency field inhomogeneity. *Magn. Reson. Med.* **2006**, *55*, 566–574. [CrossRef]
111. Hurley, S.A.; Yarnykh, V.L.; Johnson, K.M.; Field, A.S.; Alexander, A.L.; Samsonov, A. Simultaneous variable flip angle-actual flip angle imaging method for improved accuracy and precision of three-dimensional T1 and B1 measurements. *Magn. Reson. Med.* **2012**, *68*, 54–64. [CrossRef]
112. Yarnykh, V.L. Optimal radiofrequency and gradient spoiling for improved accuracy of T1 and B1 measurements using fast steady-state techniques. *Magn. Reson. Med.* **2010**, *63*, 1610–1626. [CrossRef]
113. Eggenschwiler, F.; Kober, T.; Magill, A.W.; Gruetter, R.; Marques, J.P. SA2RAGE: A new sequence for fast B1+-mapping. *Magn. Reson. Med.* **2011**, *67*, 1609–1619. [CrossRef] [PubMed]
114. Karger, C.P.; Höss, A.; Bendl, R.; Canda, V.; Schad, L. Accuracy of device-specific 2D and 3D image distortion correction algorithms for magnetic resonance imaging of the head provided by a manufacturer. *Phys. Med. Biol.* **2006**, *51*, N253–N261. [CrossRef] [PubMed]
115. Tustison, N.J.; Avants, B.B.; Cook, P.A.; Zheng, Y.; Egan, A.; Yushkevich, P.A.; Gee, J.C. N4ITK: Improved N3 bias correction. *IEEE Trans. Med. Imaging* **2010**, *29*, 1310–1320. [CrossRef] [PubMed]
116. Zhang, Y.; Brady, M.; Smith, S.M. Segmentation of brain MR images through a hidden Markov random field model and the expectation-maximization algorithm. *IEEE Trans. Med. Imaging* **2001**, *20*, 45–57. [CrossRef] [PubMed]
117. Sled, J.G.; Zijdenbos, A.; Evans, A. A nonparametric method for automatic correction of intensity nonuniformity in MRI data. *IEEE Trans. Med. Imaging* **1998**, *17*, 87–97. [CrossRef]
118. Ganzetti, M.; Wenderoth, N.; Mantini, D. Quantitative evaluation of intensity inhomogeneity correction methods for structural MR brain images. *Neuroinformatics* **2016**, *14*, 5–21. [CrossRef]
119. Delgado, A.; Van Westen, D.; Nilsson, M.; Knutsson, L.; Sundgren, P.C.; Larsson, E.M.; Delgado, A.F. Diagnostic value of alternative techniques to gadolinium-based contrast agents in MR neuroimaging-a comprehensive overview. *Insights Imaging* **2019**, *10*, 84. [CrossRef]

120. Oliveira, I.S.; Hedgire, S.S.; Li, W.; Ganguli, S.; Prabhakar, A.M. Blood pool contrast agents for venous magnetic resonance imaging. *Cardiovasc. Diagn. Ther.* **2016**, *6*, 508–518. [CrossRef]
121. Bloem, J.L.; Reijnierse, M.; Huizinga, T.W.J.; Van Der Helm-Van Mil, A.H.M. MR signal intensity: Staying on the bright side in MR image interpretation. *RMD Open* **2018**, *4*, e000728. [CrossRef]
122. Vymazal, J.; Hajek, M.; Patronas, N.; Giedd, J.N.; Bulte, J.W.; Baumgarner, C.; Brooks, R.A. The quantitative relation between T1-weighted and T2-weighted MRI of normal gray matter and iron concentration. *J. Magn. Reason. Imaging* **1995**, *5*, 554–560. [CrossRef]
123. Barral, J.K.; Gudmundson, E.; Stikov, N.; Etezadi-Amoli, M.; Stoica, P.; Nishimura, D.G. A robust methodology for in vivo T1 mapping. *Magn. Reson. Med.* **2010**, *64*, 1057–1067. [CrossRef]
124. Beriault, S.; Sadikot, A.F.; Alsubaie, F.; Drouin, S.; Collins, D.L.; Pike, G.B. Neuronavigation using susceptibility-weighted venography: Application to deep brain stimulation and comparison with gadolinium contrast: Technical note. *J. Neurosurg.* **2014**, *121*, 131–141. [CrossRef] [PubMed]
125. Ko, S.B.; Kim, S.H.; Kim, N.E.; Roh, J.K. Visualization of venous systems by time-of-flight magnetic resonance angiography. *J. Neuroimaging* **2006**, *16*, 353–356. [CrossRef] [PubMed]
126. Barnes, S.R.; Haacke, E.M. Susceptibility-weighted imaging: Clinical angiographic applications. *Magn. Reson. Imaging Clin. N. Am.* **2009**, *17*, 47–61. [CrossRef]
127. Dormont, D.; Ricciardi, K.G.; Tandé, D.; Parain, K.; Menuel, C.; Galanaud, D.; Navarro, S.; Cornu, P.; Agid, Y.; Yelnik, J. Is the subthalamic nucleus hypointense on T2-weighted images? A correlation study using MR imaging and stereotactic atlas data. *Am. J. Neuroradiol.* **2004**, *25*, 1516–1523.
128. Aquino, D.; Bizzi, A.; Grisoli, M.; Garavaglia, B.; Bruzzone, M.G.; Nardocci, N.; Savoiardo, M.; Chiapparini, L. Age-related iron deposition in the basal ganglia: Quantitative analysis in healthy subjects. *Radiology* **2009**, *252*, 165–172. [CrossRef]
129. Drayer, B.P. Basal ganglia: Significance of signal hypointensity on T2-weighted MR images. *Radiology* **1989**, *173*, 311–312. [CrossRef]
130. Keuken, M.C.; Isaacs, B.R.; Trampel, R.; Van Der Zwaag, W.; Forstmann, B.U. Visualizing the human subcortex using ultra-high field magnetic resonance imaging. *Brain Topogr.* **2018**, *31*, 513–545. [CrossRef]
131. Marques, J.P.; Norris, D.G. How to choose the right MR sequence for your research question at 7 T and above? *NeuroImage* **2018**, *168*, 119–140. [CrossRef]
132. Chavhan, G.B.; Babyn, P.S.; Jankharia, B.; Cheng, H.-L.M.; Shroff, M. Steady-state MR imaging sequences: Physics, classification, and clinical applications. *Radiographics* **2008**, *28*, 1147–1160. [CrossRef] [PubMed]
133. Hargreaves, B. Rapid gradient-echo imaging. *J. Magn. Reson. Imaging* **2012**, *36*, 1300–1313. [CrossRef] [PubMed]
134. Tang, M.Y.; Chen, T.W.; Zhang, X.M.; Huang, X.H. GRE T2*-weighted MRI: Principles and clinical applications. *BioMed Res. Int.* **2014**, *2014*, 312142. [CrossRef]
135. Chavhan, G.B.; Babyn, P.S.; Thomas, B.; Shroff, M.M.; Haacke, E.M. Principles, techniques, and applications of T2*-based MR imaging and its special applications. *Radiographics* **2009**, *29*, 1433–1449. [CrossRef] [PubMed]
136. Haacke, E.M.; Tkach, J.A.; Parrish, T.B. Reduction of T2* dephasing in gradient field-echo imaging. *Radiology* **1989**, *170*, 457–462. [CrossRef] [PubMed]
137. Pyatigorskaya, N.; Gallea, C.; Garcia-Lorenzo, D.; Vidailhet, M.; Lehéricy, S. A review of the use of magnetic resonance imaging in Parkinson's disease. *Ther. Adv. Neurol. Disord.* **2013**, *7*, 206–220. [CrossRef]
138. Kosta, P.; Argyropoulou, M.I.; Markoula, S.; Konitsiotis, S. MRI evaluation of the basal ganglia size and iron content in patients with Parkinson's disease. *J. Neurol.* **2006**, *253*, 26–32. [CrossRef] [PubMed]
139. Keuken, M.C.; Bazin, P.-L.; Schäfer, A.; Neumann, J.; Turner, R.; Forstmann, B.U. Ultra-high 7T MRI of structural age-related changes of the subthalamic nucleus. *J. Neurosci.* **2013**, *33*, 4896–4900. [CrossRef] [PubMed]
140. Abosch, A.; Yacoub, E.; Ugurbil, K.; Harel, N. An assessment of current brain targets for deep brain stimulation surgery with susceptibility-weighted imaging at 7 tesla. *Neurosurgery* **2010**, *67*, 1745–1756. [CrossRef]
141. Haacke, E.M.; Mittal, S.; Wu, Z.; Neelavalli, J.; Cheng, Y.C. Susceptibility-weighted imaging: Technical aspects and clinical applications, part 1. *Am. J. Neuroradiol.* **2008**, *30*, 19–30. [CrossRef]
142. Ishimori, Y.; Monma, M.; Kohno, Y. Artifact reduction of susceptibility-weighted imaging using a short-echo phase mask. *Acta Radiol.* **2009**, *50*, 1027–1034. [CrossRef]
143. Rauscher, A.; Sedlacik, J.; Barth, M.; Mentzel, H.-J.; Reichenbach, J.R. Magnetic susceptibility-weighted MR phase imaging of the human brain. *Am. J. Neuroradiol.* **2005**, *26*, 736–742. [PubMed]

144. Elolf, E.; Bockermann, V.; Gringel, T.; Knauth, M.; Dechent, P.; Helms, G. Improved visibility of the subthalamic nucleus on high-resolution stereotactic MR imaging by added susceptibility (T2*) contrast using multiple gradient echoes. *Am. J. Neuroradiol.* **2007**, *28*, 1093–1094. [CrossRef] [PubMed]
145. Bot, M.; Verhagen, O.; Caan, M.; Potters, W.; Dilai, J.; Odekerken, V.; Dijk, J.; De Bie, R.; Schuurman, R.; Munckhof, P.V.D. Defining the dorsal STN border using 7.0-Tesla MRI: A comparison to microelectrode recordings and lower field strength MRI. *Brain Stimul.* **2019**, *97*, 587. [CrossRef]
146. O'Gorman, R.; Shmueli, K.; Ashkan, K.; Samuel, M.; Lythgoe, D.J.; Shahidiani, A.; Wastling, S.J.; Footman, M.; Selway, R.P.; Jarosz, J. Optimal MRI methods for direct stereotactic targeting of the subthalamic nucleus and globus pallidus. *Eur. Radiol.* **2011**, *21*, 130–136. [CrossRef] [PubMed]
147. Keuken, M.C.; Schäfer, A.; Forstmann, B.U. Can we rely on susceptibility-weighted imaging (SWI) for subthalamic nucleus identification in deep brain stimulation surgery? *Neurosurgery* **2016**, *79*, e945–e946. [CrossRef]
148. Bot, M.; Bour, L.; De Bie, R.; Contarino, M.F.; Schuurman, R.; Munckhof, P.V.D. Can we rely on susceptibility-weighted imaging (SWI) for subthalamic nucleus identification in deep brain stimulation surgery? *Neurosurgery* **2016**, *78*, 353–359. [CrossRef]
149. Bus, S.; Munckhof, P.V.D.; Bot, M.; Pal, G.; Ouyang, B.; Sani, S.; Metman, L.V. Borders of STN determined by MRI versus the electrophysiological STN. A comparison using intraoperative CT. *Acta Neurochir.* **2018**, *160*, 373–383. [CrossRef]
150. Vertinsky, A.; Coenen, V.; Lang, D.J.; Kolind, S.; Honey, C.; Li, D.; Rauscher, A. Localization of the subthalamic nucleus: Optimization with susceptibility-weighted phase MR imaging. *Am. J. Neuroradiol.* **2009**, *30*, 1717–1724. [CrossRef]
151. Eckstein, K.; Dymerska, B.; Bachrata, B.; Bogner, W.; Poljanc, K.; Trattnig, S.; Robinson, S. Computationally efficient combination of multi-channel phase data from multi-echo acquisitions (ASPIRE). *Magn. Reson. Med.* **2018**, *79*, 2996–3006. [CrossRef]
152. Weiskopf, N.; Mohammadi, S.; Lutti, A.; Callaghan, M.F. Advances in MRI-based computational neuroanatomy: From morphometry to in-vivo histology. *Curr. Opin. Neurol.* **2015**, *28*, 313–322. [CrossRef] [PubMed]
153. Shin, W.; Shin, T.; Oh, S.-H.; Lowe, M.J. CNR improvement of MP2RAGE from slice encoding directional acceleration. *Magn. Reson. Imaging* **2016**, *34*, 779–784. [CrossRef] [PubMed]
154. Tsialios, P.; Thrippleton, M.; Pernet, C. Evaluation of MRI sequences for quantitative T1 brain mapping. *bioRxiv* **2017**, *931*, 195859. [CrossRef]
155. Sun, H.; Cleary, J.O.; Glarin, R.; Kolbe, S.C.; Ordidge, R.J.; Moffat, B.A.; Pike, G.B. Extracting more for less: Multi-echo MP2RAGE for simultaneous T1-weighted imaging, T1 mapping, R2* mapping, SWI, and QSM from a single acquisition. *Magn. Reson. Med.* **2020**, *83*, 1178–1191. [CrossRef] [PubMed]
156. Choi, U.S.; Kawaguchi, H.; Matsuoka, Y.; Kober, T.; Kida, I. Brain tissue segmentation based on MP2RAGE multi-contrast images in 7 T MRI. *PLoS ONE* **2019**, *14*, e0210803. [CrossRef]
157. Kerl, H.U.; Gerigk, L.; Pechlivanis, I.; Al-Zghloul, M.; Groden, C.; Nolte, I. The subthalamic nucleus at 3.0 Tesla: Choice of optimal sequence and orientation for deep brain stimulation using a standard installation protocol: Clinical article. *J. Neurosurg.* **2012**, *117*, 1155–1165. [CrossRef]
158. Marques, J.P.; Kober, T.; Krueger, G.; Van Der Zwaag, W.; Van De Moortele, P.F.; Gruetter, R. MP2RAGE, a self bias-field corrected sequence for improved segmentation and T1-mapping at high field. *NeuroImage* **2010**, *49*, 1271–1281. [CrossRef]
159. Metere, R.; Kober, T.; Möller, H.E.; Schäfer, A. Simultaneous quantitative MRI mapping of T1, T2* and magnetic susceptibility with multi-echo MP2RAGE. *PLoS ONE* **2017**, *12*, e0169265. [CrossRef]
160. Bazin, P.L.; Alkemade, A.; Van Der Zwaag, W.; Caan, M.; Mulder, M.; Forstmann, B.U. Denoising high-field multi-dimensional MRI with local complex PCA. *Front. Neurosci.* **2019**, *13*, 1066. [CrossRef]
161. Visser, E.; Keuken, M.C.; Douaud, G.; Gaura, V.; Bachoud-Lévi, A.C.; Rémy, P.; Forstmann, B.U.; Jenkinson, M. Automatic segmentation of the striatum and globus pallidus using MIST: Multimodal image segmentation tool. *NeuroImage* **2016**, *125*, 479–497. [CrossRef]
162. Visser, E.; Keuken, M.C.; Forstmann, B.U.; Jenkinson, M. Automated segmentation of the substantia nigra, subthalamic nucleus and red nucleus in 7 T data at young and old age. *NeuroImage* **2016**, *139*, 324–336. [CrossRef] [PubMed]

163. Isaacs, B.R.; Mulder, M.J.; Groot, J.; Van Berendonk, N.; Lute, N.; Bazin, P.L.; Forstmann, B. 3 versus 7 Tesla MRI for parcellations of subcortical brain structures. *bioRxiv* **2020**. under review.
164. Somasundaram, K.; Kalavathi, P. Analysis of imaging artifacts in MR brain images. *Orient J. Comput. Sci. Technol.* **2012**, *5*, 135–141.
165. Mulder, M.J.; Keuken, M.C.; Bazin, P.L.; Alkemade, A.; Forstmann, B.U. Size and shape matter: The impact of voxel geometry on the identification of small nuclei. *PLoS ONE* **2019**, *14*, e0215382. [CrossRef]
166. Van Reeth, E.; Tham, I.W.K.; Tan, C.H.; Poh, C.L. Super-resolution in magnetic resonance imaging: A review. *Concepts Magn. Reson. Part. A* **2012**, *40A*, 306–325. [CrossRef]
167. Chen, S.Y.; Tsai, S.T.; Li, S.H. Controversial issues in deep brain stimulation in Parkinson's disease. *Towar. New Ther. Park. Dis.* **2011**, *2*, 1–20. [CrossRef]
168. Chen, T.; Mirzadeh, Z.; Chapple, K.M.; Lambert, M.; Shill, H.A.; Moguel-Cobos, G.; Tröster, A.I.; Dhall, R.; Ponce, F.A. Clinical outcomes following awake and asleep deep brain stimulation for Parkinson disease. *J. Neurosurg.* **2018**, *130*, 109–120. [CrossRef]
169. Hardaway, F.A.; Raslan, A.M.; Burchiel, K.J. Deep brain stimulation-related infections: Analysis of rates, timing, and Seasonality. *Neurosurgery* **2017**, *83*, 540–547. [CrossRef]
170. Pouratian, N. *Stereotactic and Functional Neurosurgery: Principles and Applications*; Springer: Cham, Switzerland, 2020.
171. Aman, J.E.; Johnson, L.; Sanabria, D.E.; Wang, J.; Patriat, R.; Hill, M.; Marshall, E.; MacKinnon, C.D.; Cooper, S.E.; Schrock, L.E.; et al. Directional deep brain stimulation leads reveal spatially distinct oscillatory activity in the globus pallidus internus of Parkinson's disease patients. *Neurobiol. Dis.* **2020**, *139*, 104819. [CrossRef]
172. Tinkhauser, G.; Pogosyan, A.; Debove, I.; Nowacki, A.; Shah, S.A.; Seidel, K.; Tan, H.; Brittain, J.S.; Petermann, K.; Di Biase, L.; et al. Directional local field potentials: A tool to optimize deep brain stimulation. *Mov. Disord.* **2017**, *33*, 159–164. [CrossRef]
173. Anderson, D.N.; Anderson, C.; Lanka, N.; Sharma, R.; Butson, C.R.; Baker, B.W.; Dorval, A.D. The μDBS: Multiresolution, directional deep brain stimulation for improved targeting of small diameter fibers. *Front. Neurosci.* **2019**, *13*, 1152. [CrossRef] [PubMed]
174. Budrys, T.; Veikutis, V.; Lukosevicius, S.; Gleizniene, R.; Monastyreckiene, E.; Kulakienė, I. Artifacts in magnetic resonance imaging: How it can really affect diagnostic image quality and confuse clinical diagnosis? *J. Vibroengineering* **2018**, *20*, 1202–1213. [CrossRef]
175. Brau, A. New Parallel Imaging Method Enhances Imaging Speed and Accuracy. *A GE Healthc MR Publ.* **2007**, 36–38.
176. Deshmane, A.; Gulani, V.; Griswold, M.A.; Seiberlich, N. Parallel MR imaging. *J. Magn. Reson. Imaging* **2012**, *36*, 55–72. [CrossRef]
177. Brau, A.C.; Beatty, P.J.; Skare, S.; Bammer, R. Comparison of reconstruction accuracy and efficiency among autocalibrating data-driven parallel imaging methods. *Magn. Reson. Med.* **2008**, *59*, 382–395. [CrossRef] [PubMed]
178. Blaimer, M.; Breuer, F.; Mueller, M.; Heidemann, R.; Griswold, M.A.; Jakob, P. SMASH, SENSE, PILS, GRAPPA. How to Choose the Optimal Method. *Top. Magn. Reson. Imaging* **2004**, *15*, 223–236. [CrossRef] [PubMed]
179. Griswold, M.A.; Fromm, M.; Heidemann, R.; Nittka, M.; Jellus, V.; Wang, J.; Kiefer, B.; Haase, A. Generalized autocalibrating partially parallel acquisitions (GRAPPA). *Magn. Reson. Med.* **2002**, *47*, 1202–1210. [CrossRef] [PubMed]
180. Zaitsev, M.; MacLaren, J.; Herbst, M. Motion artifacts in MRI: A complex problem with many partial solutions. *J. Magn. Reson. Imaging* **2015**, *42*, 887–901. [CrossRef]
181. Havsteen, I.; Ohlhues, A.; Madsen, K.H.; Nybing, J.D.; Christensen, H.; Christensen, A. Are movement artifacts in magnetic resonance imaging a real problem? A narrative review. *Front. Neurol.* **2017**, *8*, 232. [CrossRef]
182. Noël, P.; Bammer, R.; Reinhold, C.; Haider, M.A. Parallel imaging artifacts in body magnetic resonance imaging. *Can. Assoc. Radiol. J.* **2009**, *60*, 91–98. [CrossRef]
183. Godenschweger, F.; Kägebein, U.; Stucht, D.; Yarach, U.; Sciarra, A.; Yakupov, R.; Lüsebrink, F.; Schulze, P.; Speck, O. Motion correction in MRI of the brain. *Phys. Med. Biol.* **2016**, *61*, R32–R56. [CrossRef] [PubMed]

184. Callaghan, M.F.; Ejosephs, O.; Eherbst, M.; Ezaitsev, M.; Etodd, N.; Eweiskopf, N. An evaluation of prospective motion correction (PMC) for high resolution quantitative MRI. *Front. Neuroscience* **2015**, *9*, 97. [CrossRef] [PubMed]
185. MacLaren, J.; Herbst, M.; Speck, O.; Zaitsev, M. Prospective motion correction in brain imaging: A review. *Magn. Reson. Med.* **2012**, *69*, 621–636. [CrossRef] [PubMed]
186. Wadghiri, Y.Z.; Johnson, G.; Turnbull, D.H. Sensitivity and performance time in MRI dephasing artifact reduction methods. *Magn. Reson. Med.* **2001**, *45*, 470–476. [CrossRef]
187. Duerk, J.L.; Simonetti, O.P. Theoretical aspects of motion sensitivity and compensation in echo-planar imaging. *J. Magn. Reson. Imaging* **1991**, *1*, 643–650. [CrossRef]
188. Felmlee, J.P.; Ehman, R.L.; Riederer, S.J.; Korin, H.W. Adaptive motion compensation in MRI: Accuracy of motion measurement. *Magn. Reson. Med.* **1991**, *18*, 207–213. [CrossRef]
189. Mirzadeh, Z.; Chapple, K.; Lambert, M.; Dhall, R.; Ponce, F.A. Validation of CT-MRI fusion for intraoperative assessment of stereotactic accuracy in DBS surgery. *Mov. Disord.* **2014**, *29*, 1788–1795. [CrossRef]
190. Geevarghese, R.; O'Gorman, R.; Lumsden, D.E.; Samuel, M.; Ashkan, K. Registration accuracy of CT/MRI fusion for localisation of deep brain stimulation electrode position: An imaging study and systematic review. *Ster. Funct. Neurosurg.* **2016**, *94*, 159–163. [CrossRef]
191. Nandish, S.; Prabhu, K.G.; Rajagopal, K.V. Multiresolution image registration for multimodal brain images and fusion for better neurosurgical planning. *Biomed. J.* **2017**, *40*, 329–338. [CrossRef]
192. Doltra, A.; Stawowy, P.; Dietrich, T.; Schneeweis, C.; Fleck, E.; Kelle, S. Magnetic resonance imaging of cardiovascular fibrosis and inflammation: From clinical practice to animal studies and back cardiovascular MRI view project magnetic resonance imaging of cardiovascular fibrosis and inflammation: From clinical practice to ani. *Biomed Res Int.* **2013**, *2013*, 676489. [CrossRef]
193. Charles Stud, A.; Ramamurthy, N. Interpolation of the histogramed MR brain images for resolution enhancement. *Int. J. Innov. Technol. Explor. Eng.* **2019**, *8*, 1253–1256. [CrossRef]
194. Woods, R.P.; Grafton, S.T.; Holmes, C.J.; Cherry, S.R.; Mazziotta, J.C. Automated image registration: I. general methods and intrasubject, intramodality validation. *J. Comput. Assist. Tomogr.* **1998**, *22*, 139–152. [CrossRef] [PubMed]
195. Glasser, M.F.; Sotiropoulos, S.; Wilson, J.A.; Coalson, T.S.; Fischl, B.; Andersson, J.L.; Xu, J.; Jbabdi, S.; Webster, M.; Polimeni, J.R.; et al. The minimal preprocessing pipelines for the human connectome project. *NeuroImage* **2013**, *80*, 105–124. [CrossRef]
196. Greve, D.N.; Fischl, B. Accurate and robust brain image alignment using boundary-based registration. *NeuroImage* **2009**, *48*, 63–72. [CrossRef] [PubMed]
197. Iglesias, J.E.; Sabuncu, M.R. Multi-atlas segmentation of biomedical images: A survey. *Med. Image Anal.* **2015**, *24*, 205–219. [CrossRef] [PubMed]
198. Ou, Y.; Sotiras, A.; Paragios, N.; Davatzikos, C. DRAMMS: Deformable registration via attribute matching and mutual-saliency weighting. *Med. Image Anal.* **2011**, *15*, 622–639. [CrossRef] [PubMed]
199. El-Gamal, F.E.Z.A.; Elmogy, M.; Atwan, A. Current trends in medical image registration and fusion. *Egypt. Inform. J.* **2016**, *17*, 99–124. [CrossRef]
200. De Hollander, G.; Keuken, M.C.; Forstmann, B.U. The subcortical cocktail problem; mixed signals from the subthalamic nucleus and substantia nigra. *PLoS ONE* **2015**, *10*, e0120572. [CrossRef]
201. Alkemade, A.; Mulder, M.J.; Groot, J.M.; Isaacs, B.R.; van Berendonk, N.; Lute, N.; Isherwood, S.J.S.; Bazin, P.-L.; Forstmann, B.U. The Amsterdam Ultra-high field adult lifespan database (AHEAD): A freely available multimodal 7 Tesla submillimeter magnetic resonance imaging database. *NeuroImage* **2002**, *221*, 117200. [CrossRef]
202. Lambert, C.; Lutti, A.; Helms, G.; Frackowiak, R.; Ashburner, J. Multiparametric brainstem segmentation using a modified multivariate mixture of Gaussians. *NeuroImage Clin.* **2013**, *2*, 684–694. [CrossRef]
203. Jara, H. *Theory of Quantitative Magnetic Resonance Imaging*; World Scientific Publishing Co.: New Jersey, NJ, USA, 2013.
204. Stüber, C.; Morawski, M.; Schäfer, A.; Labadie, C.; Wähnert, M.; Leuze, C.; Streicher, M.; Barapatre, N.; Reimann, K.; Geyer, S.; et al. Myelin and iron concentration in the human brain: A quantitative study of MRI contrast. *Neuroimage* **2014**, *93*, 95–106. [CrossRef] [PubMed]

205. Harkins, K.D.; Xu, J.; Dula, A.N.; Li, K.; Valentine, W.M.; Gochberg, D.F.; Gore, J.C.; Does, M.D. The microstructural correlates of T1 in white matter. *Magn Reson Med.* **2016**, *75*, 1341–1345. [CrossRef] [PubMed]
206. Polders, D. Quantitative MRI of the Human Brain at 7 tesla. Ph.D. Thesis, Utrecht University, Utrecht, The Netherlands, 2012.
207. Deoni, S.C.; Peters, T.M.; Rutt, B.K. High-resolutionT1 andT2 mapping of the brain in a clinically acceptable time with DESPOT1 and DESPOT2. *Magn. Reson. Med.* **2005**, *53*, 237–241. [CrossRef] [PubMed]
208. Deoni, S.C. High-resolution T1 mapping of the brain at 3T with driven equilibrium single pulse observation of T1 with high-speed incorporation of RF field inhomogeneities (DESPOT1-HIFI). *J. Magn. Reson. Imaging* **2007**, *26*, 1106–1111. [CrossRef] [PubMed]
209. Dekkers, I.A.; De Boer, A.; Sharma, K.; Cox, E.F.; Lamb, H.J.; Buckley, D.L.; Bane, O.; Morris, D.M.; Prasad, P.V.; Semple, S.I.K.; et al. Consensus-based technical recommendations for clinical translation of renal T1 and T2 mapping MRI. *Magn. Reson. Mater. Physics Biol. Med.* **2020**, *33*, 163–176. [CrossRef] [PubMed]
210. Keuken, M.C.; Bazin, P.-L.; Backhouse, K.; Beekhuizen, S.; Himmer, L.; Kandola, A.; Lafeber, J.J.; Prochazkova, L.; Trutti, A.C.; Schäfer, A.; et al. Effects of aging on T_1, T_2^*, and QSM MRI values in the subcortex. *Brain Struct. Funct.* **2017**, *222*, 2487–2505. [CrossRef]
211. Milford, D.; Rosbach, N.; Bendszus, M.; Heiland, S. Mono-exponential fitting in T2-relaxometry: Relevance of offset and first echo. *PLoS ONE* **2015**, *10*, e0145255. [CrossRef]
212. Schweser, F.; Sommer, K.; Deistung, A.; Reichenbach, J.R. Quantitative susceptibility mapping for investigating subtle susceptibility variations in the human brain. *NeuroImage* **2012**, *62*, 2083–2100. [CrossRef]
213. Cronin, M.J.; Wharton, S.; Al-Radaideh, A.; Constantinescu, C.S.; Evangelou, N.; Bowtell, R.; Gowland, P. A comparison of phase imaging and quantitative susceptibility mapping in the imaging of multiple sclerosis lesions at ultrahigh field. *Magn. Reson. Mater. Physics Biol. Med.* **2016**, *29*, 543–557. [CrossRef]
214. Acosta-Cabronero, J.; Milovic, C.; Mattern, H.; Tejos, C.; Speck, O.; Callaghan, M.F. A robust multi-scale approach to quantitative susceptibility mapping. *NeuroImage* **2018**, *183*, 7–24. [CrossRef]
215. Liu, C.; Li, W.; Tong, K.A.; Yeom, K.W.; Kuzminski, S. Susceptibility-weighted imaging and quantitative susceptibility mapping in the brain. *J. Magn. Reson. Imaging* **2014**, *42*, 23–41. [CrossRef] [PubMed]
216. Langkammer, C.; Schweser, F.; Krebs, N.; Deistung, A.; Goessler, W.; Scheurer, E.; Sommer, K.; Reishofer, G.; Yen, K.; Fazekas, F.; et al. Quantitative susceptibility mapping (QSM) as a means to measure brain iron? A post mortem validation study. *NeuroImage* **2012**, *62*, 1593–1599. [CrossRef] [PubMed]
217. Fang, J.; Bao, L.; Li, X.; Van Zijl, P.C.; Chen, Z. Background field removal for susceptibility mapping of human brain with large susceptibility variations. *Magn. Reson. Med.* **2019**, *81*, 2025–2037. [CrossRef] [PubMed]
218. Fortier, V.; Levesque, I.R. Phase processing for quantitative susceptibility mapping of regions with large susceptibility and lack of signal. *Magn. Reson. Med.* **2017**, *79*, 3103–3113. [CrossRef]
219. Wang, Y.; Liu, T. Quantitative susceptibility mapping (QSM): Decoding MRI data for a tissue magnetic biomarker. *Magn. Reson. Med.* **2014**, *73*, 82–101. [CrossRef]
220. Zhou, N.; Liu, T.; Spincemaille, P.; Wang, Y. Background field removal by solving the Laplacian boundary value problem. *NMR Biomed.* **2014**, *27*, 312–319. [CrossRef]
221. Li, W.; Avram, A.V.; Wu, B.; Xiao, X.; Liu, C. Integrated Laplacian-based phase unwrapping and background phase removal for quantitative susceptibility mapping. *NMR Biomed.* **2013**, *27*, 219–227. [CrossRef]
222. Liu, T.; Spincemaille, P.; De Rochefort, L.; Kressler, B.; Wang, Y. Calculation of susceptibility through multiple orientation sampling (COSMOS): A method for conditioning the inverse problem from measured magnetic field map to susceptibility source image in MRI. *Magn. Reson. Med.* **2009**, *61*, 196–204. [CrossRef]
223. Schäfer, A.; Forstmann, B.U.; Neumann, J.; Wharton, S.; Mietke, A.; Bowtell, R.; Turner, R. Direct visualization of the subthalamic nucleus and its iron distribution using high-resolution susceptibility mapping. *Neuroimage* **2012**, *46*, 2831–2842. [CrossRef]
224. Schweser, F.; Zivadinov, R. Quantitative susceptibility mapping (QSM) with an extended physical model for MRI frequency contrast in the brain: A proof-of-concept of quantitative susceptibility and residual (QUASAR) mapping. *NMR Biomed.* **2018**, *31*, e3999. [CrossRef]
225. Chatnuntawech, I.; McDaniel, P.; Cauley, S.F.; Gagoski, B.A.; Langkammer, C.; Martin, A.; Grant, P.E.; Wald, L.L.; Setsompop, K.; Adalsteinsson, E.; et al. Single-step quantitative susceptibility mapping with variational penalties. *NMR Biomed.* **2017**, *30*, e3570. [CrossRef] [PubMed]

226. Langkammer, C.; Schweser, F.; Shmueli, K.; Kames, C.; Li, X.; Guo, L.; Milovic, C.; Kim, J.; Wei, H.; Bredies, K.; et al. Quantitative susceptibility mapping: Report from the 2016 reconstruction challenge. *Magn. Reson. Med.* **2017**, *79*, 1661–1673. [CrossRef] [PubMed]
227. Tabelow, K.; Balteau, E.; Ashburner, J.; Callaghan, M.F.; Draganski, B.; Helms, G.; Kherif, F.; Leutritz, T.; Lutti, A.; Phillips, C.; et al. hMRI—A toolbox for quantitative MRI in neuroscience and clinical research. *NeuroImage* **2019**, *194*, 191–210. [CrossRef]
228. Wang, Y.; Spincemaille, P.; Liu, Z.; Dimov, A.; Deh, K.; Li, J.; Zhang, Y.; Yao, Y.; Gillen, K.M.; Wilman, A.H.; et al. Clinical quantitative susceptibility mapping (QSM): Biometal imaging and its emerging roles in patient care. *J. Magn. Reson. Imaging* **2017**, *46*, 951–971. [CrossRef] [PubMed]
229. Fan, A.P.; Bilgic, B.; Gagnon, L.; Witzel, T.; Bhat, H.; Rosen, B.R.; Adalsteinsson, E. Quantitative oxygenation venography from MRI phase. *Magn. Reson. Med.* **2014**, *72*, 149–159. [CrossRef] [PubMed]
230. Wharton, S.; Bowtell, R. Effects of white matter microstructure on phase and susceptibility maps. *Magn. Reson. Med.* **2015**, *73*, 1258–1269. [CrossRef]
231. Alkemade, A.; De Hollander, G.; Keuken, M.C.; Schäfer, A.; Ott, D.V.M.; Schwarz, J.; Weise, D.; Kotz, S.A.; Forstmann, B.U. Comparison of T2*-weighted and QSM contrasts in Parkinson's disease to visualize the STN with MRI. *PLoS ONE* **2017**, *12*, e0176130. [CrossRef]
232. Schweser, F.; Deistung, A.; Lehr, B.W.; Reichenbach, J.R. Differentiation between diamagnetic and paramagnetic cerebral lesions based on magnetic susceptibility mapping. *Med. Phys.* **2010**, *37*, 5165–5178. [CrossRef]
233. Lönnfors-Weitzel, T.; Weitzel, T.; Slotboom, J.; Kiefer, C.; Pollo, C.; Schüpbach, M.; Oertel, M.; Kaelin, A.; Wiest, R. T2-relaxometry predicts outcome of DBS in idiopathic Parkinson's disease. *NeuroImage: Clin.* **2016**, *12*, 832–837. [CrossRef]
234. Xiao, Y.; Lau, J.C.; Hemachandra, D.; Gilmore, G.; Khan, A.; Peters, T.M. Image guidance in deep brain stimulation surgery to treat Parkinson's disease: A review. *arXiv preprint* **2020**, arXiv:2003.04822. [CrossRef]
235. Bernstein, J.E.; Kashyap, S.; Ray, K.; Ananda, A.K. Infections in Deep Brain Stimulator Surgery. *Cureus* **2019**, *11*, e5440. [CrossRef] [PubMed]
236. Vedam-Mai, V.; Rodgers, C.; Gureck, A.; Vincent, M.; Ippolito, G.; Elkouzi, A.; Yachnis, A.T.; Foote, K.D.; Okun, M. Deep Brain Stimulation associated gliosis: A post-mortem study. *Park. Relat. Disord.* **2018**, *54*, 51–55. [CrossRef] [PubMed]
237. Park, C.K.; Jung, N.Y.; Kim, M.; Chang, J.W. Analysis of delayed intracerebral hemorrhage associated with deep brain stimulation surgery. *World Neurosurg.* **2017**, *104*, 537–544. [CrossRef] [PubMed]
238. Albano, L.; Rohatgi, P.; Kashanian, A.; Bari, A.; Pouratian, N. Symptomatic pneumocephalus after deep brain stimulation surgery: Report of 2 cases. *Ster. Funct. Neurosurg.* **2020**, *98*, 30–36. [CrossRef] [PubMed]
239. Mao, Z.; Ling, Z.; Pan, L.; Xu, X.; Cui, Z.; Liang, S.; Yu, X. Comparison of efficacy of deep brain stimulation of different targets in Parkinson's disease: A network meta-analysis. *Front. Aging Neurosci.* **2019**, *11*, 23. [CrossRef] [PubMed]
240. Anderson, D.; Beecher, G.; Ba, F. Deep brain stimulation in Parkinson's disease: New and emerging targets for refractory motor and nonmotor symptoms. *Park. Dis.* **2017**, *2017*, 5124328. [CrossRef] [PubMed]

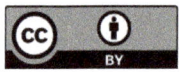

© 2020 by the authors. Licensee MDPI, Basel, Switzerland. This article is an open access article distributed under the terms and conditions of the Creative Commons Attribution (CC BY) license (http://creativecommons.org/licenses/by/4.0/).

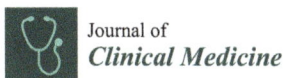

Article

Illness Representations and Coping Strategies in Patients Treated with Deep Brain Stimulation for Parkinson's Disease

Marc Baertschi [1,2,*], Nicolas Favez [1], João Flores Alves Dos Santos [3], Michalina Radomska [1], François Herrmann [4], Pierre R. Burkhard [5], Alessandra Canuto [6], Kerstin Weber [6] and Paolo Ghisletta [1,7,8]

1. Faculty of Psychology and Educational Sciences, University of Geneva, Boulevard du Pont-d'Arve 40, 1205 Geneva, Switzerland; nicolas.favez@unige.ch (N.F.); Michalina.Radomska@etu.unige.ch (M.R.); Paolo.Ghisletta@unige.ch (P.G.)
2. Nant Foundation, Service of General Psychiatry and Psychotherapy, Avenue des Alpes 66, 1820 Montreux, Switzerland
3. Service of Liaison Psychiatry and Crisis Intervention, Geneva University Hospitals, Rue Gabrielle-Perret-Gentil 4, 1205 Geneva, Switzerland; Joao.FloresAlvesDosSantos@hcuge.ch
4. Division of Geriatrics, Geneva University Hospitals, Chemin du Pont-Bochet 3, 1226 Thônex, Switzerland; Francois.Herrmann@hcuge.ch
5. Service of Neurology, Geneva University Hospitals, Rue Gabrielle-Perret-Gentil 4, 1205 Geneva, Switzerland; Pierre.Burkhard@hcuge.ch
6. Faculty of Medicine, University of Geneva, Rue Michel Servet 1, 1206 Geneva, Switzerland; Alessandra.Canuto@unige.ch (A.C.); kerstin.weber@hcuge.ch (K.W.)
7. Swiss Distance Learning University, Überlandstrasse 12, 3900 Brig, Switzerland
8. Swiss National Centre of Competence in Research LIVES—Overcoming Vulnerability: Life Course Perspectives, Universities of Lausanne and of Geneva, CH-1015 Lausanne, Switzerland
* Correspondence: Marc.Baertschi@nant.ch; Tel.: +41-21-965-76-00

Received: 26 March 2020; Accepted: 16 April 2020; Published: 21 April 2020

Abstract: There is a debate on possible alterations of self-identity following deep brain stimulation for neurological disorders including Parkinson's disease. Among the psychological variables likely to undergo changes throughout such a medical procedure, illness representations and coping strategies have not been the target of much research to this day. In order to remedy this, we investigated the dynamics of illness representations and coping strategies in an 18-month longitudinal study involving 45 patients undergoing deep brain stimulation for idiopathic Parkinson's disease. Two research hypotheses were formulated and investigated through repeated measures of ANOVAs and structural equation modelling with full information maximum likelihood and Bayesian estimations. Representations of Parkinson's disease as a cyclical condition and perception of control over the disease diminished after surgery. Use of instrumental coping strategies was not modified after deep brain stimulation. These changes were identified by SEM but not ANOVAs; their magnitude was nevertheless relatively small, implying general stability in representations. These findings suggest that psychological variables do not undergo major changes after deep brain stimulation for Parkinson's disease.

Keywords: deep brain stimulation; Parkinson's disease; illness representations; illness perceptions; coping strategies

1. Introduction

A chronic and degenerative condition without a widely available curative treatment, Parkinson's disease (PD) is characterized by a complex constellation of motor and non-motor symptoms [1,2].

Preferential treatment targets motor symptoms and consists in substitutive dopaminergic therapy. Yet, when disabling symptoms persist despite optimal medical treatment, patients may be proposed to undergo deep brain stimulation (DBS), a stereotactic neurosurgical procedure during which electrodes are implanted into strategic deep nuclei of the brain [3]. DBS results in rapid motor improvement, in some cases immediately observable after the stimulation is switched on [4]. In addition, DBS allows neurologists to drastically decrease patients' dopaminergic medication, leading to a positive impact on drug-induced motor and non-motor symptoms [5,6]. Beneficial effects on motor symptoms and medication decrease for patients treated with DBS over those only treated with medication had large size effects with a Cohen's d approaching 1.35 in both cases [7].

As illustrated by the therapeutic objectives of DBS, there is a medical focus on motor symptoms in PD that underscores the under-appreciation of health professionals and researchers regarding non-motor symptoms [8]. This factual situation is nevertheless paradoxical as, in the long run, patients consider non-motor symptoms as more disabling than motor symptoms [9]. In this regard, it should be mentioned that recent research points out the importance to consider non-motor symptoms along with motor symptoms in the development of future treatments such as closed-loop DBS [10]. Among the numerous non-motor symptoms of PD identified in the literature, some are related to mental health such as depression, apathy, anxiety, or hallucinations [1,8]. Although a leading treatment like DBS provides moderate improvement ($d \approx 0.30$) on variables related to mental health and quality of life [7], it is unsurprising that a range of non-motor symptoms remain in the patients' clinical picture even after a medically successful DBS.

The paradox of patients experiencing a medically successful DBS, objectively assessed in measuring the pre/post-operative difference of motor functioning, but nevertheless, a psychosocially unsuccessful DBS characterized by dissatisfaction regarding the everyday life was pictured as a 'burden of health' by Burkhard et al. [11]. Progressively, the concept of social or psychosocial adjustment has emerged as a pivotal theme in the post-DBS rehabilitation of PD patients [12,13]. More recently, a study has provided empirical data supporting the beneficial effects of designing specific rehabilitation programs based on psychosocial adjustment [14]. In this context, researchers have suggested that the burden of normality, a model of psychosocial adjustment initially developed for epilepsy surgery [15,16], could relevantly describe the ins and outs of psychosocial adjustment difficulties throughout the DBS process provided that characteristics inherent to PD (e.g., symptoms continuing to develop post-surgery) are taken into account [17–19]. Among the various difficulties listed in the burden of normality regarding the post-surgical adjustment process, patients may encounter psychological changes and notably feelings of self-transformation [16]. In PD, patients have indeed reported identity-related complains following DBS surgery, such as feelings of strangeness, loss of body control and dehumanization [12,20–23], which were associated with life adjustment difficulties. As patients undergoing DBS for PD expect improvement of their motor symptoms, unexpected side effects of brain surgery leading to psychological changes would constitute, in addition to adjustment problems, an ethical issue: Indeed, such involuntary changes would possibly induce more harm than benefits and therefore be experienced negatively because they are undesired [24–26]. In a recent literature review, Gilbert et al. [27] have nevertheless pointed out the lack of empirical data supporting changes after DBS in variables that could labelled 'psychological' such as personality, self-identity, agency, authenticity and autonomy. This publication has given rise to a scientific debate that is still ongoing [28,29]. Among similar psychological types of variables, neither illness representations nor coping strategies have been widely studied in the context of DBS, notably for PD.

Both illness representations and coping strategies are psychological constructs pivotal to understand the dynamics that are in play in the patients' subjective perception of their clinical condition. The common sense model [30,31] indeed posits that internal or external stimuli (e.g., appearance of clinical symptoms) generate cognitive and emotional representations of what is associated with a potential danger (e.g., an illness). These representations are addressed with coping strategies, whose efficiency in the symptom/illness management is appraised, leading to possible changes to better

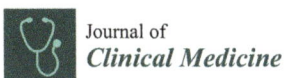

Article

Illness Representations and Coping Strategies in Patients Treated with Deep Brain Stimulation for Parkinson's Disease

Marc Baertschi [1,2,*], Nicolas Favez [1], João Flores Alves Dos Santos [3], Michalina Radomska [1], François Herrmann [4], Pierre R. Burkhard [5], Alessandra Canuto [6], Kerstin Weber [6] and Paolo Ghisletta [1,7,8]

1. Faculty of Psychology and Educational Sciences, University of Geneva, Boulevard du Pont-d'Arve 40, 1205 Geneva, Switzerland; nicolas.favez@unige.ch (N.F.); Michalina.Radomska@etu.unige.ch (M.R.); Paolo.Ghisletta@unige.ch (P.G.)
2. Nant Foundation, Service of General Psychiatry and Psychotherapy, Avenue des Alpes 66, 1820 Montreux, Switzerland
3. Service of Liaison Psychiatry and Crisis Intervention, Geneva University Hospitals, Rue Gabrielle-Perret-Gentil 4, 1205 Geneva, Switzerland; Joao.FloresAlvesDosSantos@hcuge.ch
4. Division of Geriatrics, Geneva University Hospitals, Chemin du Pont-Bochet 3, 1226 Thônex, Switzerland; Francois.Herrmann@hcuge.ch
5. Service of Neurology, Geneva University Hospitals, Rue Gabrielle-Perret-Gentil 4, 1205 Geneva, Switzerland; Pierre.Burkhard@hcuge.ch
6. Faculty of Medicine, University of Geneva, Rue Michel Servet 1, 1206 Geneva, Switzerland; Alessandra.Canuto@unige.ch (A.C.); kerstin.weber@hcuge.ch (K.W.)
7. Swiss Distance Learning University, Überlandstrasse 12, 3900 Brig, Switzerland
8. Swiss National Centre of Competence in Research LIVES—Overcoming Vulnerability: Life Course Perspectives, Universities of Lausanne and of Geneva, CH-1015 Lausanne, Switzerland
* Correspondence: Marc.Baertschi@nant.ch; Tel.: +41-21-965-76-00

Received: 26 March 2020; Accepted: 16 April 2020; Published: 21 April 2020

Abstract: There is a debate on possible alterations of self-identity following deep brain stimulation for neurological disorders including Parkinson's disease. Among the psychological variables likely to undergo changes throughout such a medical procedure, illness representations and coping strategies have not been the target of much research to this day. In order to remedy this, we investigated the dynamics of illness representations and coping strategies in an 18-month longitudinal study involving 45 patients undergoing deep brain stimulation for idiopathic Parkinson's disease. Two research hypotheses were formulated and investigated through repeated measures of ANOVAs and structural equation modelling with full information maximum likelihood and Bayesian estimations. Representations of Parkinson's disease as a cyclical condition and perception of control over the disease diminished after surgery. Use of instrumental coping strategies was not modified after deep brain stimulation. These changes were identified by SEM but not ANOVAs; their magnitude was nevertheless relatively small, implying general stability in representations. These findings suggest that psychological variables do not undergo major changes after deep brain stimulation for Parkinson's disease.

Keywords: deep brain stimulation; Parkinson's disease; illness representations; illness perceptions; coping strategies

1. Introduction

A chronic and degenerative condition without a widely available curative treatment, Parkinson's disease (PD) is characterized by a complex constellation of motor and non-motor symptoms [1,2].

Preferential treatment targets motor symptoms and consists in substitutive dopaminergic therapy. Yet, when disabling symptoms persist despite optimal medical treatment, patients may be proposed to undergo deep brain stimulation (DBS), a stereotactic neurosurgical procedure during which electrodes are implanted into strategic deep nuclei of the brain [3]. DBS results in rapid motor improvement, in some cases immediately observable after the stimulation is switched on [4]. In addition, DBS allows neurologists to drastically decrease patients' dopaminergic medication, leading to a positive impact on drug-induced motor and non-motor symptoms [5,6]. Beneficial effects on motor symptoms and medication decrease for patients treated with DBS over those only treated with medication had large size effects with a Cohen's d approaching 1.35 in both cases [7].

As illustrated by the therapeutic objectives of DBS, there is a medical focus on motor symptoms in PD that underscores the under-appreciation of health professionals and researchers regarding non-motor symptoms [8]. This factual situation is nevertheless paradoxical as, in the long run, patients consider non-motor symptoms as more disabling than motor symptoms [9]. In this regard, it should be mentioned that recent research points out the importance to consider non-motor symptoms along with motor symptoms in the development of future treatments such as closed-loop DBS [10]. Among the numerous non-motor symptoms of PD identified in the literature, some are related to mental health such as depression, apathy, anxiety, or hallucinations [1,8]. Although a leading treatment like DBS provides moderate improvement ($d \approx 0.30$) on variables related to mental health and quality of life [7], it is unsurprising that a range of non-motor symptoms remain in the patients' clinical picture even after a medically successful DBS.

The paradox of patients experiencing a medically successful DBS, objectively assessed in measuring the pre/post-operative difference of motor functioning, but nevertheless, a psychosocially unsuccessful DBS characterized by dissatisfaction regarding the everyday life was pictured as a 'burden of health' by Burkhard et al. [11]. Progressively, the concept of social or psychosocial adjustment has emerged as a pivotal theme in the post-DBS rehabilitation of PD patients [12,13]. More recently, a study has provided empirical data supporting the beneficial effects of designing specific rehabilitation programs based on psychosocial adjustment [14]. In this context, researchers have suggested that the burden of normality, a model of psychosocial adjustment initially developed for epilepsy surgery [15,16], could relevantly describe the ins and outs of psychosocial adjustment difficulties throughout the DBS process provided that characteristics inherent to PD (e.g., symptoms continuing to develop post-surgery) are taken into account [17–19]. Among the various difficulties listed in the burden of normality regarding the post-surgical adjustment process, patients may encounter psychological changes and notably feelings of self-transformation [16]. In PD, patients have indeed reported identity-related complains following DBS surgery, such as feelings of strangeness, loss of body control and dehumanization [12,20–23], which were associated with life adjustment difficulties. As patients undergoing DBS for PD expect improvement of their motor symptoms, unexpected side effects of brain surgery leading to psychological changes would constitute, in addition to adjustment problems, an ethical issue: Indeed, such involuntary changes would possibly induce more harm than benefits and therefore be experienced negatively because they are undesired [24–26]. In a recent literature review, Gilbert et al. [27] have nevertheless pointed out the lack of empirical data supporting changes after DBS in variables that could labelled 'psychological' such as personality, self-identity, agency, authenticity and autonomy. This publication has given rise to a scientific debate that is still ongoing [28,29]. Among similar psychological types of variables, neither illness representations nor coping strategies have been widely studied in the context of DBS, notably for PD.

Both illness representations and coping strategies are psychological constructs pivotal to understand the dynamics that are in play in the patients' subjective perception of their clinical condition. The common sense model [30,31] indeed posits that internal or external stimuli (e.g., appearance of clinical symptoms) generate cognitive and emotional representations of what is associated with a potential danger (e.g., an illness). These representations are addressed with coping strategies, whose efficiency in the symptom/illness management is appraised, leading to possible changes to better adapt the situation. Thus, patients' subjective representations of their illness are closely intertwined with the way they attempt to cope with the stress related to their clinical condition, as both illness representations and coping strategies are likely to be modified depending on the perceived outcome on health [30–32]. From this perspective, one may wonder whether DBS could constitute a life experience disruptive enough to elicit psychological changes in patients; such kinds of changes would besides have a potential impact on psychosocial adjustment as illness representations and coping strategies have been associated to a variety of adaptive and maladaptive outcomes in terms of well-being and social functioning [33].

To our knowledge, no research has been published on the illness representations of patients undergoing DBS for PD. Nevertheless, based on the common sense model, one might expect that DBS would bring in changes in patients' feelings of personal control over their symptoms. Indeed, in advanced PD, patients look to gain a certain degree of control over their symptoms, including motor and non-motor fluctuations, by managing themselves medication intake [12,22,34–37]. Yet, DBS requires active and regular neurologist intervention to adjust stimulation parameters to PD continuous development, which might lead patients to experience feelings of increased dependence on external intervention in their postsurgical disease management. In line with this, one may wonder whether DBS would lead patients to consider PD as more cyclical with regard to the regular search for stimulation adjustment. On the other hand, it is likely that PD would remain identified as such and associated with severe consequences despite the motor improvement brought in by DBS, as the diseased continues to develop and is frequently associated with psychosocial symptoms [20,23,38].

In contrast, a limited number of studies have longitudinally addressed coping strategies before and after surgery, yielding contradictory findings. While some found that patients use more frequently instrumental coping strategies (i.e., task-oriented responses, such as looking for information or for efficient treatment) before than after surgery [14,39,40], others noted that coping strategies were not employed differently over this period [41]. When observed, changes in coping strategies were associated with patients' situation regarding their illness. Those about to undergo surgery or who could possibly be treated by DBS in the future sought out further information on this procedure, hence a more frequent recourse to instrumental strategies. Yet, patients already operated appeared to be concerned by new life issues and, accordingly, adjusted their ways of coping; they nevertheless kept using more instrumental strategies than those not selected for DBS, who employed predominantly emotional coping strategies (e.g., avoidance, emotional preoccupation) [39,40].

In light of the above, the present study aimed to address, at least partially, the current lack of empirical data regarding potential changes in the psychological experience of patients undergoing DBS highlighted by Gilbert et al. [27]. This study focused on two specific aspects, namely illness representations and coping strategies, in patients treated with DBS for idiopathic PD through an 18-month longitudinal investigation. Taking limitations of our methodological design into account, we decided to preferentially test hypotheses underlying potential pre/post-DBS changes. Thus, based on the existing literature, we assumed that patients should consider PD after surgery as more cyclical and less controllable in comparison with the pre-DBS period (Hypothesis 1). Second, as all patients included in the study knew that they were about to undergo surgery, they should have resorted to instrumental strategies more frequently before DBS than after (Hypothesis 2).

2. Materials and Methods

2.1. Procedure

Forty-five patients diagnosed with PD and treated at the Geneva University Hospitals were included between 31 January 2013 and 8 June 2017 in a global study investigating the possible determinants of quality of life after DBS. The study procedure consisted in filling out a series of self-reported questionnaires 2 weeks before DBS surgery (T0), as well as 6 (T1), 12 (T2) and 18 (T3) months after. Inclusion criteria were a DBS medical indication for idiopathic PD collaboratively established by senior neurologist, neurosurgeon, neuropsychologist and consultation-liaison psychiatrist; a sufficient French level to read and understand a series of self-administered questionnaires; and agreement to sign a consent form. Participation was proposed to all patients clinically accepted for DBS, which includes capacity of discernment, and all participants agreed with the study procedure.

The present study received approval from the Canton of Geneva ethics committee under the registration number 14-182.

2.2. Participants

At study inclusion, patients were aged 60.6 ± 8.6 years and most of them (60.0%) were males. The majority (66.7%) had been in a couple relationship for a long time (on average 33.1 ± 13.0 years), and 71.4% had children (1.5 ± 1.2 on average). Patients had a school background of 12.1 ± 5.3 years and had been diagnosed with PD for 9.8 ± 4.0 years. Patients score at the third part of the Movement Disorder Society Unified Parkinson's Disease Rating Scale (MDS-UPDRS), a clinician-administered measurement of motor functioning standard in PD, was 21.105 ± 11.347 at T0, 11.419 ± 7.244 at T2 (corresponding to a 45.9% improvement), and 14.720 ± 6.921 at T3 (corresponding to a 30.3% improvement compared to T0). No measure was available at T1, post-DBS scores correspond to an on-medication and on-stimulation condition.

2.3. Instruments

The revised version of the Illness Perception Questionnaire (IPQ-R) [42] assesses attributes of illness representations based on the common sense model of Leventhal et al. [30,31]. This instrument proposes a self-evaluation of the main attributes defined by the common sense model, that is the identity of the illness (i.e., the observed symptoms, which may form a label—typically, the name of a disease), the possible causes of the illness, the timeline defining an acute, chronic or cyclic perception of the illness course, the consequences of the illness on daily living, the representations of the controllability or curability of the illness, the perception of the illness as a more or less coherent entity, and the emotional impact of illness representations. For the specific need of this study, we focused on two types of illness representations, namely cyclical timeline and curability/controllability.

The IPQ-R proposes scales to measure separately each of these attributes. Timeline is assessed with one scale whereas curability/controllability is evaluated with two scales (i.e., personal control and treatment control). These scales are designed with Likert-type items proposing five response possibilities (score range per item: 1–5). Test-retest reliability for the two illness representations considered in this study (i.e., cyclical timeline, and personal control and treatment control) showed mixed stability at 3 weeks (correlations from 0.46 to 0.72) and 6 months (correlations from 0.35 to 0.57) [42]. A version of the scale in French language is available on its official website (http://www.uib.no/ipq/).

The Brief COPE [43] is a questionnaire assessing 14 coping strategies with two items for each, leading to a total of 28 items. Coping strategies are evaluated using four-point Likert scales. The score range for each coping strategy is 2–8, with high scores indicating frequent use of the strategy in question. In order to investigate the use of instrumental coping strategies before and after DBS (Hypothesis 2), we created a composite variable by adding the scores of three subscales of the Brief COPE, namely active coping (e.g., item 7: "I've been taking action to try to make the situation better"), use of instrumental support (e.g., item 10: "I've been getting help and advice from other people"), and planning (e.g., item 25: "I've been thinking hard about what steps to take"). This composite variable had a score range of 6–24, with higher scores suggesting greater use of instrumental coping strategies. Like the IPQ-R, internal reliability of the Brief COPE scales was mixed with correlations ranging from 0.50 to 0.90 [43].

2.4. Statistical Analyses

After computing descriptive statistics for all variables of interest, we attempted to test our two hypotheses by a series of inferential analyses. As these hypotheses were all based on mean comparisons, we initially conducted repeated measures analyzes of variance (rANOVA). Yet, ANOVA deals with missing data through pairwise or listwise deletion, which increases the likelihood to lose information on participants notably in a longitudinal design. For this reason, we ran additional analyses with structural equation modelling (SEM), a statistical method offering better options with regard to missing data. Three nested models were built for model comparison, namely; a level model assuming no change between before and after DBS (i.e., T0 = T1 = T2 = T3); a step model assuming a change between before and after DBS (i.e., T0 ≠ T1 = T2 = T3), and; a model allowing a free slope estimation so that possible changes within post-DBS measurement times can be taken into consideration. This procedure was repeated to address each research hypothesis.

In the present study, the initial sample size ($n = 45$) increases to a potential $n = 180$ because of its longitudinal design comprising four measurement times. Although SEM is generally used with larger sample sizes, it can be applied to smaller samples starting from 30 depending on the model tested [44]. Notably, Bayesian estimation has been found adapted to small samples [45,46]. Thus, we conducted SEM analyses by comparing models estimated; first, with the traditionally used full information maximum likelihood (FIML) and; second, with Bayesian estimation of probability. In order to assess the latter, we examined the following attributes: convergence statistic (acceptable if < 1.002), trace plots stability, convergence in the comparison of first and last third of each parameter's posterior distribution, stability of autocorrelation plots, and comparison of value estimates with those obtained from FIML analyses. In addition, we provided the deviance information criterion (DIC) and the effective number of parameters (enp) in tables.

All statistical analyses were conducted with IBM SPSS Statistics version 25.0 (IBM Corp., Armonk, NY, USA) and IBM SPSS Amos version 25.0 (IBM SPSS, Chicago, IL, USA). A significance threshold of 0.05 was adopted for inferential statistics. All the data were normally distributed.

3. Results

Hypothesis 1. *We tested this hypothesis by using three illness representations variables, that is cyclical timeline, personal control and treatment control.*

First, cyclical timeline representations of PD were stable between pre- and post-DBS assessments as showed by a rANOVA, $F(2.025, 32.397) = 0.867$, $p = 0.431$, $\eta^2 = 0.020$, $\omega^2 = 0.000$. Because of sphericity violation (Greenhouse-Geisser $\varepsilon = 0.675$), we used Greenhouse-Geisser correction to interpret the analyses.

In contrast with the rANOVA above, SEM analyses showed that patients perceived PD as less cyclical after surgery than before, as demonstrated with significant global mean slope changes in both the step ($b = -1.482$, SE = 0.536, $p = 0.006$) and the free ($b = -0.556$, SE = 0.235, $p = 0.018$) models. The latter model showed a significant change between T0 and T1 ($b = 3.122$, SE = 0.523, $p < 0.001$) with an effect size ($d = 0.540$) estimated as medium to large according to the criteria of Cohen [47]. In FIML estimation, the free model obtained the best statistical fit to the data as depicted in Table 1; yet using Bayesian estimation the step model was better adjusted. Considering that the magnitude of the T1-T2 change was, although significant, very small ($b = 2.804$, SE = 0.528, $p < 0.001$, $d = 0.053$), our data suggest that the change toward less cyclical representations of PD after DBS does not reinforce but stabilizes in the later post-surgical assessment sessions.

Second, patients did not report change in their representation of personal control over PD between pre- and post-DBS assessments as showed by a rANOVA, $F(3, 48) = 0.044$, $p = 0.987$, $\eta^2 = 0.001$, $\omega^2 = 0.000$. Because of sphericity violation (Greenhouse-Geisser $\varepsilon = 0.867$), we used Huynh-Feldt correction to interpret the analyses.

In the SEM analyses, although the three tested models showed good statistical fit (see Table 2), the step model was significantly better than the level, suggesting that representations of personal control over PD decreased after surgery ($b = -1.393$, SE = 0.627, $p = 0.026$). The free model specified that this diminution had a small to medium effect size in the DBS pre-post transition ($\beta_{T1} = 1.776$, SE = 0.687, $p = 0.010$, $d = 0.267$) and continued after surgery, albeit with a much smaller amplitude, $\beta_{T2} = 2.026$, SE = 0.774, $p = 0.009$, $d = 0.039$. Bayesian analyses were adequate for all models, except for the slightly unstable autocorrelation trace plots of the free model.

Third, patients did not report change in their representations of treatment control on PD between pre- and post-DBS assessments as showed by a rANOVA, F (2.197, 35.146) = 0.1.195, $p = 0.318$, $\eta^2 = 0.001$, $\omega^2 = 0.000$. Because of sphericity violation (Greenhouse–Geisser $\varepsilon = 0.732$), we used Greenhouse–Geisser correction to interpret the analyses.

In the SEM analyses, the free model best fitted the data, as shown in Table 2, with significant mean slope change ($b = -0.312$, SE = 0.145, $p = 0.030$) and interindividual variability ($b = -1.066$, SE = 0.411, $p = 0.010$). This suggests that treatment control was perceived as weaker after DBS than before. Yet, slope estimations were not significantly different from 0 at any specific measurement session; in addition, Bayesian analyses showed that the level and step models were better adjusted to the data than the free. Overall, it implies that representations of treatment control did not undergo significant changes over DBS surgery.

Hypothesis 2. *Recourse to instrumental coping was stable over the pre- and post-DBS period, as showed by a rANOVA, F (23, 51) = 2.774, $p = 0.051$, $\eta^2 = 0.032$, $\omega^2 = 0.007$. Because of sphericity violation (Greenhouse–Geisser $\varepsilon = 0.851$), we used Huynh–Feldt correction to interpret the analyses.*

In line with this and as summarized in Table 3, the three models designed through SEM did not differ significantly from one another and were very similar in terms of fit indices. However, the Bayesian solution for the free model was not adequate, contrary to these of the level and the step. Detailed analyses of the step model showed that the global mean slope did not change significantly ($b = -0.562$, SE = 0.501, $p = 0.262$).

Table 1. Comparisons of latent growth curve models estimating growth trajectory for a cyclical representation of PD over an 18-month follow-up (T0–T3).

#	n	Mean	SD	Skewness	SE Skewness	Excess Kurtosis	SE Kurtosis
T0	39	13.564	3.307	-0.473	0.378	0.357	0.741
T1	30	11.833	3.495	0.144	0.427	-0.693	0.833
T2	20	11.600	3.050	0.065	0.512	-0.616	0.992
T3	23	12.522	3.475	-0.156	0.481	-0.277	0.935

#	Tested models	χ^2	df	p-value	χ^2/df	CFI	TLI	RMSEA (90% CI), pclose
1	Level	35.053	11	<0.001	3.187	0.281	0.346	0.226 (0.144–0.311), 0.001
2	Step	27.668	10	0.002	2.767	0.472	0.472	0.203 (0.115–0.295), 0.005
3	Free	14.880	6	0.021	2.480	0.734	0.557	0.186 (0.067–0.307), 0.036

Model comparison	$\Delta \chi^2$	Δdf	p-value	DIC	enp
1 vs 2	7.385	1	0.007	416.67	2.78
1 vs 3	20.173	5	0.001	411.16	3.78
2 vs 3	12.788	4	0.012	406.08	7.05

Note: SD = standard deviation, SE = standard error, p = probability, χ^2 = chi-squared, df = degrees of freedom, CFI = comparative fit index, pclose = probability that the RMSEA value is below .05, TLI = Tucker-Lewis index, RMSEA = root mean square error of approximation, CI = confidence intervals, DIC = deviance information criterion, enp = effective number of parameters

Table 2. (a)Comparisons of latent growth curve models estimating growth trajectory for the representation of a personal control of PD over an 18-month follow-up (T0–T3). (b) Comparisons of latent growth curve models estimating growth trajectory for the representation of a control of PD by treatment over an 18-month follow-up (T0–T3).

(a)

#	n	Mean	SD	Skewness	SE Skewness	Excess Kurtosis	SE Kurtosis
T0	39	20.026	4.374	−0.945	0.378	1.274	0.741
T1	30	18.900	4.302	−0.531	0.427	0.745	0.833
T2	20	19.300	4.256	−0.604	0.512	−0.642	0.992
T3	23	17.609	4.356	−0.209	0.481	−0.973	0.935

#	Tested models	χ^2	df	p-value	χ^2/df	CFI	TLI	RMSEA (90% CI), pclose	Model comparison	$\Delta\chi^2$	Δ df	p-value	DIC	emp
1	Level	9.675	11	0.560	0.880	1.000	1.055	0.000 (0.000–0.145), 0.648	1 vs 2	4.799	1	0.028	460.35	2.82
2	Step	4.876	10	0.89	0.488	1.000	1.232	0.000 (0.000–0.072), 0.928	1 vs 3	8.586	5	0.127	457.35	3,76
3	Free	1.089	6	0.982	0.181	1.000	1.371	0.000 (0.000–0.000), 0.986	2 vs 3	3.787	4	0.436	461.72	7.20

(b)

#	N	Mean	SD	Skewness	SE skewness	Excess kurtosis	SE kurtosis
T0	39	16.923	3.800	0.342	0.378	−0.129	0.741
T1	30	15.333	4.063	−0.986	0.427	0.826	0.833
T2	20	16.650	3.588	−0.526	0.512	−0.629	0.992
T3	23	15.739	2.942	−1.139	0.481	2.512	0.935

#	Tested models	χ^2	df	p-value	χ^2/df	CFI	TLI	RMSEA (90% CI), pclose	Model comparison	$\Delta\chi^2$	Δ df	p-value	DIC	emp
1	Level	17.399	11	0.097	1.582	0.649	0.681	0.116 (0.000–0.215), 0.152	1 vs 2	3.094	1	0.079	432.83	2.78
2	Step	14.305	10	0.160	1.431	0.764	0.764	0.100 (0.000–0.207), 0.228	1 vs 3	11.61	5	0.041	431.77	3.79
3	Free	5.789	6	0.447	2.480	0.734	0.557	0.000 (0.000–0.194), 0.516	2 vs 3	8.516	4	0.074	-	-

Table 3. Comparisons of latent growth curve models estimating growth trajectory for a cyclical representation of PD over an 18-month follow-up (T0-T3).

#	n	Mean	SD	Skewness	SE Skewness	Excess Kurtosis	SE Kurtosis
T0	42	14.000	4.283	0.274	0.365	−0.408	0.717
T1	31	13.097	3.581	0.051	0.421	−0.659	0.821
T2	24	14.333	3.795	−0.750	0.472	0.063	0.918
T3	24	13.417	3.944	−0.047	0.472	−0.875	0.918

#	Tested models	χ^2	df	p-value	χ^2/df	CFI	TLI	RMSEA (90% CI), pclose	Model comparison	$\Delta \chi^2$	Δ df	p-value	DIC	emp
1	Level	17.093	11	0.105	1.554	0.868	0.955	0.112 (0.000–0.210), 0.164	1 vs 2	1.245	1	0.265	457.12	2.85
2	Step	15.848	10	0.104	1.585	0.874	0.874	0.115 (0.000–0.217), 0.160	1 vs 3	7.326	5	0.198	457.77	3.80
3	Free	9.767	6	0.135	1.628	0.919	0.551	0.119 (0.000–0.250), 0.185	2 vs 3	6.081	4	0.193	-	-

4. Discussion

In this study, we attempted to provide empirical evidence on the question of whether DBS may induce psychological changes using an empirical, inferential approach with patients diagnosed with idiopathic PD. To this end, we targeted two specific variables, namely illness representations and coping strategies.

Based on the existing literature, we had expectations of various kinds of change that DBS would bring in as formulated in two research hypotheses. Yet, globally, our results did not provide confirmation of these expected changes. The first hypothesis, related to illness representations, was partly invalidated as PD was perceived as less cyclical after surgery than before, although patients had lower representations of personal control on PD post-surgically, this latter finding being expected. Regarding the second hypothesis, we observed that the use of instrumental coping strategies was not modified by DBS, which invalidates our initial assumption.

These results suggest that PD remains globally perceived as the same medical entity after DBS, despite the important reduction of motor symptoms induced by brain surgery. Patients' representations of control on PD decreased after surgery, and this was notably the case for personal control. The notion of control is ethically important as it is associated with autonomy, which, in this context, relates to the patient's right to decide about his/her treatment [26]. In this regard, feelings of self-estrangement reported from testimonies of operated patients were associated with the impression of losing the control over one's emotions and capabilities [48]. More generally, a loss of personal control in illness management was expected as it has been well illustrated by testimonies of operated patients [12,49]. In terms of adjustment, this is problematic as subjective perception of control over a chronic disease was associated with adaptive outcomes [33]. This association was notably established in PD patients not treated with DBS [50]. It was however surprising to observe a diminution in representations of treatment control of PD—although this was weak and suggests that, globally, perceptions of treatment control remain similar before and after surgery. One might have indeed imagined that the necessity to rely on neurologists to adapt stimulation parameters would have led to an impression that health professionals may manage the disease efficiently. Possibly related to this latter issue, patients had a less cyclical representation of PD after DBS than before. This suggests that regular appointments with a neurologist to adapt stimulations parameters are not sufficient to create a cyclical representation of PD; however, stabilization of motor fluctuations induced by DBS surgery [51] may have instilled the feelings of a medical condition having become less cyclical after surgery. Representations of PD as becoming more stable after DBS may be related to better psychological well-being, as it was measured in non-DBS patients diagnosed with PD [52].

Finally, we found that use of instrumental coping strategies to deal with stressful situations was not reduced after DBS. This result, which adds to some previous findings [41] but stands in contradiction to others [14,39,40], suggests that DBS does not deeply modify strategies of stress management, the latter being not exclusively dependent on situational issues (e.g., intensity of motor symptoms before vs. after DBS).

Overall, the findings of this study highlight the stability in illness representations and coping strategies throughout the DBS process and rehabilitation. Although significant changes were found here and there, their magnitude was generally small. The only notable exception was representations of PD as being less cyclical after DBS than before. Yet, even in this specific case, magnitude of change should be interpreted with caution. For instance, the implied mean at T0 retrieved from the free model was 13.515 and that at T1 was 11.779. As representations of cyclical timeline are assessed in the IPQ-R with four items, these means correspond to an item mean score of 3.379 at T0 and 2.945 at T1. In other words, representations of cyclical timeline remain around a mean item score of 3 corresponding to a "neither agree nor disagree" response anchor at each measurement time. Thus, even significant and with a medium to large effect size, changes in representations of cyclical timeline remain globally stable over the DBS process and should not be associated with a major alteration in patients' perception of PD. Interestingly, these small changes were all identified by a critical examination of both FIML and

Bayesian estimations in SEM, a method that does not suppress missing data from analyses; on the contrary, rANOVA analyses did not find any significant difference between measurement sessions. Methodologically, this observation implies that SEM remains discriminant with small-size samples, which is a scenario likely to happen frequently in heavy medical situations such as DBS surgery.

Our results should be considered with caution because of limitations inherent to the study design. First, illness representations and coping strategies are not representative of all psychological aspects of the DBS experience. Besides, we decided to focus our analyses on a limited number of illness representations and coping strategies, based on assumptions from the literature and methodological limitations of our experimental design; it remains nevertheless possible that other kinds of illness representations and coping strategies are significantly altered after DBS. Finally, the findings of the current study stand for patients undergoing DBS for PD; it cannot be ruled out that individuals treated with DBS for other medical conditions would experience different outcomes regarding the variables investigated in this research.

5. Conclusions

In conclusion, our study suggests that DBS does not induce major psychological changes as measured in terms of illness representations and coping strategies. These conclusions are in line with those of Gilbert et al. [27], who pointed out the lack of current empirical data showing significant changes in personality, self-identity, agency, authenticity, autonomy and self after DBS. Yet, we advocate that future studies continue exploring how psychological variables may impact the acceptation process of life with DBS. In this regard, the burden of normality model may be useful to identify and address the non-motor issues occurring after DBS in PD patients [17]. In addition, and as illustrated in a recent qualitative study [53], considering data related to psychological aspects before surgical implantation may be predictive of post-operative outcome. This implies that a complete psychological assessment taking place before surgery would help clinicians identify risks of developing post-surgical psychosocial complications.

Author Contributions: Conceptualization, M.B., N.F. and P.G.; methodology, M.B., N.F., F.H. and P.G.; software, M.B. and P.G.; validation, M.B., N.F. and P.G.; formal analysis, M.B., F.H. and P.G.; investigation, M.B., J.F.A.D.S., M.R., P.R.B., A.C. and K.W. ; resources, M.B., J.F.A.D.S., K.W.; data curation, J.F.A.D.S. and M.R.; writing—Original draft preparation, M.B.; writing—Review and editing, M.B., N.F. and P.G.; visualization, M.B., N.F., K.W. and P.G.; supervision, N.F. and P.G.; project administration, P.R.B., A.C. and K.W.; funding acquisition, P.R.B. and A.C. All authors have read and agreed to the published version of the manuscript.

Funding: This research was funded by the Swiss National Science Foundation, grant number CR31I3_149578/1.

Acknowledgments: We are thankful to Bernard Baertschi from the Institute for Biomedical Ethics of the University of Geneva for his precious advice during the construction of the manuscript.

Conflicts of Interest: The authors declare no conflict of interest.

References

1. Chaudhuri, K.R.; Healy, D.G.; Schapira, A.H. Non-motor symptoms of Parkinson's disease: Diagnosis and management. *Lancet Neurol.* **2006**, *5*, 235–245. [CrossRef]
2. Jankovic, J. Parkinson's disease: Clinical features and diagnosis. *J. Neurol. Neurosurg. Psychiatry* **2008**, *79*, 368–376. [CrossRef] [PubMed]
3. Pollak, P. Deep brain stimulation for Parkinson's disease—Patient selection. In *Handbook of Clinical Neurology*, 1st ed.; Elsevier: Amsterdam, The Netherlands, 2013; Volume 116. [CrossRef]
4. Castrioto, A.; Volkmann, J.; Krack, P. Postoperative management of deep brain stimulation in Parkinson's disease. *Handb. Clin. Neurol.* **2013**, *116*, 129–146. [CrossRef] [PubMed]
5. Lhommée, E.; Klinger, H.; Thobois, S.; Schmitt, E.; Ardouin, C.; Bichon, A.; Krack, P. Subthalamic stimulation in Parkinson's disease: Restoring the balance of motivated behaviours. *Brain J. Neurol.* **2012**, *135*, 1463–1477. [CrossRef]

6. Thobois, S.; Ardouin, C.; Lhommée, E.; Klinger, H.; Lagrange, C.; Xie, J.; Krack, P. Non-motor dopamine withdrawal syndrome after surgery for Parkinson's disease: Predictors and underlying mesolimbic denervation. *Brain* **2010**, *133*, 1111–1127. [CrossRef]
7. Perestelo-Pérez, L.; Rivero-Santana, A.; Pérez-Ramos, J.; Serrano-Pérez, P.; Panetta, J.; Hilarion, P. Deep brain stimulation in Parkinson's disease: Meta-analysis of randomized controlled trials. *J. Neurol.* **2014**, *261*, 2051–2060. [CrossRef]
8. Chaudhuri, K.R.; Odin, P.; Antonini, A.; Martinez-Martin, P. Parkinson's disease: The non-motor issues. *Parkinsonism Relat. Disord.* **2011**, *17*, 717–723. [CrossRef]
9. Hely, M.A.; Morris, J.G.L.; Reid, W.G.J.; Trafficante, R. Sydney multicenter study of Parkinson's disease: Non-L-dopa-responsive problems dominate at 15 years. *Mov. Disord.* **2005**, *20*, 190–199. [CrossRef]
10. Bouthour, W.; Mégevand, P.; Donoghue, J.; Lüscher, C.; Birbaumer, N.; Krack, P. Biomarkers for closed-loop deep brain stimulation in Parkinson disease and beyond. *Nat. Rev. Neurol.* **2019**, *15*, 343–352. [CrossRef]
11. Burkhard, P.R.; Vingerhoets, F.J.G.G.; Berney, A.; Bogousslavsky, J.; Villemure, J.-G.; Ghika, J. Suicide after successful deep brain stimulation for movement disorders. *Neurology* **2004**, *63*, 2170–2172. [CrossRef]
12. Haahr, A.; Kirkevold, M.; Hall, E.O.C.; Østergaard, K. From miracle to reconciliation: A hermeneutic phenomenological study exploring the experience of living with Parkinson's disease following deep brain stimulation. *Int. J. Nurs. Stud.* **2010**, *47*, 1228–1236. [CrossRef] [PubMed]
13. Meyer, M.; Montel, S.R.; Colnat-Coulbois, S.; Lerond, J.; Potheegadoo, J.; Vidailhet, P.; Schwan, R. Neurosurgery in Parkinson's disease: Social adjustment, quality of life and coping strategies. *Neural Regen. Res.* **2013**, *8*, 2856–2867. [CrossRef]
14. Flores Alves Dos Santos, J.; Tezenas du Montcel, S.; Gargiulo, M.; Behar, C.; Montel, S.; Hergueta, T.; Welter, M.-L. Tackling psychosocial maladjustment in Parkinson's disease patients following subthalamic deep-brain stimulation: A randomised clinical trial. *PLoS ONE* **2017**, *12*, e0174512. [CrossRef] [PubMed]
15. Bladin, P.F. Psychosocial difficulties and outcome after temporal lobectomy. *Epilepsia* **1992**, *33*, 898–907. [CrossRef]
16. Wilson, S.J.; Bladin, P.; Saling, M. The "burden of normality": Concepts of adjustment after surgery for seizures. *J. Neurol. Neurosurg. Psychiatry* **2001**, *70*, 649–656. [CrossRef] [PubMed]
17. Baertschi, M.; Favez, N.; Radomska, M.; Herrmann, F.; Burkhard, P.R.; Weber, K.; Flores Alves Dos Santos, J. An empirical study on the application of the burden of normality to patients undergoing deep brain stimulation for Parkinson's disease. *J. Psychosoc. Rehabil. Ment. Health* **2019**, *6*, 175–186. [CrossRef]
18. Baertschi, M.; Flores Alves Dos Santos, J.; Burkhard, P.; Weber, K.; Canuto, A.; Favez, N. The burden of normality as a model of psychosocial adjustment after deep brain stimulation for Parkinson's disease: A systematic investigation. *Neuropsychology* **2019**, *33*, 178–194. [CrossRef] [PubMed]
19. Gilbert, F. The burden of normality: From "chronically ill" to "symptom free". New ethical challenges for deep brain stimulation postoperative treatment. *J. Med Ethics* **2012**, *38*, 408–412. [CrossRef]
20. Agid, Y.; Schüpbach, M.; Gargiulo, M.; Mallet, L.; Houeto, J.L.; Behar, C.; Welter, M.L. Neurosurgery in Parkinson's disease: The doctor is happy, the patient less so? *J. Neural Transm.* **2006**, (Suppl. 70), 409–414. [CrossRef]
21. Hariz, G.-M.; Hamberg, K. Perceptions of living with a device-based treatment: An account of patients treated with deep brain stimulation for Parkinson's disease. *Neuromodulation J. Int. Neuromodulation Soc.* **2014**, *17*, 272–277, discussion 277–278. [CrossRef]
22. Perozzo, P.; Rizzone, M.; Bergamasco, B.; Castelli, L.; Lanotte, M.; Tavella, A.; Lopiano, L. Deep brain stimulation of subthalamic nucleus: Behavioural modifications and familiar relations. *Neurol. Sci.* **2001**, *22*, 81–82. [CrossRef] [PubMed]
23. Schüpbach, W.M.M.; Gargiulo, M.; Welter, M.L.; Mallet, L.; Béhar, C.; Houeto, J.L.; Agid, Y. Neurosurgery in Parkinson disease: A distressed mind in a repaired body? *Neurology* **2006**, *66*, 1811–1816. [CrossRef] [PubMed]
24. Baertschi, B. Intended changes are not always good, and unintended changes are not always bad—Why? *Am. J. Bioeth.* **2009**, *9*, 39–40. [CrossRef] [PubMed]
25. Baertschi, B.; Hurst, S.A.; Mauron, A. It's not who you are. *AJOB Neurosci.* **2010**, *1*, 18–19. [CrossRef]
26. Müller, S.; Christen, M. Deep brain stimulation in parkinsonian patients—Ethical evaluation of cognitive, affective, and behavioral sequelae. *AJOB Neurosci.* **2011**, *2*, 3–13. [CrossRef]
27. Gilbert, F.; Viaña, J.N.M.; Ineichen, C. Deflating the "DBS causes personality changes" bubble. *Neuroethics* **2018**, 1–17. [CrossRef]

28. Kubu, C.S.; Ford, P.J.; Wilt, J.A.; Merner, A.R.; Montpetite, M.; Zeigler, J.; Racine, E. Pragmatism and the importance of interdisciplinary teams in investigating personality changes following DBS. *Neuroethics* **2019**, 1–10. [CrossRef]
29. Thomson, C.J.; Segrave, R.A.; Carter, A. Changes in personality associated with deep brain stimulation: A qualitative evaluation of clinician perspectives. *Neuroethics* **2019**. [CrossRef]
30. Leventhal, H.; Bodnar-Deren, S.; Breland, J.Y.; Hash-Converse, J.; Phillips, L.A.; Leventhal, E.A.; Cameron, L.D. Modeling health and illness behavior: The approach of the commonsense model. In *Handbook of Health Psychology*, 2nd ed.; Baum, A., Revenson, T.A., Singer, J., Eds.; Taylor Francis Inc.: Philadelphia, PA, USA, 2012; pp. 3–35.
31. Leventhal, H.; Meyer, D.; Nerenz, D. The common sense representation of illness danger. In *Medical Psychology*; Rachman, S., Ed.; Pergamon Press: New York, NY, USA, 1980; Volume 2, pp. 7–30.
32. Leventhal, H.; Benyamini, Y.; Brownlee, S.; Diefenbach, M.; Leventhal, E.A.; Patrick-Miller, L.; Robitaille, C. Illness representations: Theoretical foundations. In *Perceptions of Health and Illness*; Weinman, J., Petrie, K., Eds.; Harwood: London, UK, 1997; pp. 19–45.
33. Hagger, M.S.; Orbell, S. A meta-analytic review of the common-sense model of illness representations. *Psychol. Health* **2003**, *18*, 141–184. [CrossRef]
34. Caap-Ahlgren, M.; Lannerheim, L. Older Swedish women's experiences of living with symptoms related to Parkinson's disease. *J. Adv. Nurs.* **2002**, *39*, 87–95. [CrossRef]
35. Gisquet, E. Cerebral implants and Parkinson's disease: A unique form of biographical disruption? *Soc. Sci. Med.* **2008**, *67*, 1847–1851. [CrossRef]
36. Haahr, A.; Kirkevold, M.; Hall, E.O.C.; Østergaard, K. Living with advanced Parkinson's disease: A constant struggle with unpredictability. *J. Adv. Nurs.* **2011**, *67*, 408–417. [CrossRef]
37. Van der Bruggen, H.; Widdershoven, G. Being a Parkinson's patient: Immobile and unpredictably whimsical. Literature and existential analysis. *Med. Health Care Philos.* **2004**, *7*, 289–301. [CrossRef] [PubMed]
38. Maier, F.; Lewis, C.J.; Horstkoetter, N.; Eggers, C.; Kalbe, E.; Maarouf, M.; Timmermann, L. Patients' expectations of deep brain stimulation, and subjective perceived outcome related to clinical measures in Parkinson's disease: A mixed-method approach. *J. Neurol. Neurosurg. Psychiatry* **2013**, *84*, 1273–1281. [CrossRef] [PubMed]
39. Montel, S.R.; Bungener, C. What relation is there between deep brain stimulation and coping strategies in Parkinson's disease? *Mov. Disord. Off. J. Mov. Disord. Soc.* **2008**, *23*, 1780–1784. [CrossRef] [PubMed]
40. Montel, S.R.; Bungener, C. Coping and quality of life of patients with Parkinson disease who have undergone deep brain stimulation of the subthalamic nucleus. *Surg. Neurol.* **2009**, *72*, 105–110, discussion 110–111. [CrossRef] [PubMed]
41. Soulas, T.; Sultan, S.; Gurruchaga, J.; Palfi, S.; Fénelon, G. Depression and coping as predictors of change after deep brain stimulation in Parkinson's disease. *World Neurosurg.* **2011**, *75*, 525–532. [CrossRef] [PubMed]
42. Moss-Morris, R.; Weinman, J.; Petrie, K.; Horne, R.; Cameron, L.; Buick, D. The revised illness perception questionnaire (IPQ-R). *Psychol. Health* **2002**, *17*, 1–16. [CrossRef]
43. Carver, C.S. You want to measure coping but your protocol's too long: Consider the brief COPE. *Int. J. Behav. Med.* **1997**, *4*, 92–100. [CrossRef]
44. Wolf, E.J.; Harrington, K.M.; Clark, S.L.; Miller, M.W. Sample size requirements for structural equation models: An evaluation of power, bias, and solution propriety. *Educ. Psychol. Meas.* **2013**, *73*, 913–934. [CrossRef]
45. Lee, S.-Y.; Song, X.-Y. Evaluation of the bayesian and maximum likelihood approaches in analyzing structural equation models with small sample sizes. *Multivar. Behav. Res.* **2004**, *39*, 653–686. [CrossRef]
46. Spiegelhalter, A.R.; Abrams, K.R.; Myles, J.P. *Bayesian Approaches to Clinical Trials and Health-Care Evaluation*; John Wiley Sons: Chichester, UK, 2004.
47. Cohen, J. *Statistical Power Analysis for the Behavioral Sciences*, 2nd ed.; Lawrence Erlbaum Associates: Hillsdale, NJ, USA, 1988.
48. Gilbert, F. Deep brain stimulation: Inducing self-estrangement. *Neuroethics* **2018**, *11*, 157–165. [CrossRef]
49. Gilbert, F.; Goddard, E.; Viaña, J.N.M.; Carter, A.; Horne, M. I miss being me: Phenomenological effects of deep brain stimulation. *AJOB Neurosci.* **2017**, *8*, 96–109. [CrossRef]
50. Evans, D.; Norman, P. Illness representations, coping and psychological adjustment to Parkinson's disease. *Psychol. Health* **2009**, *24*, 1181–1196. [CrossRef] [PubMed]

51. Schüpbach, W.M.M.; Chastan, N.; Welter, M.L.; Houeto, J.L.; Mesnage, V.; Bonnet, A.M.; Agid, Y. Stimulation of the subthalamic nucleus in Parkinson's disease: A 5 year follow up. *J. Neurol. Neurosurg. Psychiatry* **2005**, *76*, 1640–1644. [CrossRef] [PubMed]
52. Hurt, C.S.; Burn, D.J.; Hindle, J.; Samuel, M.; Wilson, K.; Brown, R.G. Thinking positively about chronic illness: An exploration of optimism, illness perceptions and well-being in patients with Parkinson's disease. *Br. J. Health Psychol.* **2014**, *19*, 363–379. [CrossRef]
53. Gilbert, F.; Cook, M.; O'Brien, T.; Illes, J. Embodiment and estrangement: Results from a first-in-human "Intelligent BCI" trial. *Sci. Eng. Ethics* **2019**, *25*, 83–96. [CrossRef] [PubMed]

© 2020 by the authors. Licensee MDPI, Basel, Switzerland. This article is an open access article distributed under the terms and conditions of the Creative Commons Attribution (CC BY) license (http://creativecommons.org/licenses/by/4.0/).

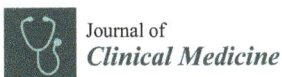

Review

Deep Brain Stimulation Selection Criteria for Parkinson's Disease: Time to Go beyond CAPSIT-PD

Carlo Alberto Artusi [1,*], Leonardo Lopiano [1] and Francesca Morgante [2,3]

1. Department of Neuroscience 'Rita Levi Montalcini', University of Torino, 10126 Torino, Italy; Leonardo.lopiano@unito.it
2. Neurosciences Research Centre, Molecular and Clinical Sciences Research Institute, St George's University of London, London SW17 0RE, UK; fmorgante@gmail.com
3. Department of Clinical and Experimental Medicine, University of Messina, 98125 Messina, Italy
* Correspondence: caartusi@gmail.com; Tel.: +39-011-6709366

Received: 15 November 2020; Accepted: 2 December 2020; Published: 4 December 2020

Abstract: Despite being introduced in clinical practice more than 20 years ago, selection criteria for deep brain stimulation (DBS) in Parkinson's disease (PD) rely on a document published in 1999 called 'Core Assessment Program for Surgical Interventional Therapies in Parkinson's Disease'. These criteria are useful in supporting the selection of candidates. However, they are both restrictive and out-of-date, because the knowledge on PD progression and phenotyping has massively evolved. Advances in understanding the heterogeneity of PD presentation, courses, phenotypes, and genotypes, render a better identification of good DBS outcome predictors a research priority. Additionally, DBS invasiveness, cost, and the possibility of serious adverse events make it mandatory to predict as accurately as possible the clinical outcome when informing the patients about their suitability for surgery. In this viewpoint, we analyzed the pre-surgical assessment according to the following topics: early versus delayed DBS; the evolution of the levodopa challenge test; and the relevance of axial symptoms; patient-centered outcome measures; non-motor symptoms; and genetics. Based on the literature, we encourage rethinking of the selection process for DBS in PD, which should move toward a broad clinical and instrumental assessment of non-motor symptoms, quantitative measurement of gait, posture, and balance, and in-depth genotypic and phenotypic characterization.

Keywords: Parkinson's disease; deep brain stimulation; selection; levodopa; axial symptoms; non motor symptoms; genetics

1. Introduction

Despite having being introduced in clinical practice more than 20 years ago, selection criteria for deep brain stimulation (DBS) as an effective treatment for advanced Parkinson's disease (PD) still rely on the 'Core Assessment Program for Surgical Interventional Therapies in Parkinson's Disease' (CAPSIT-PD) published in 1999 [1]. These criteria were primarily designed to facilitate clinical research, harmonizing the cohorts of clinical trials. However, most of the indications provided in the CAPSIT-PD document were introduced as guidance into the clinical practice of DBS centers worldwide, being extremely useful in supporting the selection of candidates [2]. Twenty years later, these indications could be considered both restrictive and out-of-date, because the knowledge on PD progression, phenotyping, and genotyping has strongly evolved over the last 20 years. Indeed, according to CAPSIT-PD, only 1.6% of PD subjects would be eligible for DBS, rising to 4.5% when applying more flexible criteria [3].

Moreover, a growing number of studies have reported novel data on the outcome of DBS in the short- and long-term follow-up and proposed predictors of DBS response [4,5]. However, evidence on how to improve and refine the selection process based on these insights for candidates to DBS is still lacking. Finally, despite the consolidated efficacy of DBS in improving PD cardinal symptoms and motor complications, the factors predicting a successful outcome on activities of daily living (ADL) and quality of life (QoL) have been addressed only by a few studies so far [6].

Advances in understanding the heterogeneity of PD presentation, courses, phenotypes, and genotypes impose a better identification of DBS candidates as a research priority. Additionally, DBS invasiveness, cost, and the possibility of serious adverse events make it mandatory to predict as accurately as possible the clinical outcome when informing the patients about their suitability for surgery.

Here, we appraised the DBS pre-surgical assessment for PD starting from the original CAPSIT-PD document and addressed the following topics which may impact on the selection process: early versus delayed DBS; the evolution of the levodopa challenge test; the relevance of axial symptoms; new focus on patient-centered outcome measures; the relevance of non-motor symptoms; and a new role for genetics. Our main aim was to highlight current pitfalls and potentialities in the DBS selection process, stimulating future randomized control trials (RCT) to address specific needs.

2. Early Versus Delayed DBS: How Early?

2.1. The Standard Rule

The CAPSIT-PD document recommended that a patient considered for interventional surgery should have a diagnosis of idiopathic PD and a minimum disease duration of five years [1]. These requirements were developed to exclude people with atypical parkinsonism, given the absence of benefits and the risk to harm patients with no idiopathic PD [7].

2.2. Pros and Cons

The concept of a five-year disease duration has been challenged upon the results of a large RCT published in 2013 (the EARLY-STIM trial) [8]. In this trial demonstrating the superiority of subthalamic (STN) DBS compared to medical therapy alone, patients were included when having a PD diagnosis of ≥4 years, and fluctuations or dyskinesia present for four years or less [8].

The EARLY-STIM trial endorsed a conceptual change about the use of DBS for PD favoring a paradigm shift from DBS as the last therapeutic option for advanced disease stages toward an earlier approach for patients experiencing motor complications. This paradigm change is based on three relevant points: (1) the confirmation of DBS safety over the years, even in the long term; (2) the great efficacy of DBS in improving the QoL of patients, even superior to levodopa alone [9]; (3) an earlier intervention could preserve functional capacity. The evidence of efficacy provided by the EARLY-STIM trial led the U.S. Food and Drug Administration (FDA) to extend the DBS indication to patients with a four year PD diagnosis in the presence of at least four months of uncontrolled motor complications [10].

The EARLY-STIM trial has triggered discussion as to whether its findings should be translated into clinical practice [11]. Firstly, the shorter disease duration at the time of surgery might pose the risks of including subjects with atypical parkinsonism for which the five-year rule has been developed for CAPSIT-PD. However, in the EARLY-STIM cohort, the mean disease duration of the surgically-treated group was 7.3 ± 3.1 years and only three cases (0.8% of the cohort) were re-diagnosed as non-idiopathic PD eight years after the first randomization and approximately 15 years after diagnosis [12]. However, it should be noted that the issue of a shorter disease duration at the time of surgery might mirror a greater and faster burden of disability which is also associated with specific genotypes associated to PD, such as severe and complex glucocerobrosidase (*GBA*) gene variants [13], which have been associated to poor DBS functional outcome [14].

A related matter is the difficulty in predicting the trajectory of disease progression at such an early stage, either for more benign or rapidly progressing phenotypes [15], with the consequent risk of referring to surgery patients whose motor fluctuations could remain mild for a long time, or vice-versa, those who may develop symptoms non-responsive to DBS and severely impacting ADL and QoL.

However, when looking carefully into the EARLY-STIM cohort, all patients had experienced either motor or psychiatric disability due to PD. Accordingly, further analyses on this population have demonstrated that STN-DBS was successful in improving freezing of gait (FoG) in OFF medication condition [16], which affected 52% of the patients at baseline. Remarkably, behavioral complications linked to dopaminergic overmedication had a better outcome in the neurostimulation group [17].

How early should DBS be considered in PD? A pilot open label study on 28 patients suggested to consider DBS even earlier, before motor complications arose [18]. However, despite long term follow-up data on the same cohort [19], the impact of early surgical intervention in such earlier stages is still unknown and should be carefully interpreted including the risks we mentioned above but also a presumptive neuroprotective effect [20]. Finally, it should be taken into account that DBS (STN-DBS in particular) allows a reduction in dose of dopaminergic therapies in most patients [21]. Although favoring the improvement of dyskinesia, the reduction in antiparkinsonian drugs could have role in improving impulsive-compulsive behaviors and obsessive-compulsive and paranoid traits [22,23].

2.3. Recommendations

There is evidence for an earlier use of DBS as a treatment option to improve patients' QoL and early levodopa-responsive axial symptoms, while minimizing the psychiatric consequences of overtreatment. Long-term results from the EARLY-STIM trial would allow the better defining of which PD features are associated to a long-term successful outcome. However, there is not enough knowledge on how early into the disease history DBS should be considered, given the paucity of published data and the current lack of knowledge on how to predict disease progression and DBS response in such early stages. We recommend considering each case singularly, according to the patient's phenotype, age, needs, and expectations in patients whose symptoms significantly impact ADL and QoL despite a reasonable number of attempts to provide the best medical therapy.

3. The Evolution of the Levodopa Challenge Test

3.1. The Standard Rule

The second recommendation of CAPSIT-PD is dopaminergic responsiveness confirmed by a levodopa/apomorphine challenge test (LCT). Accordingly, the test has to demonstrate at least a 33% decrease in the Unified Parkinson's Disease Rating Scale (UPDRS) part III score in the "defined-on condition" (best therapeutic effect after medication agreed by patient and physician) compared to the "defined-off condition" (at least 12 h after receiving the last medication dose).

3.2. Pros and Cons

The threshold of 33% for UPDRS improvement is considered relevant to rule out possible misdiagnoses (i.e., identifying atypical parkinsonism for which DBS is not recommended). The LCT is also important to inform the possible outcome of surgery, showing the likely extent of symptom improvement after surgery, and to establish realistic expectations from DBS [24]. Indeed, it is generally accepted that symptoms improving with levodopa are likely to respond to DBS [25]. However, there are some exceptions and caveats to these widely accepted concepts. Firstly, levodopa-resistant tremor represents one of the indications of DBS, even in the absence of disabling motor fluctuations [26,27], given its excellent effect in controlling or even suppressing tremors, regardless of the deep nuclei targeted [28].

Another relevant challenge related to the LCT is the cut-off of 33%. This value has been validated by a study based on its ability to predict chronic levodopa responsiveness, with a positive predictive value for the PD diagnosis of 88.6% [29]. Notably, the Movement Disorders Society (MDS)-sponsored UPDRS scale introduced in 2008 has some differences in the scoring of the part-III (motor part), and a study analyzing the MDS-UPDRS scores with the old UPDRS [30] ones after an acute LCT found an excellent correlation between the two scales, with the 30% UPDRS score variation used for predicting sustained long-term levodopa response equivalent to 24% in MDS-UPDRS [31]. However, data from STN-DBS clinical trials seems to indicate that an excellent response to levodopa (i.e., >50% UPDRS part-III improvement) could be associated with a better DBS motor outcome [32]. A meta-analysis published in 2006 on the STN-DBS outcomes supports this hypothesis, demonstrating that the magnitude of decrease in both UPDRS part-II and part-III scores exhibits a dose–response relationship with the presurgical response to the levodopa challenge test [33]. However, it is unknown whether the magnitude of response at the LCT may predict better ADL and Qol after DBS. Moreover, the relevance of axial symptoms as a source of disability, their heterogenous response to dopaminergic therapies, and their influence on the trajectory of the PD course put in light further considerations on the usefulness of the presurgical LCT simplistically considered as a >30% motor response.

3.3. Recommendations

We recommend using LCT as a key tool to obtain relevant presurgical information on the patient's status and the possibility of improvement after DBS. However, the rule of UPDRS part-III improvement >30% should not be strictly applied. Although patients affected by disabling dopa-resistant tremor could represent an exception to this rule, improvement >50% can be associated with greater overall benefit in most patients. The LCT response of disabling axial symptoms, such as FoG, is important and should be weighted independently from the percentage UPDRS part-III total score improvement.

4. The Relevance of Axial Symptoms: How Sensitive Is Current Clinical Assessment?

4.1. The Standard Rule

The term 'axial symptoms' is commonly referred to as a group of PD motor features encompassing gait impairment, postural instability, postural abnormalities, and speech disorders, especially dysarthria and stuttering. These are a major source of disability because they are associated with reduced mobility, communication difficulties, recurrent falls, and subsequent injuries [34]. Moreover, they are markers of advanced disease and are often resistant to dopaminergic therapies or exhibit an heterogenous pattern of response to levodopa [35]. There are no precise indications on how to consider these symptoms and their pre-surgical response to levodopa in the clinical practice.

4.2. Pros and Cons

The evidence on the effect of DBS on axial symptoms is controversial. A meta-analysis published in 2004 showed that one year after surgery, STN-DBS or globus pallidus pars interna (GPi) DBS can improve gait and balance symptoms, with an effect size similar to the preoperative effects of dopaminergic medication [36]. However, the improvement provided by DBS seems not sustained over the years. Evidence for axial symptom progression, despite a good control of PD appendicular motor symptoms, has been shown in open-label, long-term follow-up studies, although some extent of axial improvement related to stimulation is reported in the first years after surgery [37–40].

The relevance of axial symptoms as a marker of disease progression was disclosed in a cohort of 143 PD patients treated with STN-DBS [5], in whom axial disability during the follow-up period was strongly associated with an increased risk of death (hazard ratio of 4.3), proving to be the most accurate mortality predictor, even superior to the cognitive status.

Axial symptoms track disease progression and disability, therefore an accurate presurgical evaluation of levodopa-responsiveness would be necessary for estimating the extent of response after DBS. Indeed, worsening or amelioration after DBS of speech, posture and gait disorders is multifactorial and depends upon clinical variables such as disease duration [16,41], the type of axial symptom (gait often improves after DBS, speech may worsen as a stimulus-related side effect), their interplay with dopaminergic medications [42,43], the brain target employed for DBS, the frequency [44,45] and distribution of stimulation [46], and placement of active electrode contact [41].

Levodopa-resistant axial symptoms are considered a relative contraindication for surgery [47]; however, the current pre-surgical clinical examination is unable to detect early axial signs which may foster worse DBS outcomes. In particular, FoG evaluation poses great challenges, given the episodic nature of this phenomenon and the complex relationship with dopaminergic medications. Trunk postural abnormalities also represent a source of difficulty at the time of DBS selection (including on which target to choose), because camptocormia and Pisa syndrome might be responsive to STN-DBS, even with poor or no amelioration after LCT [48,49].

These difficulties which impact on the selection process might be overcome by integrating objective evaluation involving kinematic analysis and wearable sensors to the pre-operative clinical examination. Specifically, novel technological developments on wearable sensors for home-monitoring have the potential to provide a measure of axial symptoms and their relation to levodopa intake in a naturalistic way [50,51]. These technologies should be employed to detect early axial signs which might predict worsening after DBS and assist the identification of the best candidates. Indeed, a study employing kinematic assessment of gait demonstrated a correlation between presurgical levodopa response of stride length and range of motion and FoG outcome after DBS [52].

4.3. Recommendations

The global burden of axial symptoms can be considered a proxy for disease stage because of their correlation with disability and death. A fine-grained assessment of each axial symptom, the accurate evaluation of their relationship with dopaminergic therapy, and the integration of technology outcome measures into the clinical practice should favor a better understanding of candidates to DBS, with the potential to predict their disease course and the probability to improve after DBS. Pending clinical trials aiming at the evaluation of the effect of DBS on PD-related axial symptoms, we recommend to accurately evaluate in clinical practice the presence, severity, and impact on patient's daily life and independence of axial symptoms before surgery, and discuss the weight of each symptom with the patient, clarifying its poor, good, or indeterminate probability of improvement after DBS. Severe FoG and speech issues, in particular, represent a potential challenge in the management of patients undergoing DBS, while camptocormia and Pisa syndrome could have good chances of improvement and should not be considered contraindications for DBS.

5. The Need for Patient-Centered Outcome Measures

5.1. The Standard Rule

From a regulatory point of view, the FDA and European Medicine Agency (EMA) request the presence of motor fluctuations as a mandatory criterion for DBS indication in PD [10]. Reduction in severity and frequency of motor fluctuations represents one of the most relevant achievements obtained by DBS, which translates into the improvement of QoL revealed by randomized controlled trials [8,53].

5.2. Pros and Cons

In CAPSIT-PD, it is recommended that the patients perform the self-reporting diary one week per month during the three preoperative months, indicating the presence of four conditions: complete OFF, partial OFF, complete ON, and ON with dyskinesias [1]. However, these measures are highly subjective, and wrong or missed entries may occur in about one third of cases—also when using electronic motor diaries [54]. That is, objective home-based quantification by wearable sensors of PD motor symptoms [55], including FoG [56], should be explored carefully in patients considered for DBS, also with respect to the predictive value of these measures. Indeed, when it comes to predicting the outcome of DBS in PD and patient-centered outcome measures are employed, some discrepancies arise. Patient-centered outcome measures are represented by QoL, evaluated by the validated Parkinson's Disease Questionnaire 39 (PDQ-39) [57] or by its short form (PDQ-8) [58], and ADL functioning or independence, typically measured by UPDRS part-II and the Schwab and England (S&E) scale [59]. The importance of measuring patient-centered outcomes relates to the discrepancy between the judgment made in-clinic by the neurologist and the degree of satisfaction [60] and independence obtained by the patient during daily life [54]. Two key factors may account for this discrepancy: (1) motor symptoms observed by clinicians explain only a small part of the complex picture of PD, which encompasses several non-motor symptoms; (2) the standardized tasks assessed during in-clinic visits and the non-quantitative, non-continuous, non-ecologic in-clinic examinations may not represent a comprehensive measure of the patient situation and condition during daily life. This last aspect is true even when limiting the evaluation to motor symptoms, in particular episodic motor symptoms such as FoG [61], which are not adequately captured during in-clinic standard assessments [54].

When it comes to analyzing determinants of improvement in QoL after STN DBS, a post-hoc analysis of the EARLY-STIM trial found smaller QoL improvement at 24-months follow-up in patients with better pre-surgical PDQ-39 scores [6]. Interestingly, patients with pre-surgical PDQ-39 scores ≤ 15 had no significant change in QoL following surgery. This finding is not meant to be caused by a ceiling effect of STN-DBS to improve motor symptoms in the EARLY-STIM cohort, because the change in QoL over the two years was independent of the severity of parkinsonian motor signs assessed by UPDRS-III [8]. Accordingly, in another study analyzing a cohort of 85 PD patients treated with DBS, the magnitude of motor symptom improvement with a pre-surgical LCT was only borderline associated with improvement of QoL after DBS ($p = 0.053$) [62].

A systematic review [63] demonstrated that higher baseline QoL predicted larger QoL changes after surgery in three out of four studies. The analysis of the 18 studies included in this review yielded mixed results with respect to the predictive value of other clinical and demographical features. There are two main explanations for such discrepant findings: (1) most of these studies were not primarily designed to detect predictors of QoL change after DBS and results are influenced by the main a priori hypothesis tested in each study; (2) factors contributing to QoL in PD include not only motor disability but also non-motor symptoms [64], and the interplay between these domains might be individualized and have a different weight in each subject. Moreover, among motor symptoms, axial disability (and its response to therapies) might have a high impact, which has not been yet explored carefully in regard to QoL or ADL outcome after DBS.

5.3. Recommendations

Future studies should be designed to capture predictors of QoL and ADL improvements after DBS, taking into account the heterogeneity of the disease, the contribution of non-motor symptoms, and the impact of axial symptoms. We recommend evaluating both the ADL and QoL of candidates for DBS by means of validated scales (e.g., UPDRS part-II and PDQ-39 or PDQ-8) and carefully discuss with patients the disease burden and their determinants. After surgery, these scales can inform more than the in-clinic motor assessment about the clinical status of the patient and the impact of stimulation on their functioning in daily life, guiding possible changes in stimulation parameters, medical therapy or non-medical interventions, such as psychological support, physiotherapy, and emotional and social stimulation.

6. The Complexity of PD Spectrum Integrated into the Selection Process: Relevance of Non-Motor Symptoms

6.1. The Standard Rule

Despite the fact that DBS was developed to treat motor symptoms, the growing relevance given to non-motor symptoms (NMS) in the last 15 years fostered investigations into the effect of DBS for these features as well [65,66]. There are no indications nor clues so far on how to consider the presence and burden of non-motor symptoms in PD candidates for DBS.

6.2. Pros and Cons

A few studies have demonstrated the improvement of different NMS (cardiovascular, sleep/fatigue, perceptual problems/hallucinations, gastrointestinal, urinary, and miscellaneous domains) six months after surgery [65], which were maintained at 24 months for the sleep/fatigue, urinary and miscellaneous domains [66], and at 36 months for the sleep domain [67]. These findings were confirmed in a small cohort of young onset PD patients, for whom STN-DBS provided sustained improvement of the sleep domain of the Non-Motor Symptoms Scale and Parkinson's disease sleep scale-2 up to 24 months and correlated to the decrease in dopamine-agonist medication [68].

Remarkably, change in NMS frequency and severity after STN-DBS is strongly correlated to the improvement in QoL both in uncontrolled [66] and controlled studies [67,69] performed in the same STN-treated cohort at different follow-up.

In the attempt to define profiles for the best DBS candidates which may encompass the complexity of PD clinical spectrum and its heterogeneity, a new data-driven approach to PD, supported by biomarkers and neuropathology, disclosed three different PD subtypes: mild-motor predominant, intermediate, and diffuse malignant [70,71]. These three groups, defined based on the progression of disability and mortality, differ in the presentation of motor and non-motor symptoms at onset, in particular for the contribution of three types of NMS: cognitive impairment, rapid eye movement sleep behavior disorder, and dysautonomia. When the same subtyping criteria were applied to a cohort of STN-DBS patients at the time of the surgical selection, the mild phenotype seem to perform better on ADL independence at the short and long-term follow-up compared to the malignant phenotype, despite similar efficacy of stimulation on motor symptoms, fluctuations, and ambulatory capacity [72].

6.3. Recommendations

More efforts are needed to understand which NMS are predictors of good or poor outcome, how different targets of DBS (STN or GPi) should be indicated to treat different NMS based on the ability to decrease total LEDD and dopamine-agonists LEDD [17], or directly treat particular symptoms by means of the stimulation of specific networks involved in pain or mood, apathy and attention [73]. We recommend to carefully assess the presence and severity of non-motor symptoms before surgery and explain to the patients that when the disease burden is mainly driven by non-motor symptoms, DBS might not be the best therapeutic option to consider.

7. A New Role for Genetics

7.1. The Standard Rule

One of the most remarkable advances in our understanding of PD pathogenesis in the last 20 years is represented by genetics. The increasing power of genetic analyses led to the identification of several chromosomal loci that cause or modulate the risk for PD [74]. Moreover, specific genetic mutations have been associated to specific clinical features and different disease courses, which could have an impact on the selection for DBS.

That is, only some evidence on the differential DBS response in different forms of monogenic PD has been put forward, suggesting some differences in the magnitude of response [14,75–77]. However, in this case there are no specific recommendations on the use of genetics in the clinical practice of DBS centers.

7.2. Pros and Cons

The main advantage of knowing the genotype of a PD patient appraised for DBS is related to the knowledge of disease evolution associated to a particular gene variant. However, despite the effort of systematic reviews [76,77] and one meta-analysis [14], the small size of the cohorts reported and the paucity of data on different gene variants and brain targets other than STN, do not allow researchers to reach firm conclusions. For example, *LRRK2*-G2019S variant carriers, described in 44 out of 50 *LRRK2* subjects with DBS reported in the literature, show an excellent response to STN DBS, which is also the most reported target [76]. G2019S is the most frequent *LRRK2* variant and produces a phenotype overlapping to late-onset, non-mutated PD with frequent presence of tremor and good response to dopaminergic medications [78]. However, in three out of four reported cases with *LRRK2*-R1441G variant, a mutation variant rarely found outside northern Spain, poor response to STN-DBS was reported [76]. The paucity of data characterizing the phenotype of *LRRK2*-R1441G variant makes it impossible to assume that the poor DBS outcome was due to more severe disease progression and development of DBS resistant features. A similar issue applies to carriers of glucocerebrosidase (*GBA*) gene variants which have a high prevalence of neuropsychiatric symptoms, especially impulsive compulsive behavior and hallucinations, and a higher risk to develop early over disease course cognitive disturbances [13]. Indeed, *GBA*-associated PD showed worse cognitive and functional performances and lower reductions in dopaminergic medication after surgery [14]. However, it is unknown which variants mostly contribute to this result. Remarkably, the risk of hallucinations and cognitive impairment, as well as survival, differs across *GBA* subjects, being higher in subjects carrying complex and severe variants [13,79].

7.3. Recommendations

Genetic testing is becoming accessible and affordable in clinical practice in many countries and may be used to inform PD candidates for their suitability for DBS. Evidence is still weak to opt for either endorsing DBS or not for a certain patient only relying on the genetic background, but in the future it is probable that certain genotypes will be considered not suitable for DBS on the basis of their improbability to benefit from the effects. To date, genetic testing of patients undergoing DBS might be proposed in those manifesting specific phenotype features (e.g., rapid development of disability, susceptibility to behavioral complications and hallucinations) consistent with particular gene variants, such as severe *GBA* mutations, which may determine possible issues presented in the post-operative follow-up (Figure 1).

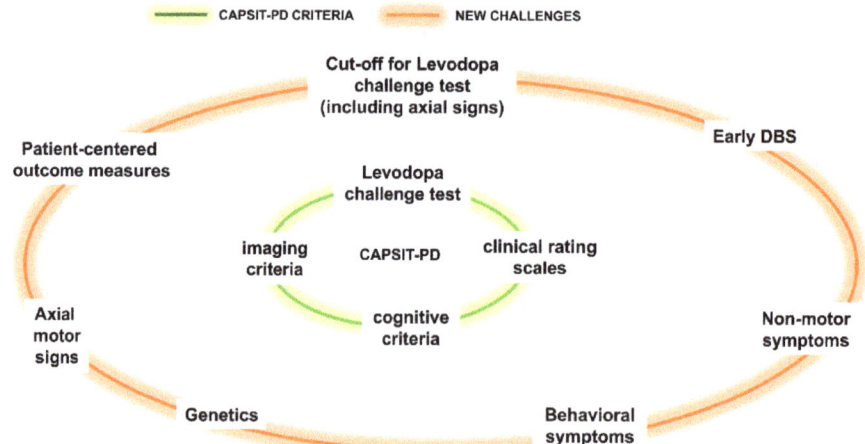

Figure 1. Core Assessment Program for Surgical Interventional Therapies in Parkinson's Disease (CAPSIT-PD) and recommendations on challenging areas related to the deep brain stimulation (DBS) selection.

8. Conclusions

Advances in understanding both the complexity of PD and the effect of DBS in PD patients have provided new evidence for a better stratification of patients and a more conscious use of this therapeutic option.

It is critical to take into account that the multifaceted symptomatology of PD, encompassing motor, non-motor, and behavioral issues, makes a candidate's selection for advanced therapies a process difficult to fit in fixed and precise borders. Additionally, the probability of improving or worsening certain symptoms according to clinical trials (or to post-hoc analysis of trials) cannot capture the full clinical complexity and heterogeneity of the PD clinical spectrum and should be used cautiously for making a decision at a single level. To date, in addition to studies supporting a better comprehension of pre-surgical predictors of DBS outcomes, we also need a shift in the statistical approach to improve the decision-making from a group to an individual level.

In conclusion, the improvement in the stratification of PD patients according to their clinical features and genetic background can inform the disease course, and more-in-depth knowledge on patients most probable to benefit from DBS. A redefinition of CAPSIT-PD criteria for DBS should be pursued based on the new knowledge gained on PD clinical spectrum and DBS long term follow-up studies. This would allow surgical centers to be more accurate in predicting the outcome after functional neurosurgery and choosing the best target for stimulation. We can now estimate the probability to improve specific disabling symptoms and choose integrated approaches, combining stimulation of specific targets according to patients' issues (e.g., ventral STN for high non-motor burden [73]) with other therapeutic options (e.g., rehabilitation), with the ultimate goal of improving ADL, mental wellbeing, and eventually the QoL of PD patients. This viewpoint provided updated recommendations for a more accurate and fine-grained assessment of PD patients considered as potential candidates for DBS and highlighted the need for further studies to strengthen the evidence on predictors of DBS outcomes at an individual level, encompassing the complex and multifaceted syndromic picture of the disease and the new possibilities offered by validated clinical scales, technological devices, and genetic analysis.

Author Contributions: C.A.A.: conception, design and organization of the study, literature search, writing of the first draft; L.L.: data interpretation, review and critique; F.M.: conception, design and organization of the study, literature search, review and critique. All authors have read and agreed to the published version of the manuscript.

Funding: This research received no external funding.

Conflicts of Interest: The authors declare no conflict of interest.

Financial Disclosures: Carlo Alberto Artusi: received travel grants from Zambon and Abbvie, and educational grants from Ralpharma and Neuraxpharm. Leonardo Lopiano: speaking honoraria from UCB Pharma, AbbVie, DOC, Zambon and Bial. Francesca Morgante: speaking honoraria from Abbvie, Medtronic, Zambon, Bial, Merz; Travel grants from the International Parkinson's disease and Movement Disorder Society; advisory board fees from Merz; consultancy fees from Boston Scientific, Merz and Bial; research support from Boston Scientific, Merz and Global Kynetic; royalties for the book "Disorders of Movement" from Springer; member of the editorial board of Movement Disorders, Movement Disorders Clinical Practice, European Journal of Neurology.

References

1. Defer, G.L.; Widner, H.; Marie, R.M.; Remy, P.; Levivier, M. Core assessment program for surgical interventional therapies in Parkinson's disease (CAPSIT-PD). *Mov. Disord.* **1999**, *14*, 572–584. [CrossRef]
2. Munhoz, R.P.; Picillo, M.; Fox, S.H.; Bruno, V.; Panisset, M.; Honey, C.R.; Fasano, A. Eligibility Criteria for Deep Brain Stimulation in Parkinson's Disease, Tremor, and Dystonia. *Can. J. Neurol. Sci.* **2016**, *43*, 462–471. [CrossRef]
3. Morgante, L.; Morgante, F.; Moro, E.; Epifanio, A.; Girlanda, P.; Ragonese, P.; Antonini, A.; Barone, P.; Bonuccelli, U.; Contarino, M.F.; et al. How many parkinsonian patients are suitable candidates for deep brain stimulation of subthalamic nucleus? Results of a questionnaire. *Parkinsonism Relat. Disord.* **2007**, *13*, 528–531. [CrossRef] [PubMed]

4. Abboud, H.; Genc, G.; Thompson, N.R.; Oravivattanakul, S.; Alsallom, F.; Reyes, D.; Wilson, K.; Cerejo, R.; Yu, X.X.; Floden, D.; et al. Predictors of Functional and Quality of Life Outcomes following Deep Brain Stimulation Surgery in Parkinson's Disease Patients: Disease, Patient, and Surgical Factors. *Parkinsons Dis.* **2017**, *2017*, 5609163. [CrossRef] [PubMed]
5. Lau, B.; Meier, N.; Serra, G.; Czernecki, V.; Schuepbach, M.; Navarro, S.; Cornu, P.; Grabli, D.; Agid, Y.; Vidailhet, M.; et al. Axial symptoms predict mortality in patients with Parkinson disease and subthalamic stimulation. *Neurology* **2019**, *92*, e2559–e2570. [CrossRef] [PubMed]
6. Schuepbach, W.M.M.; Tonder, L.; Schnitzler, A.; Krack, P.; Rau, J.; Hartmann, A.; Halbig, T.D.; Pineau, F.; Falk, A.; Paschen, L.; et al. Quality of life predicts outcome of deep brain stimulation in early Parkinson disease. *Neurology* **2019**, *92*, e1109–e1120. [CrossRef] [PubMed]
7. Lopez-Cuina, M.; Fernagut, P.O.; Canron, M.H.; Vital, A.; Lannes, B.; De Paula, A.M.; Streichenberger, N.; Guehl, D.; Damier, P.; Eusebio, A.; et al. Deep brain stimulation does not enhance neuroinflammation in multiple system atrophy. *Neurobiol. Dis.* **2018**, *118*, 155–160. [CrossRef]
8. Schuepbach, W.M.; Rau, J.; Knudsen, K.; Volkmann, J.; Krack, P.; Timmermann, L.; Halbig, T.D.; Hesekamp, H.; Navarro, S.M.; Meier, N.; et al. Neurostimulation for Parkinson's disease with early motor complications. *N. Engl. J. Med.* **2013**, *368*, 610–622. [CrossRef]
9. Vizcarra, J.A.; Situ-Kcomt, M.; Artusi, C.A.; Duker, A.P.; Lopiano, L.; Okun, M.S.; Espay, A.J.; Merola, A. Subthalamic deep brain stimulation and levodopa in Parkinson's disease: A meta-analysis of combined effects. *J. Neurol.* **2019**, *266*, 289–297. [CrossRef]
10. Cabrera, L.Y.; Goudreau, J.; Sidiropoulos, C. Critical appraisal of the recent US FDA approval for earlier DBS intervention. *Neurology* **2018**, *91*, 133–136. [CrossRef]
11. Mestre, T.A.; Espay, A.J.; Marras, C.; Eckman, M.H.; Pollak, P.; Lang, A.E. Subthalamic nucleus-deep brain stimulation for early motor complications in Parkinson's disease-the EARLYSTIM trial: Early is not always better. *Mov. Disord.* **2014**, *29*, 1751–1756. [CrossRef] [PubMed]
12. Schupbach, W.M.; Rau, J.; Houeto, J.L.; Krack, P.; Schnitzler, A.; Schade-Brittinger, C.; Timmermann, L.; Deuschl, G. Myths and facts about the EARLYSTIM study. *Mov. Disord.* **2014**, *29*, 1742–1750. [CrossRef] [PubMed]
13. Petrucci, S.; Ginevrino, M.; Trezzi, I.; Monfrini, E.; Ricciardi, L.; Albanese, A.; Avenali, M.; Barone, P.; Bentivoglio, A.R.; Bonifati, V.; et al. GBA-Related Parkinson's Disease: Dissection of Genotype-Phenotype Correlates in a Large Italian Cohort. *Mov. Disord.* **2020**. [CrossRef] [PubMed]
14. Artusi, C.A.; Dwivedi, A.K.; Romagnolo, A.; Pal, G.; Kauffman, M.; Mata, I.; Patel, D.; Vizcarra, J.A.; Duker, A.; Marsili, L.; et al. Association of Subthalamic Deep Brain Stimulation With Motor, Functional, and Pharmacologic Outcomes in Patients With Monogenic Parkinson Disease: A Systematic Review and Meta-analysis. *JAMA Netw. Open* **2019**, *2*, e187800. [CrossRef] [PubMed]
15. Merola, A.; Romagnolo, A.; Dwivedi, A.K.; Padovani, A.; Berg, D.; Garcia-Ruiz, P.J.; Fabbri, M.; Artusi, C.A.; Zibetti, M.; Lopiano, L.; et al. Benign versus malignant Parkinson disease: The unexpected silver lining of motor complications. *J. Neurol.* **2020**. [CrossRef]
16. Barbe, M.T.; Tonder, L.; Krack, P.; Debu, B.; Schupbach, M.; Paschen, S.; Dembek, T.A.; Kuhn, A.A.; Fraix, V.; Brefel-Courbon, C.; et al. Deep Brain Stimulation for Freezing of Gait in Parkinson's Disease With Early Motor Complications. *Mov. Disord.* **2020**, *35*, 82–90. [CrossRef]
17. Lhommee, E.; Wojtecki, L.; Czernecki, V.; Witt, K.; Maier, F.; Tonder, L.; Timmermann, L.; Halbig, T.D.; Pineau, F.; Durif, F.; et al. Behavioural outcomes of subthalamic stimulation and medical therapy versus medical therapy alone for Parkinson's disease with early motor complications (EARLYSTIM trial): Secondary analysis of an open-label randomised trial. *Lancet Neurol.* **2018**, *17*, 223–231. [CrossRef]
18. Charles, D.; Konrad, P.E.; Neimat, J.S.; Molinari, A.L.; Tramontana, M.G.; Finder, S.G.; Gill, C.E.; Bliton, M.J.; Kao, C.; Phibbs, F.T.; et al. Subthalamic nucleus deep brain stimulation in early stage Parkinson's disease. *Parkinsonism Relat. Disord.* **2014**, *20*, 731–737. [CrossRef]
19. Hacker, M.L.; Turchan, M.; Heusinkveld, L.E.; Currie, A.D.; Millan, S.H.; Molinari, A.L.; Konrad, P.E.; Davis, T.L.; Phibbs, F.T.; Hedera, P.; et al. Deep brain stimulation in early-stage Parkinson disease: Five-year outcomes. *Neurology* **2020**, *95*, e393–e401. [CrossRef]
20. Fasano, A.; Merello, M. Fading of Deep Brain Stimulation Efficacy Versus Disease Progression: Untangling a Gordian Knot. *Mov. Disord. Clin. Pract.* **2020**, *7*, 747–749. [CrossRef]

21. Zibetti, M.; Pesare, M.; Cinquepalmi, A.; Rosso, M.; Bergamasco, B.; Ducati, A.; Lanotte, M.; Lopiano, L. Antiparkinsonian therapy modifications in PD patients after STN DBS: A retrospective observational analysis. *Parkinsonism Relat. Disord.* **2008**, *14*, 608–612. [CrossRef] [PubMed]
22. Castelli, L.; Perozzo, P.; Zibetti, M.; Crivelli, B.; Morabito, U.; Lanotte, M.; Cossa, F.; Bergamasco, B.; Lopiano, L. Chronic deep brain stimulation of the subthalamic nucleus for Parkinson's disease: Effects on cognition, mood, anxiety and personality traits. *Eur. Neurol.* **2006**, *55*, 136–144. [CrossRef] [PubMed]
23. Merola, A.; Romagnolo, A.; Rizzi, L.; Rizzone, M.G.; Zibetti, M.; Lanotte, M.; Mandybur, G.; Duker, A.P.; Espay, A.J.; Lopiano, L. Impulse control behaviors and subthalamic deep brain stimulation in Parkinson disease. *J. Neurol.* **2017**, *264*, 40–48. [CrossRef] [PubMed]
24. Saranza, G.; Lang, A.E. Levodopa challenge test: Indications, protocol, and guide. *J. Neurol.* **2020**. [CrossRef]
25. Machado, A.G.; Deogaonkar, M.; Cooper, S. Deep brain stimulation for movement disorders: Patient selection and technical options. *Clevel. Clin. J. Med.* **2012**, *79* (Suppl. S2), S19–S24. [CrossRef]
26. Bronstein, J.M.; Tagliati, M.; Alterman, R.L.; Lozano, A.M.; Volkmann, J.; Stefani, A.; Horak, F.B.; Okun, M.S.; Foote, K.D.; Krack, P.; et al. Deep brain stimulation for Parkinson disease: An expert consensus and review of key issues. *Arch. Neurol.* **2011**, *68*, 165. [CrossRef]
27. Armstrong, M.J.; Okun, M.S. Choosing a Parkinson Disease Treatment. *JAMA* **2020**, *323*, 1420. [CrossRef]
28. Benabid, A.L.; Benazzouz, A.; Hoffmann, D.; Limousin, P.; Krack, P.; Pollak, P. Long-term electrical inhibition of deep brain targets in movement disorders. *Mov. Disord.* **1998**, *13* (Suppl. S3), 119–125. [CrossRef]
29. Merello, M.; Nouzeilles, M.I.; Arce, G.P.; Leiguarda, R. Accuracy of acute levodopa challenge for clinical prediction of sustained long-term levodopa response as a major criterion for idiopathic Parkinson's disease diagnosis. *Mov. Disord.* **2002**, *17*, 795–798. [CrossRef]
30. Fahn, S.; Elton, R.; Members of the UPDRS Development Committee. The Unified Parkinson's Disease Rating Scale. In *Recent Developments in Parkinson's Disease*; Fahn, S., Marsden, C.D., Calne, D.B., Goldstein, M., Eds.; Macmillan Health Care Information: Florham Park, NJ, USA, 1987; Volume 2, pp. 153–163, 293–304.
31. Merello, M.; Gerschcovich, E.R.; Ballesteros, D.; Cerquetti, D. Correlation between the Movement Disorders Society Unified Parkinson's Disease rating scale (MDS-UPDRS) and the Unified Parkinson's Disease rating scale (UPDRS) during L-dopa acute challenge. *Parkinsonism Relat. Disord.* **2011**, *17*, 705–707. [CrossRef]
32. Deuschl, G.; Follett, K.A.; Luo, P.; Rau, J.; Weaver, F.M.; Paschen, S.; Steigerwald, F.; Tonder, L.; Stoker, V.; Reda, D.J. Comparing two randomized deep brain stimulation trials for Parkinson's disease. *J. Neurosurg.* **2019**, 1–9. [CrossRef] [PubMed]
33. Kleiner-Fisman, G.; Herzog, J.; Fisman, D.N.; Tamma, F.; Lyons, K.E.; Pahwa, R.; Lang, A.E.; Deuschl, G. Subthalamic nucleus deep brain stimulation: Summary and meta-analysis of outcomes. *Mov. Disord.* **2006**, *21* (Suppl. S14), S290–S304. [CrossRef]
34. Fasano, A.; Aquino, C.C.; Krauss, J.K.; Honey, C.R.; Bloem, B.R. Axial disability and deep brain stimulation in patients with Parkinson disease. *Nat. Rev. Neurol.* **2015**, *11*, 98–110. [CrossRef] [PubMed]
35. Fasano, A.; Bloem, B.R. Gait disorders. *Contin. Lifelong Learn. Neurol.* **2013**, *19*, 1344–1382. [CrossRef] [PubMed]
36. Bakker, M.; Esselink, R.A.; Munneke, M.; Limousin-Dowsey, P.; Speelman, H.D.; Bloem, B.R. Effects of stereotactic neurosurgery on postural instability and gait in Parkinson's disease. *Mov. Disord.* **2004**, *19*, 1092–1099. [CrossRef] [PubMed]
37. Zibetti, M.; Merola, A.; Rizzi, L.; Ricchi, V.; Angrisano, S.; Azzaro, C.; Artusi, C.A.; Arduino, N.; Marchisio, A.; Lanotte, M.; et al. Beyond nine years of continuous subthalamic nucleus deep brain stimulation in Parkinson's disease. *Mov. Disord.* **2011**, *26*, 2327–2334. [CrossRef] [PubMed]
38. Rizzone, M.G.; Fasano, A.; Daniele, A.; Zibetti, M.; Merola, A.; Rizzi, L.; Piano, C.; Piccininni, C.; Romito, L.M.; Lopiano, L.; et al. Long-term outcome of subthalamic nucleus DBS in Parkinson's disease: From the advanced phase towards the late stage of the disease? *Parkinsonism Relat. Disord.* **2014**, *20*, 376–381. [CrossRef]
39. Castrioto, A.; Lozano, A.M.; Poon, Y.Y.; Lang, A.E.; Fallis, M.; Moro, E. Ten-year outcome of subthalamic stimulation in Parkinson disease: A blinded evaluation. *Arch. Neurol.* **2011**, *68*, 1550–1556. [CrossRef] [PubMed]
40. Fasano, A.; Romito, L.M.; Daniele, A.; Piano, C.; Zinno, M.; Bentivoglio, A.R.; Albanese, A. Motor and cognitive outcome in patients with Parkinson's disease 8 years after subthalamic implants. *Brain* **2010**, *133*, 2664–2676. [CrossRef]

41. Tripoliti, E.; Limousin, P.; Foltynie, T.; Candelario, J.; Aviles-Olmos, I.; Hariz, M.I.; Zrinzo, L. Predictive factors of speech intelligibility following subthalamic nucleus stimulation in consecutive patients with Parkinson's disease. *Mov. Disord.* **2014**, *29*, 532–538. [CrossRef]
42. Mei, S.; Li, J.; Middlebrooks, E.H.; Almeida, L.; Hu, W.; Zhang, Y.; Ramirez-Zamora, A.; Chan, P. New Onset On-Medication Freezing of Gait After STN-DBS in Parkinson's Disease. *Front. Neurol.* **2019**, *10*, 659. [CrossRef] [PubMed]
43. Vercruysse, S.; Vandenberghe, W.; Munks, L.; Nuttin, B.; Devos, H.; Nieuwboer, A. Effects of deep brain stimulation of the subthalamic nucleus on freezing of gait in Parkinson's disease: A prospective controlled study. *J. Neurol. Neurosurg. Psychiatry* **2014**, *85*, 871–877. [CrossRef] [PubMed]
44. Moreau, C.; Pennel-Ployart, O.; Pinto, S.; Plachez, A.; Annic, A.; Viallet, F.; Destee, A.; Defebvre, L. Modulation of dysarthropneumophonia by low-frequency STN DBS in advanced Parkinson's disease. *Mov. Disord.* **2011**, *26*, 659–663. [CrossRef] [PubMed]
45. Zibetti, M.; Moro, E.; Krishna, V.; Sammartino, F.; Picillo, M.; Munhoz, R.P.; Lozano, A.M.; Fasano, A. Low-frequency Subthalamic Stimulation in Parkinson's Disease: Long-term Outcome and Predictors. *Brain Stimul.* **2016**, *9*, 774–779. [CrossRef] [PubMed]
46. Golfre Andreasi, N.; Rispoli, V.; Contaldi, E.; Colucci, F.; Mongardi, L.; Cavallo, M.A.; Sensi, M. Deep brain stimulation and refractory freezing of gait in Parkinson's disease: Improvement with high-frequency current steering co-stimulation of subthalamic nucleus and substantia Nigra. *Brain Stimul.* **2020**, *13*, 280–283. [CrossRef]
47. Antonini, A.; Stoessl, A.J.; Kleinman, L.S.; Skalicky, A.M.; Marshall, T.S.; Sail, K.R.; Onuk, K.; Odin, P.L.A. Developing consensus among movement disorder specialists on clinical indicators for identification and management of advanced Parkinson's disease: A multi-country Delphi-panel approach. *Curr. Med. Res. Opin.* **2018**, *34*, 2063–2073. [CrossRef]
48. Artusi, C.A.; Zibetti, M.; Romagnolo, A.; Rizzone, M.G.; Merola, A.; Lopiano, L. Subthalamic deep brain stimulation and trunk posture in Parkinson's disease. *Acta Neurol. Scand.* **2018**, *137*, 481–487. [CrossRef]
49. Roediger, J.; Artusi, C.A.; Romagnolo, A.; Boyne, P.; Zibetti, M.; Lopiano, L.; Espay, A.J.; Fasano, A.; Merola, A. Effect of subthalamic deep brain stimulation on posture in Parkinson's disease: A blind computerized analysis. *Parkinsonism Relat. Disord.* **2019**, *62*, 122–127. [CrossRef]
50. Silva de Lima, A.L.; Evers, L.J.W.; Hahn, T.; Bataille, L.; Hamilton, J.L.; Little, M.A.; Okuma, Y.; Bloem, B.R.; Faber, M.J. Freezing of gait and fall detection in Parkinson's disease using wearable sensors: A systematic review. *J. Neurol.* **2017**, *264*, 1642–1654. [CrossRef]
51. Silva de Lima, A.L.; Smits, T.; Darweesh, S.K.L.; Valenti, G.; Milosevic, M.; Pijl, M.; Baldus, H.; de Vries, N.M.; Meinders, M.J.; Bloem, B.R. Home-based monitoring of falls using wearable sensors in Parkinson's disease. *Mov. Disord.* **2020**, *35*, 109–115. [CrossRef]
52. Cebi, I.; Scholten, M.; Gharabaghi, A.; Weiss, D. Clinical and Kinematic Correlates of Favorable Gait Outcomes From Subthalamic Stimulation. *Front. Neurol.* **2020**, *11*, 212. [CrossRef] [PubMed]
53. Deuschl, G.; Schade-Brittinger, C.; Krack, P.; Volkmann, J.; Schafer, H.; Botzel, K.; Daniels, C.; Deutschlander, A.; Dillmann, U.; Eisner, W.; et al. A randomized trial of deep-brain stimulation for Parkinson's disease. *N. Engl. J. Med.* **2006**, *355*, 896–908. [CrossRef] [PubMed]
54. Erb, M.K.; Karlin, D.R.; Ho, B.K.; Thomas, K.C.; Parisi, F.; Vergara-Diaz, G.P.; Daneault, J.F.; Wacnik, P.W.; Zhang, H.; Kangarloo, T.; et al. mHealth and wearable technology should replace motor diaries to track motor fluctuations in Parkinson's disease. *NPJ Digit. Med.* **2020**, *3*, 6. [CrossRef] [PubMed]
55. Espay, A.J.; Hausdorff, J.M.; Sanchez-Ferro, A.; Klucken, J.; Merola, A.; Bonato, P.; Paul, S.S.; Horak, F.B.; Vizcarra, J.A.; Mestre, T.A.; et al. A roadmap for implementation of patient-centered digital outcome measures in Parkinson's disease obtained using mobile health technologies. *Mov. Disord.* **2019**, *34*, 657–663. [CrossRef]
56. Capecci, M.; Pepa, L.; Verdini, F.; Ceravolo, M.G. A smartphone-based architecture to detect and quantify freezing of gait in Parkinson's disease. *Gait Posture* **2016**, *50*, 28–33. [CrossRef]
57. Jenkinson, C.; Fitzpatrick, R.; Peto, V.; Greenhall, R.; Hyman, N. The Parkinson's Disease Questionnaire (PDQ-39): Development and validation of a Parkinson's disease summary index score. *Age Ageing* **1997**, *26*, 353–357. [CrossRef]

58. Jenkinson, C.; Fitzpatrick, R. Cross-cultural evaluation of the short form 8-item Parkinson's Disease Questionnaire (PDQ-8): Results from America, Canada, Japan, Italy and Spain. *Parkinsonism Relat. Disord.* **2007**, *13*, 22–28. [CrossRef]
59. Schwab, R.S.; England, A.C. Projection techniques for evaluating surgery in Parkinson's Disease. In Proceedings of the Third Symposium on Parkinson's Disease, Royal College of Surgeons in Edinburgh, Edinburgh, UK, 20–22 May 1968.
60. Karl, J.A.; Ouyang, B.; Colletta, K.; Verhagen Metman, L. Long-Term Satisfaction and Patient-Centered Outcomes of Deep Brain Stimulation in Parkinson's Disease. *Brain Sci.* **2018**, *8*, 60. [CrossRef]
61. Barthel, C.; Mallia, E.; Debu, B.; Bloem, B.R.; Ferraye, M.U. The Practicalities of Assessing Freezing of Gait. *J. Parkinsons Dis.* **2016**, *6*, 667–674. [CrossRef]
62. Floden, D.; Cooper, S.E.; Griffith, S.D.; Machado, A.G. Predicting quality of life outcomes after subthalamic nucleus deep brain stimulation. *Neurology* **2014**, *83*, 1627–1633. [CrossRef]
63. Geraedts, V.J.; Feleus, S.; Marinus, J.; van Hilten, J.J.; Contarino, M.F. What predicts quality of life after subthalamic deep brain stimulation in Parkinson's disease? A systematic review. *Eur. J. Neurol.* **2020**, *27*, 419–428. [CrossRef]
64. Barone, P.; Antonini, A.; Colosimo, C.; Marconi, R.; Morgante, L.; Avarello, T.P.; Bottacchi, E.; Cannas, A.; Ceravolo, G.; Ceravolo, R.; et al. The PRIAMO study: A multicenter assessment of nonmotor symptoms and their impact on quality of life in Parkinson's disease. *Mov. Disord.* **2009**, *24*, 1641–1649. [CrossRef] [PubMed]
65. Dafsari, H.S.; Reddy, P.; Herchenbach, C.; Wawro, S.; Petry-Schmelzer, J.N.; Visser-Vandewalle, V.; Rizos, A.; Silverdale, M.; Ashkan, K.; Samuel, M.; et al. Beneficial Effects of Bilateral Subthalamic Stimulation on Non-Motor Symptoms in Parkinson's Disease. *Brain Stimul.* **2016**, *9*, 78–85. [CrossRef] [PubMed]
66. Dafsari, H.S.; Silverdale, M.; Strack, M.; Rizos, A.; Ashkan, K.; Mahlstedt, P.; Sachse, L.; Steffen, J.; Dembek, T.A.; Visser-Vandewalle, V.; et al. Nonmotor symptoms evolution during 24 months of bilateral subthalamic stimulation in Parkinson's disease. *Mov. Disord.* **2018**, *33*, 421–430. [CrossRef] [PubMed]
67. Jost, S.T.; Ray Chaudhuri, K.; Ashkan, K.; Loehrer, P.A.; Silverdale, M.; Rizos, A.; Evans, J.; Petry-Schmelzer, J.N.; Barbe, M.T.; Sauerbier, A.; et al. Subthalamic Stimulation Improves Quality of Sleep in Parkinson Disease: A 36-Month Controlled Study. *J. Parkinsons Dis.* **2020**, 1–13. [CrossRef]
68. Ricciardi, L.; Sorbera, C.; Barbuto, M.; Morgante, F. Sleep disturbances are mainly improved by deep brain stimulation of the subthalamic nucleus. *Mov. Disord.* **2019**, *34*, 154–155. [CrossRef]
69. Jost, S.T.; Sauerbier, A.; Visser-Vandewalle, V.; Ashkan, K.; Silverdale, M.; Evans, J.; Loehrer, P.A.; Rizos, A.; Petry-Schmelzer, J.N.; Reker, P.; et al. A prospective, controlled study of non-motor effects of subthalamic stimulation in Parkinson's disease: Results at the 36-month follow-up. *J. Neurol. Neurosurg. Psychiatry* **2020**, *91*, 687–694. [CrossRef]
70. Fereshtehnejad, S.M.; Zeighami, Y.; Dagher, A.; Postuma, R.B. Clinical criteria for subtyping Parkinson's disease: Biomarkers and longitudinal progression. *Brain* **2017**, *140*, 1959–1976. [CrossRef]
71. De Pablo-Fernandez, E.; Lees, A.J.; Holton, J.L.; Warner, T.T. Prognosis and Neuropathologic Correlation of Clinical Subtypes of Parkinson Disease. *JAMA Neurol.* **2019**, *76*, 470–479. [CrossRef]
72. Parkinson Disease Phenotype Classification Predicts the Outcome of Deep Brain Stimulation. Available online: https://www.mdsabstracts.org/abstract/parkinson-disease-phenotype-classification-predicts-the-outcome-of-deep-brain-stimulation/ (accessed on 3 December 2020).
73. Petry-Schmelzer, J.N.; Krause, M.; Dembek, T.A.; Horn, A.; Evans, J.; Ashkan, K.; Rizos, A.; Silverdale, M.; Schumacher, W.; Sack, C.; et al. Non-motor outcomes depend on location of neurostimulation in Parkinson's disease. *Brain* **2019**, *142*, 3592–3604. [CrossRef]
74. Bandres-Ciga, S.; Diez-Fairen, M.; Kim, J.J.; Singleton, A.B. Genetics of Parkinson's disease: An introspection of its journey towards precision medicine. *Neurobiol. Dis.* **2020**, *137*, 104782. [CrossRef] [PubMed]
75. Rizzone, M.G.; Martone, T.; Balestrino, R.; Lopiano, L. Genetic background and outcome of Deep Brain Stimulation in Parkinson's disease. *Parkinsonism Relat. Disord.* **2019**, *64*, 8–19. [CrossRef] [PubMed]
76. De Oliveira, L.M.; Barbosa, E.R.; Aquino, C.C.; Munhoz, R.P.; Fasano, A.; Cury, R.G. Deep Brain Stimulation in Patients With Mutations in Parkinson's Disease-Related Genes: A Systematic Review. *Mov. Disord. Clin. Pract.* **2019**, *6*, 359–368. [CrossRef] [PubMed]
77. Kuusimaki, T.; Korpela, J.; Pekkonen, E.; Martikainen, M.H.; Antonini, A.; Kaasinen, V. Deep brain stimulation for monogenic Parkinson's disease: A systematic review. *J. Neurol.* **2020**, *267*, 883–897. [CrossRef] [PubMed]

78. Marras, C.; Schule, B.; Munhoz, R.P.; Rogaeva, E.; Langston, J.W.; Kasten, M.; Meaney, C.; Klein, C.; Wadia, P.M.; Lim, S.Y.; et al. Phenotype in parkinsonian and nonparkinsonian LRRK2 G2019S mutation carriers. *Neurology* **2011**, *77*, 325–333. [CrossRef]
79. Cilia, R.; Tunesi, S.; Marotta, G.; Cereda, E.; Siri, C.; Tesei, S.; Zecchinelli, A.L.; Canesi, M.; Mariani, C.B.; Meucci, N.; et al. Survival and dementia in GBA-associated Parkinson's disease: The mutation matters. *Ann. Neurol.* **2016**, *80*, 662–673. [CrossRef]

Publisher's Note: MDPI stays neutral with regard to jurisdictional claims in published maps and institutional affiliations.

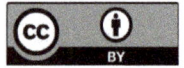
© 2020 by the authors. Licensee MDPI, Basel, Switzerland. This article is an open access article distributed under the terms and conditions of the Creative Commons Attribution (CC BY) license (http://creativecommons.org/licenses/by/4.0/).

MDPI
St. Alban-Anlage 66
4052 Basel
Switzerland
Tel. +41 61 683 77 34
Fax +41 61 302 89 18
www.mdpi.com

Journal of Clinical Medicine Editorial Office
E-mail: jcm@mdpi.com
www.mdpi.com/journal/jcm

www.ingramcontent.com/pod-product-compliance
Lightning Source LLC
LaVergne TN
LVHW070436100526
838202LV00014B/1609